NORMAL AND ABNORMAL DEVELOPMENT
OF BRAIN AND BEHAVIOUR

BOERHAAVE SERIES
FOR POSTGRADUATE
MEDICAL EDUCATION

PROCEEDINGS OF THE BOERHAAVE COURSES
ORGANIZED BY
THE FACULTY OF MEDICINE, UNIVERSITY OF LEIDEN
THE NETHERLANDS

NORMAL AND ABNORMAL DEVELOPMENT OF BRAIN AND BEHAVIOUR

EDITED BY

G. B. A. STOELINGA M. D.

J. J. VAN DER WERFF TEN BOSCH M. D.

LEIDEN UNIVERSITY PRESS

1971

SOLE DISTRIBUTOR FOR THE UNITED STATES OF AMERICA AND CANADA
THE WILLIAMS AND WILKINS COMPANY / BALTIMORE

Library of Congress Catalog Card Number 74-149161

ISBN 978-94-010-2923-0   ISBN 978-94-010-2921-6   (eBook)
DOI 10.1007/978-94-010-2921-6

Jacket design: E. Wijnans gvn

PREFACE

This volume contains the proceedings of a postgraduate course for medical practitioners of various specialties. One purpose of the course was to provide factual data on developmental aspects of the brain and behaviour, and about the possible impact of several important categories of internal and environmental factors upon neural development. Another purpose was to indicate the extent and the limitations of the methodology now available for the scientific approach of the study of the development of behaviour. In general the investigator is faced with methodological problems of two types, the proper definition and scoring of behavioural items, and the isolation of the different factors that contribute to a particular behaviour. An example of the latter is given in the very last paper, which is concerned with attempts at unravelling under experimental conditions the contributions made by various influences upon a single sequence of behaviour.

The course was held in Leiden in November 1970, and was the third in a series of Boerhaave Courses instigated by the Dutch Growth Foundation. Previous subjects have been 'Somatic growth of the child' (in 1964) and 'Human body composition' (in 1967).

The programme was planned in collaboration with Prof. Dr. H. H. van Gelderen, Dr. D. G. Lawrence, Prof. Dr. F. J. Mönks, Prof. Dr. H. F. R. Prechtl and Prof. Dr. H. K. A. Visser.

Financial support was given by the pharmaceutical firms Philips-Duphar, Sandoz and Specia, and by the Dutch Growth Foundation.

Major editorial contributions were made by Anneke Bot.

Department of Pediatrics
University Hospital, Nijmegen

G. B. A. STOELINGA M.D.

Department of Endocrinology
Medical Faculty, Rotterdam
University Hospital, Leiden

J. J. VAN DER WERFF TEN BOSCH M.D.

CONTENTS

CONTRIBUTORS

R. Ader, Rudolf Magnus Institute for Pharmacology, State University of Utrecht, The Netherlands.

Y. Akiyama, Department of Developmental Neurology, University Hospital, Groningen, The Netherlands.

J. Ariëns Kappers, The Netherlands Central Institute for Brain Research, Amsterdam, The Netherlands.

T. B. Brazelton, Committee on Human Development, The University of Chicago, Illinois, U.S.A.

P. Casaer, Department of Developmental Neurology, University Hospital, Groningen, The Netherlands.

W. Croughs, Wilhelmina Children's Hospital, State University of Utrecht, The Netherlands.

J. Dobbing, Department of Child Health, University of Manchester, U.K.

D. G. Freedman, Committee on Human Development, The University of Chicago, Illinois, U.S.A.

J. J. van Gemund, Department of Paediatrics, University Hospital, Leiden, The Netherlands.

J. F. van Gils, Sophia Children's Hospital, Rotterdam Medical Faculty, Rotterdam, The Netherlands.

D. A. Goldfoot, Department of Endocrinology, Growth and Reproduction, Rotterdam Medical Faculty, Rotterdam, The Netherlands.

M. W. van Hof, Department of Physiology, Rotterdam Medical Faculty, Rotterdam, The Netherlands.

J. Jans, Department of Psychology, University of Nijmegen, The Netherlands.

A. F. Kalverboer, Department of Developmental Neurology, University Hospital, Groningen, The Netherlands.

S. Levine, Department of Psychiatry, Stanford University Medical Center, Stanford, California, U.S.A.

M. S. Laurent de Angulo, The Netherlands Institute for Preventive Medicine – TNO, Leiden, The Netherlands.

W. A. Marshall, Department of Growth and Development, Institute of Child Health, University of London, U. K.

H. F. R. Prechtl, Department of Developmental Neurology, University Hospital, Groningen, The Netherlands.

B. C. L. Touwen, Department of Developmental Neurology, University Hospital, Groningen, The Netherlands.

A. M. J. van Uden, Institute for the Deaf, St. Michielsgestel, The Netherlands.

E. M. Widdowson, University of Cambridge and Medical Research Council, Dunn Nutritional Laboratory, Cambridge, U.K.

D. de Wied, Rudolf Magnus Institute for Pharmacology, State University of Utrecht, The Netherlands.

SOMATIC DEVELOPMENT
AND THE STUDY OF
THE CENTRAL NERVOUS SYSTEM

W. A. MARSHALL

LIMITATIONS OF CROSS-SECTIONAL DATA

The development of the body can be studied more easily than that of the central nervous system. In studying somatic growth it is usually possible to make either repeated observations on the same subjects (longitudinal study) or single observations on each one of a large number of individuals at each age (cross-sectional study). Many of the techniques used to investigate the central nervous system require destruction or injury of the subject and therefore permit only cross-sectional studies. The two methods of approach do not yield the same information and it is important that the distinction between them should be clearly understood.

For example, the average stature of children at different ages and the variation about this average could be determined by a cross-sectional study. Fig. 1 is a chart based on cross-sectional data, showing the normal variation in stature of English children at different ages. 10% fall below the 10th percentile, 90% below the 90th percentile line, etc. However, the growth curves of individuals seldom coincide with the percentile lines throughout childhood. The thick line in the centre of the chart might be obtained from repeated measurements of an individual of average stature. It follows the 50th percentile line in early childhood but at the age of about $12\frac{1}{2}$ it begins to rise more steeply than the percentile line. The steep upward slope represents the adolescent growth spurt and occurs at the average age in the subject shown in fig. 1, but it does not begin or end at the same age in all children (see fig. 2). The curve obtained by plotting the average stature at each age begins its upward inflection when the earliest children enter the adolescent growth spurt, but does not level out until the last children have reached their adult stature. It is therefore less steep than the curve describing each individual's growth.

We can obtain a graph describing the growth of a single individual only by longitudinal study. We also need longitudinal data in order to determine

1

how the rate, or velocity, of growth varies, either with age in an individual, or at any given age in a population. We express this speed in cm/yr in just the same way as we talk about the speed of a motor car in km/hr.

If a large number of individuals were each measured on two successive birthdays and each child's growth velocity between each two successive

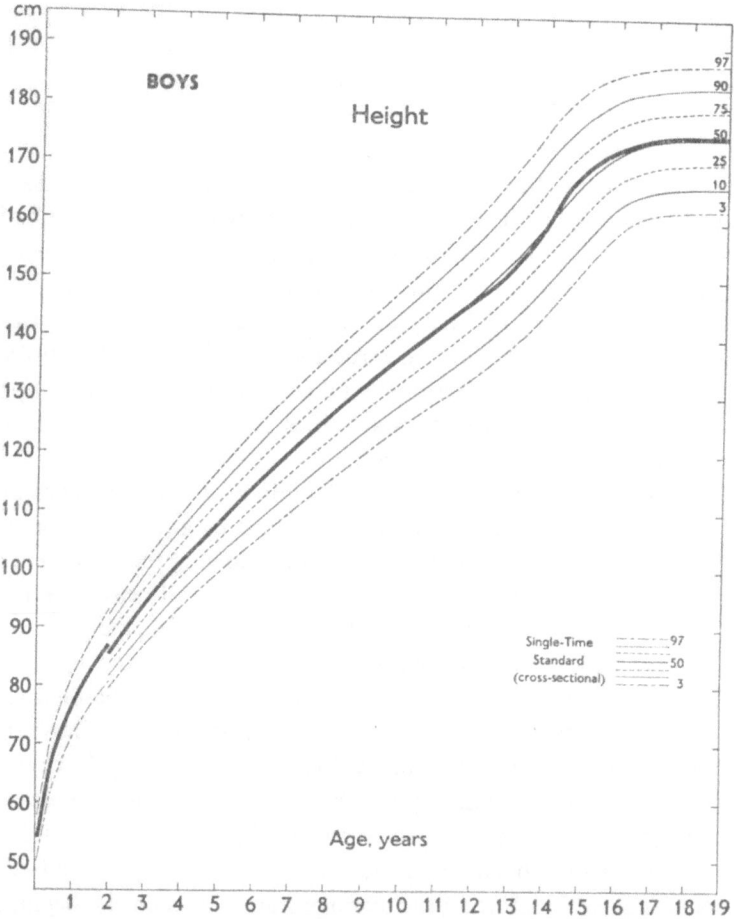

Fig. I. Chart showing the percentile distribution of stature for boys at different ages. The thick black line represents repeated measurements of an individual of average stature throughout childhood and as an adult. Note that between the ages of 12½ and 16 this line does not follow the 50th percentile line. The steeper slope at this age represents the individual's adolescent spurt and in this case is occurring at the average age. The discontinuity of the individual's line at age 2 is due to the changeover from supine length measurements to measurement of stature while standing.

measurements calculated, we could plot the mean velocity with some measure of its variability in the group (e.g. percentiles) at successive ages. The result would be the percentile distribution shown in fig. 3. The thick line shows how the speed of growth changes with age in a typical child. He grows very quickly at the beginning of life but the velocity decreases markedly in the first two or three years. It then decreases much more slowly until about the time of puberty, when there is the sudden increase in speed which we call the adolescent spurt. When the growth rate reaches its maximum during this spurt it immediately begins to slow down again. There is no plateau during which the maximal growth rate is maintained. In retrospective longitudinal data, the point at which maximal velocity is reached is a useful landmark in the growth process and we refer to it as 'peak height velocity'.

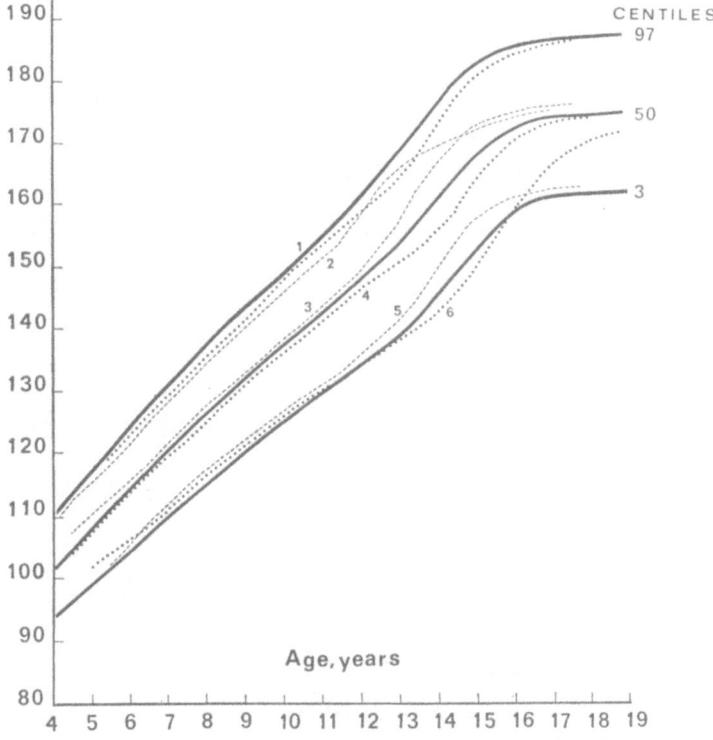

Fig. 2. Individual growth curves obtained by repeated measurements of 6 boys plotted against the background of 3rd, 50th and 97th percentiles for the population. Note that the adolescent spurt occurs at different ages and some boys continue growing for a longer period of time than others. Boys who are approximately the same stature during childhood may have quite different final statures.

This pattern of changes in growth velocity occurs in all normal children but it is not clearly revealed unless individuals are studied longitudinally. The adolescent spurt represented on the percentile chart appears to be of much longer duration and lower magnitude than it is in the individual. The reason for this is illustrated by fig. 4, which shows velocity curves which might be obtained by following five boys longitudinally throughout the age range indicated. Each boy's adolescent spurt is shown. The broken line,

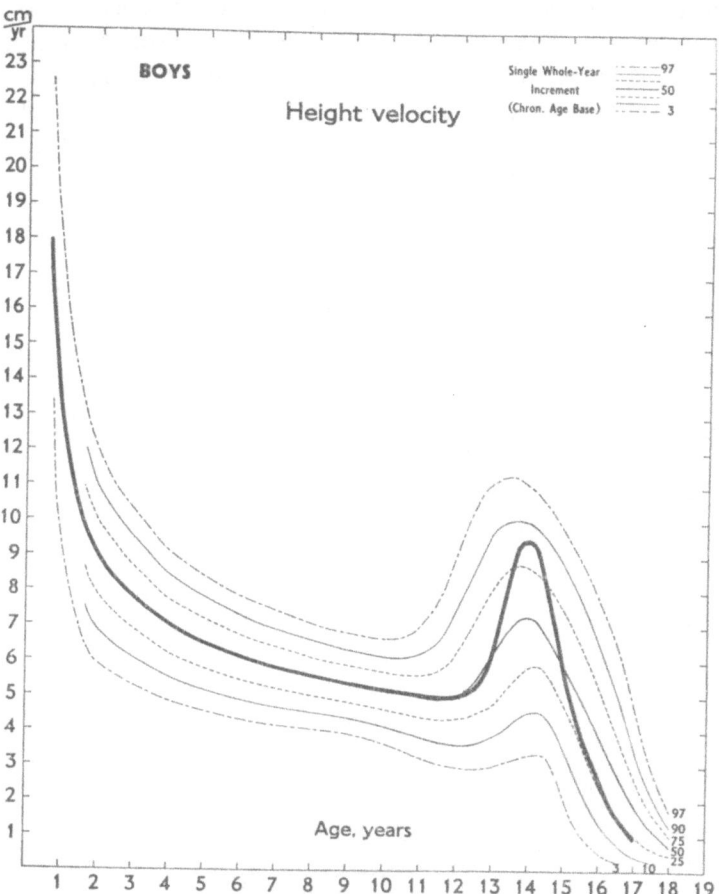

Fig. 3. Percentiles for growth velocity at different ages. The thick black line represents the change of growth velocity with age in a typical individual who has the adolescent spurt at the average age. Note that the increase in velocity during the adolescent spurt is greater than the 50th percentile line would suggest. The duration of the adolescent spurt is shorter in the individual than is suggested by the percentiles.

which indicates the average velocity for the group, gives a completely false impression of both the magnitude and duration of the adolescent spurt (1). Thus if we are to interpret longitudinal data correctly we must analyse them in such a way that we can see what happens to each individual. This may be done by methods ranging from the drawing of simple graphs by hand to complex mathematical processes.

Longitudinal studies require fewer subjects than cross-sectional ones. According to Tanner (2), it takes 20 times the number of subjects studied cross-sectionally to obtain as accurate an estimate of the mean increment over a given period of time in most body measurements as would be obtained from longitudinal data. On the other hand owing to the serial correlation between successive observations in a longitudinal study independent cross-sectional samples with the same number of subjects at each age will provide more information on the mean and variance of individual measurements at each age.

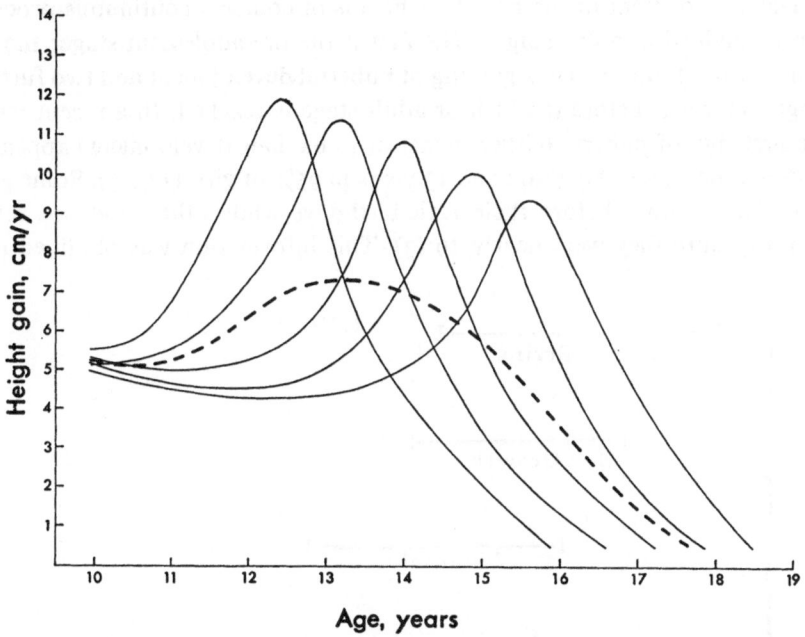

Fig. 4. Growth velocity curves of 5 individual boys during adolescence. The adolescent spurt is occurring at a different age in each and attains a different maximum velocity. The broken line represents the average velocity for the group. It does not describe the changes in velocity experienced by any individual. (From Tanner, Whitehouse and Takaishi (1). Reproduced by kind permission of the authors and the Editor, Archives of Disease in Childhood.)

Longitudinal studies need not always last throughout the entire period of maturation. Even if each subject is measured on only two or three occasions, more information can be obtained than by the cross-sectional approach, provided the data are interpreted correctly.

So far I have mentioned only growth in stature, which is a measure of overall size. This is a relatively unimportant parameter of development in the central nervous system but the arguments apply equally to any more or less continuous process of change whose rate varies with age, e.g. the increase in the quantity of a substance as estimated chemically. In the central nervous system 'stages' of development, recognised by anatomical, chemical, physiological or psychological methods are frequently studied, e.g. stage of cell multiplication then differentiation and then the development of function. Usually the so-called 'stages' are simply recognisable points or periods in a continuous process of change. The changes at puberty provide an example of a comparable process in the body.

The development of the breasts, which is of course a continuous process, can be divided into five stages. The first is the pre-adolescent stage; the second (or bud) stage is the beginning of pubertal development and two further stages intervene before the fifth or adult stage is reached. In a recent study the first sign of puberty (either breast or pubic hair development) appeared between the ages of 8.5 years and 13 years in 95% of girls (Fig. 5). Some girls were fully mature before their 12th birthdays while others did not reach maturity until they were nearly 19 (3). This information was obtained in a

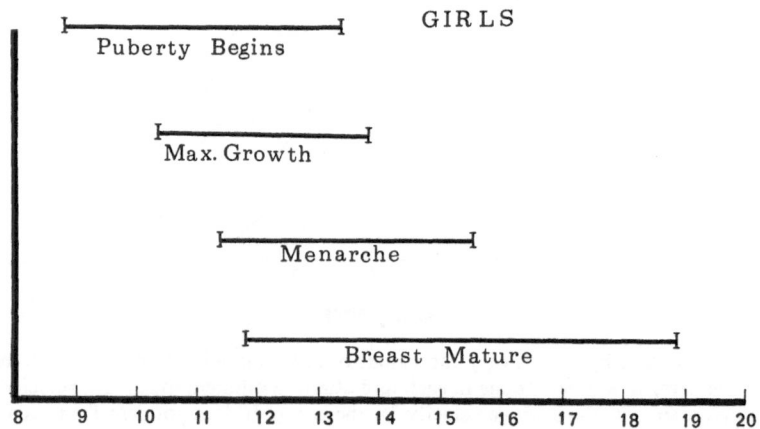

Fig. 5. Variation in ages at which different stages of puberty are reached in British girls. (Based on data from Marshall and Tanner, 3). Max. Growth = peak height velocity.

longitudinal study but similar results have been obtained from a cross-sectional study of Dutch children (4) in which data giving the number of girls who had, or had not, reached a given stage of development at each age were analysed. However, longitudinal data also show that the girls who are first to begin puberty are not necessarily the first to reach maturity. The interval from the first sign of puberty to complete maturity may be anything from 1.5 years to over 6 years. In some girls the bud stage of breast development persists for only 6 months while in others it may last for over 2 years before there is any further development of the breast. The mean interval from the beginning of breast development to menarche is 2.3 years but anything from 5 months to 5 years 9 months is within normal limits (3). The intervals between stages in development of the central nervous system may vary similarly, and only longitudinal data could reveal this.

In about 25% of girls menarche occurs while the breasts are in stage 3 but in 10% there is no menstruation until after the breasts have reached

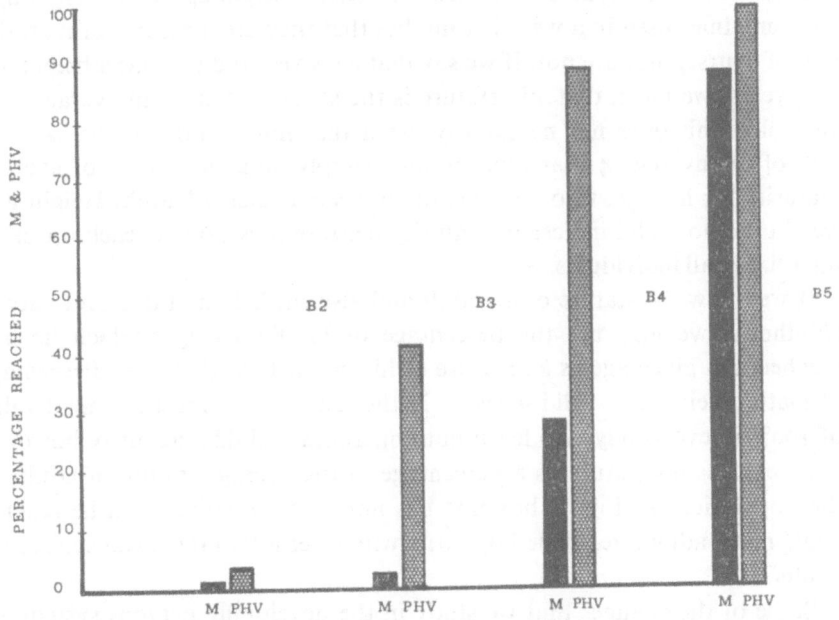

Fig. 6. Percentage of girls who had reached menarche and peak height velocity before reaching each stage of breast development. B2, B3 etc. represent the moments of reaching the corresponding breast stages. Thus the histogram between B2 and B3 shows the percentage of girls in breast Stage 2 who reached menarche or peak height velocity before they reached the 3rd breast stage. (From Marshall and Tanner (3). Reproduced by kind permission of the Editor, Archives of Disease in Childhood.)

maturity (Fig. 6). Peak height velocity may be reached in either the second, third or fourth stages of breast development. Thus in somatic development, and probably neurological development too, we cannot assume that the stage reached in one sequence of changes is necessarily reflected by the others.

MATURITY

It is certainly clear that a child's chronological age gives us very little information about the stage of sexual development which he or she may have reached or the proportion of the total somatic growth that has been completed. Individuals of the same age vary greatly in their maturity and therefore we need a measure of maturity which is independent of chronological age. We must use a parameter which reaches the same maximum value in all members of the species. Ideally it should be possible to measure it throughout the whole period of development and to study it longitudinally.

In the case of somatic development the terms 'height age' and 'weight age' are sometimes used in a way that implies that they are measures of maturity but, of course, they are not. If we say that a six year old boy has a height age of 4 years, we mean that his stature is the same as that of an average four year old. This does not necessarily mean that his maturity is the same as that of the average 4 year old. He may simply be a small boy, of average maturity for his age, who will eventually become a small adult. Height and weight are not valid indices of maturity because they do not reach the same final size in all individuals.

If we know the stature of an adult and also his height at different ages in childhood, we may use the percentage of his final height which he had reached at a given age as a measure of his maturity at that time. Percentage of mature height is a valid measure in the sense that it reaches a final value of 100% in everybody. We learn nothing about a child's maturity however, if we express his stature as a percentage of the average stature of adults in the population. In Fig. 2, boy no: 1 is not nearly mature when he reaches 100% mean adult size, while boy no: 6 will never attain the mean stature for adults.

Some of the changes that we study in the developing nervous system are similar to stature in that they do not reach the same final value in all individuals and therefore cannot be used as measures of maturity. This is obviously true of any measure of size. Estimates of cell numbers present the same problem. By various criteria we can assess the maturity of individual cells and where it is legitimate to assume that no new cells are being created, the percentage of cells at a given stage of development in the whole brain, or in specific regions, might be useful measures of maturity.

Chemical estimations of the absolute quantity of any one substance in the brain cannot indicate maturity and neither can the amount expressed as a percentage of the mean adult value. Changes in the relative amounts of different substances might be used if the relationship were nearly constant in adults. Changes in enzyme activity in relation to the quantity of another substance, e.g. the decrease in isocitric dehydrogenase per mg of protein which occurs during maturation of the rat's brain (5) might provide measures of maturity if the end result were the same in all normal animals.

The best overall measure of maturity of the body is provided by the skeleton. There are various methods of estimating skeletal maturity but the technique with the best theoretical basis (6, 7) is that of Tanner, White-house and Healy (8) which employs radiographs of only the hand and wrist. As the round bones of the wrist and the epiphyses of the long bones calcify, their radiographic shadows go through a series of changes which are essentially the same in all individuals. The development of each round bone or epiphysis can be divided into stages and can be studied longitudinally. In each centre, each stage of ossification is given a numerical score, which has its highest value when the centre has reached its adult form. When all the bones are mature, the maximum overall score is attained. This has the same value in all individuals. Before the adult stage is reached the total score of all the bones is a measure of the maturity of the individual. A similar method, but employing the whole skeleton, is available for the assessment of skeletal maturity in rats (9). Skeletal maturity is related to overall somatic development in the sense that growth, for practical purposes, ceases when the skeleton becomes mature.

It would be useful if we could develop a comparable method of assessing the maturity of the central nervous system. It might be possible to do this on a histochemical or microchemical basis. If it were shown that certain enzymes or other substances became detectable in different regions of the brain in a constant sequence, the appearance (or the disappearance) of each substance in a given region could be regarded as a stage of maturation.

For example, we have seldom been able to demonstrate acetylcholinesterase in the ventromedial nucleus of the hypothalamus in rats during the first few days after birth. In slightly older animals the enzyme is usually present in all major nuclei including the ventromedial. In most animals at a gestational age of more than 47 days the enzyme is again absent or has only very slight activity in the ventromedial nucleus although it persists in most of the others. These observations suggest a sequence of changes which might form part of a system for estimating maturity, although we have not yet studied a sufficiently large number of animals to be able to state with certainty that the sequence exists. A satisfactory scale of overall maturation would, of course, involve the study of more than one region, and probably several substances. With histochemical methods, however, we can obtain only cross-sectional data from which we cannot accurately examine a sequence of changes but it is possible to establish beyond reasonable doubt that a sequence exists and to assess its value as a maturity indicator.

Localised electrical phenomena occurring in a definite sequence might provide another basis for assessing maturity along similar lines but clearly parameters which could be studied without damaging the subject would be much more satisfactory and are essential for the study of human development.

The following might be considered:

1. Sensory motor development.
2. Overall electrical activity (the electroencephalogram).
3. Intellectual development.

There is little doubt that certain reflexes appear and disappear in a fairly constant sequence in the foetuses and young infants of most mammals. This sequence reaches a similar end point in all normal individuals in a given species and therefore is a justifiable basis for a maturity index. The end point is of course reached in very early life and the indicator is only valid during the period before this. In the human foetus and infant this aspect of development has been studied in considerable detail although longitudinal data on the subject are not nearly as plentiful as one might hope. A basis does however exist for developing a satisfactory scoring system which might be used as an index of maturity in late foetal and early postnatal life. Some authors have implied that the sequence of sensory motor development can be used to assess the chronological age of an infant (10). This would only be possible if all infants reached the same stage of maturity at the same age which, of course, they do not. We need more information about the variation in age at which a given stage of sensory motor development is reached. This will probably show that sensory motor development, like skeletal development, is useless as an index of chronological age, although both may be valuable maturity indicators.

Longitudinal electro-encephalographic data on normal subjects are also surprisingly scarce. However, if it were possible to recognise a sequence of changes which fulfilled the basic criteria of a maturity indicator this would be extremely useful.

The development of a child's ability to perform activities such as walking and talking is commonly regarded as an index of maturity. This however, is only partly justified. There is probably a clearly defined stage in the child's development at which the central nervous system becomes sufficiently mature to enable him to walk. The act of walking itself however may be delayed for some time after this stage is reached, for various reasons. The development of speech is subject to alteration by so many variables in the environment that it is of little value at all as a developmental index as far as the central nervous system is concerned.

Measurements of intellectual function are commonly misinterpreted. Even if there were an entirely satisfactory measurement of a child's intellectual ability it would not measure his maturity. It would be analogous to the measurement of stature. If we know a child's stature and skeletal maturity we can tell what portion of his ultimate growth has been completed and we can predict his final stature with reasonable accuracy. With stature alone we can do neither of these things. Similarly we shall not be able to predict a child's ultimate intellectual abilities from his ability in any stage in childhood until we have an independent measure of the maturity of the central nervous system which is relevant to the development of the intellect. The relationship between the rate of intellectual development and the rate of physical development is not close enough for us to use an individual's physical maturity as an index of his intellectual development.

THE RELATIONSHIP BETWEEN SOMATIC DEVELOPMENT AND THE CNS

The growth of the foetus and the differentiation of many organs can apparently proceed more or less normally in the absence of the brain, although certain biochemical changes which are dependent upon adrenal or other hormones do not occur (11). The influence of the central nervous system can however be seen in certain aspects of postnatal growth.

a. Growth hormone

This hormone is one of the major factors influencing somatic growth. Children who lack it are very small and their skeletal maturation is delayed, but they are normal in all other respects. If they are given replacement therapy with the hormone their development may be completely normal.

There is evidence that the output of growth hormone by the pituitary is regulated by a growth hormone releasing factor from the hypothalamus.

Feedback action of growth hormone itself, or of some secondary product, on the hypothalamus regulates the production of this factor (12). There is no direct evidence that the size of the body governs the level of hormone output to which this feedback is adjusted.

b. Catch-up growth

If growth is inhibited in childhood and the cause of the inhibition is then removed, the child will grow at a rate greater than the average until he has reached approximately the stature he would have achieved if the initial inhibition had not occurred (13). He then grows at a normal rate. Tanner has suggested that there is, within the brain, some record of the size that the body ought to have achieved after a given period of time and some signal which informs the central nervous system of the difference between the actual size of the body and its expected size at any moment (14). If growth is inhibited in utero, complete catch-up does not usually occur. In this case the growth potential may be reduced by a deficiency of somatic cells or the central mechanism controlling catch-up may not be sufficiently developed in early life to work effectively. Alternatively the amount of growth which occurs during a certain critical period in utero may play some part in programming the mechanism which regulates further growth. Abnormally slow growth at this period might then reduce the final stature to which the programme is directed.

Direct evidence for central control of catch-up growth is, however, limited and one could postulate mechanisms within the somatic cells which would account for all aspects of catch-up growth, including its uniformity throughout the body.

c. The secular trend

In many countries nowadays children are reaching physical maturity at an earlier age than they did in the past (15, 16). It is generally assumed that improved health and nutrition are major factors causing this trend but we have no information as to whether or not they act via the central nervous system.

d. Puberty

We do not know what maturational changes within the central nervous system result in the occurrence of puberty.

The well known homeostatic mechanism, by which gonadal hormones act on the hypothalamus to inhibit the output of gonadotrophins and hence the production of further gonadal hormones, apparently begins to function in early life (17). At puberty it becomes 'set' at a higher level so that the amount of circulating hormone is increased. This change apparently does not represent maturation of the central homeostatic mechanism itself, as the homeostat can be re-set to the higher level long before the normal time. Damage to the hypothalamus will do this in several species including man. Presumably the lesions damage neuronal pathways which normally inhibit the output of gonadotrophins. In rats and ferrets, exposure to additional light may accelerate the appearance of some aspects of sexual maturity although it has not yet been shown whether or not this advancement of 'puberty' is preceded by accelerated maturation of the organism as a whole.

Changes in the central mechanism governing the output of gonadotrophic hormones cannot account for all the phenomena of puberty. The output of androgens from the adrenal cortex remains unaccounted for and so do some changes which occur in the testes. The testes of pre-pubertal calves produce a considerable amount of androstenedione, a precursor of testosterone but very little testosterone. In adult animals testosterone predominates. The injection of chorionic gonadotrophin into calves causes an increase of androstenedione secretion but only after puberty does it cause increased production of testosterone (18). At puberty therefore the Leydig cells acquire the capacity to convert androstenedione to testosterone but this is apparently not the result of exposure to increased amounts of gonadotrophic hormones. There is some evidence of a similar situation in man.

e. Seasonal variations in growth rate

Children grow in stature more quickly during the spring and summer than they do in the autumn and winter. In blind children this annual cycle of growth appears to be less well synchronized with the seasons (19). This suggests that some environmental factor which synchronizes the seasonal growth cycles of normal children does not operate in those whose eyes are insensitive to light. Light itself, transmitted through the eye and acting through neuro-endocrine pathways might well be the synchronizing agent. It is certainly difficult to account for this phenomenon without implicating the central nervous system.

CONCLUSIONS

1. Many of our opinions of developmental neurology are based on cross-sectional data which cannot give us an exact picture of the pattern of deve-

lopment in individuals. There is an urgent need for greater use of techniques which can provide longitudinal data.

2. Chronological age is not an adequate measure of maturity and, in the case of the central nervous system, no satisfactory alternative has yet been found. We must use a parameter which goes through the same changes and reaches the same final value in all individuals of the species.

3. The central nervous system plays an essential role regulating the concentration in the blood of growth hormone and gonadotrophic hormones. 'Catch-up' growth and seasonal variations in growth rate may also be dependent on the central nervous system, but nothing is known of the neurological mechanism involved.

REFERENCES

1. Tanner, J. M., Whitehouse, R. H. & Takaishi, M., Standards from birth to maturity for height, weight, height velocity and weight velocity: British children 1965. *Arch. Dis. Childh.* 41, 454; 613 (1966).
2. Tanner, J. M., *Growth at adolescence*, Oxford 1962.
3. Marshall, W. A. & Tanner, J. M., Variations in the pattern of pubertal changes in girls. *Arch. Dis. Childh.* 44, 291 (1969).
4. van Wieringen, J. C., Wafelbakker, F., Verbrugge, H. P. de Haas, J. H., *Groeidiagrammen Nederland* 1965, Groningen 1968.
5. de Vellis, J., Scheide, O. A. & Clemente, C. D., Protein synthesis and enzymic patterns in the developing brain following head X-irradiation of newborn rats. *J. Neurochem.* 14, 491 (1967).
6. Acheson, R. M., Maturation of the skeleton. In: *Human development*, Philadelphia 1966.
7. Marshall, W. A., Physical growth and development. In: *Practice of pediatrics*, Washington 1970.
8. Tanner, J. M., Whitehouse, R. H. & Healy, M. J. R., A new system for estimating skeletal maturity from the hand and wrist, with standards derived from a study of 2,600 healthy British children. Parts I and II. *Centre international de l'Enfance*, Paris (1962).
9. Hughes, P. C. R. & Tanner, J. M., The assessment of skeletal maturity in the growing rat. *J. Anat.* 106, 371 (1970).
10. Dubowitz, L. M. S., Dubowitz, V. & Goldberg, C., Clinical assessment of gestational age in the newborn infant. *J. Pediat.* 77, 1 (1970).
11. Jost, A., La place de la croissance cerebrale dans la croissance corporelle. In: *Regional development of the brain in early life*, Oxford, 1967.
12. Igarishi, M., Short and auto-feedback control of the adenohypophyseal function: a review. *Endocrinol. Japon.* Suppl. 1, 63 (1969).
13. Prader, A., Tanner, J. M. & von Harnack, G. A., Catch-up growth following illness or starvation. *J. Pediat.* 62, 646 (1963).
14. Tanner, J. M., Regulation of growth in size in mammals. *Nature* 199, 845 (1963).

15. Tanner, J. M., The secular trend towards earlier physical maturation. *T. soc. Geneesk.* 44, 524 (1966).
16. Tanner, J. M., Earlier maturation in man. *Sci. Amer.* 218, 21 (1968).
17. Donovan, B. T. & van der Werff ten Bosch, J. J., *Physiology of puberty*, London 1965.
18. Lindner, H. R., Androgens and related compounds in the spermatic vein blood of domestic animals. II. Species linked differences in the metabolism of androstenedione in the blood. *J. Endocr.* 23, 161, (1961).
19. Marshall, W. A. & Swan, A. V., Seasonal variation in growth rates of normal and blind children. *Hum. Biol.* (in press).

DISCUSSION

Visser: It seemed quite logical that we should start this course on growth and development of the central nervous system by summarizing all the problems we have been faced with over the last decades in studies of somatic growth and development. Dr. Marshall has stated these problems clearly: the differences between longitudinal and cross-sectional studies, the choice of parameters, the variation in the sequence of signs, and so on. I think we will see during this course that we will have exactly the same problems in studies on the growth and development of the central nervous system.

Widdowson: What is the difference in age at which boys and girls reach skeletal maturity?

Marshall: I take it the variation within the boys and within the girls is what you mean. About two years on either side of the mean value. There are long tails to the distribution and there are individuals who develop perfectly normally and reach maturity three or four years after the mean age for their sex. But these are unusual.

Dobbing: Dr. Marshall has emphasized very correctly for us this terribly important problem of the difficulty of only being able to do cross-sectional studies in the brain, because we have to destroy the brain. I was not so happy about his rejection of chemical indices of maturity as indices of maturity. You see, I think brain size for all practical purposes is very much less variable than height. If you alter the height experimentally or if you look at different heights within the normal population, the range in brain size is very much less. The brain size parameter is buffered in some way. Now, within brains of different sizes, and I am speaking now of mature brains within one species, the total number of cells is remarkably constant. The difference in size is not due to the different number of cells. Except in certain abnormal situations it is due to a different size of the cells and in fact the

16

total number of cells fits remarkably well the criteria which Dr. Marshall uses as good indices of maturity. Furthermore, a parameter such as cholesterol concentration in the mature brain varies remarkably little within a species, very much less even than the number of cells. It even varies but little between species and this is a most remarkable thing. Cholesterol being a structural component of the brain, its concentration per gram wet weight of the brain, I would have thought, is a first class index of brain maturity. The only problem being of course that you have to take out the brain and analyze it in a test-tube in order to determine it. But as an index of maturity it is a good one in an experimental series. The alternatives to the cross-sectional approach I don't find very attractive. I don't find developmental electro-encephalography, at least in its present stage, a very accurate estimate of brain maturity, as little as I know of it. Neither do I anticipate that a growth-curve in behavioural terms might be a very much better one. So I think this is a problem that we are stuck with.

Marshall: I would largely agree with Dr. Dobbing here. Certainly I did not intend to imply that electro-encephalography or behaviour, at least in the present state of knowledge, were good maturity indicators. I was suggesting that perhaps if we could think along those lines something might come out of it. It would be nice to have something that we could study longitudinally, although we are for the time being stuck with the cross-sectional methods. I tended to over-emphasize the difficulties attached to them, because it is important that we should remember that these limitations exist and that we have not, in fact, got a clear measure of maturity. Cholesterol concentration, in fact any concentration, is essentially a relationship between one thing and another, and there are many such relationships that one might think of. There may be some which do reach constant values and which could be used as indicators of the maturity of certain functions. Equally there is no objection to measuring the absolute amount of something, provided one can establish that the value in all adults is identical, or at least sufficiently alike for our purpose at a given time. We will probably never get an ideal measure of maturity so we must constantly think of the limitations of each method that we use.

Freedman: I'd like you to please summarize current thinking as to what the cause and the possible adaptive function of the secular trend is. I have not heard it discussed for about five years, and I want to hear if any advances have been made, at the conceptual level, about this interesting phenomenon.

Marshall: There has been essentially no useful new thinking about the cause of the secular trend. It has possibly something to do with better nutrition and better social conditions. There is a whole list of other factors that might be involved and we will never really know the part played by each. I take it that you are all familiar with the term 'secular trend', which means that general maturation is speeding up, puberty is being reached at an earlier age and adult size is being reached earlier. It still seems to be happening in most of the areas where it is being studied. There is some evidence that amongst the well off in some parts of the United States the trend may be stopping, and indeed it may then even go into reversal, because historically whatever the cause of it, it must have some kind of cyclicity. Whether it will go on being cyclic or whether we will reach a condition which is optimal for us in the present state of the environment, and then stay there, I don't know.

Levine: I am afraid I have to take issue with you on the importance of the role of the central nervous system in puberty. Some of the very elegant current evidence by Ramirez & McCann and by Davidson & Smith in animals, and by Grumbach in man, indicate that in fact the central nervous system does change in its feedback aspects about the time of puberty. Indeed the feedback-system works exquisitely prepubescently and there is indeed a period of time at which the gonadostat, the sensitivity of the central nervous system, changes dramatically as a corollary of puberty. Apparently this alteration in hypothalamic sensitivity to the circulating hormones is indeed what may be one of the parameters which initiates puberty so that the nervous system is indeed playing a very central role here.

Marshall: Oh yes, I agree absolutely. What I tried to say (I quoted, in fact Van der Werff ten Bosch) was that there is a feedback working in early life and that, round about the time of puberty a 'switch' is turned so that the feedback works at a higher level. The turning of the 'switch' is an event within the central nervous system which is an essential part of puberty. What is still open to question is whether the turning of the 'switch' is a stage of maturation of the nervous system itself, or whether the 'switch' is already mature and waiting for some external stimulus (external to the central nervous system but not necessarily outside the body) to come and 'turn' it. You see, we know that it can be turned before it usually is. Certain lesions to the central nervous system will have the same effect as 'turning the switch'. Exposure of certain prepubertal animals (e.g. ferrets) to different lighting conditions will cause the first cycles to occur early. Therefore it seems to be possible to 'turn' this 'switch' at an earlier stage of development than it usually is 'turned'. What I'm questioning is not that a change within the nervous system is important for puberty. I would agree with that. What I do question is to what extent puberty, and the fact that this 'switch' does 'turn', is an index of development of the central nervous system itself as distinct from perhaps something else having impinged upon it. Follow me?

Levine: Yes. I followed you. A very difficult point to argue. We can always say something else occurs and then we don't know what that something else is indeed.

Marshall: Exactly.

Stoelinga: Dr. Marshall, what is your opinion about the value of measuring head circumference as a parameter of brain development for practical purposes?

Marshall: I would not have thought it was of great value within the normal range of variation. Clearly, if a head is very small, microcephalic, this probably means that there is something wrong. Equally, if the head is enormously macrocephalic there is probably something wrong. But within, between those limits I think it is probably of little value. Perhaps Dr. Dobbing could comment on that.

Dobbing: I think very briefly that I agree entirely with Dr. Marshall. It is much too insensitive a measure of brain size. It is very difficult to define. In solid geometrical terms it is much too insensitive a measure. It is very interesting that the latest way of measuring foetal biparietal diameter with ultra-sound which is so accurate, yields longitudinal curves of biparietal diameter development which tail off towards the end of pregnancy, at the very time when the brain is beginning to grow fast. So the whole thing is a little bedevilled by the solid geometry of the head being so complicated.

Marshall: And also there is a rather poor relationship between brain size and other aspects of brain function anyway.

UNDERNUTRITION AND THE DEVELOPING BRAIN: THE USE OF ANIMAL MODELS TO ELUCIDATE THE HUMAN PROBLEM

J. DOBBING*

INTRODUCTION

There is no longer any doubt that growth restriction due to malnutrition at certain ages is associated in many children with an irreversible deficit in higher mental function. The phenomenon is by no means confined to the underprivileged communities of developing countries, but can be found, although on a smaller scale, in similar communities in the most advanced country in the world. It may also be allied to the diminished ultimate potential of some low birth weight babies from even the most privileged homes. A constant feature appears to be the need to maintain a good growth rate at least until the eighteenth month of human postnatal life (1). By contrast, the effects of growth retardation at later ages can apparently be reversed on restoring good dietary and other conditions.

It is important to appreciate that we cannot at present distinguish between malnutrition as an aetiological factor in the mental impairment, and all the other environmental hazards of deprived socio-economic and cultural conditions. The increased exposure to infectious diseases, the general level of education and experience, and even the poor genetic endowment by which such children may also be afflicted, may also conspire in a cumulative fashion to reduce the child's eventual mental potential (2). Thus it is very probable that malnutrition is only one facet, although a central one, of a highly complex aetiology (3). Still less can we be certain that any such effect of early malnutrition is mediated by a modification of the normal physical development of the brain. To demonstrate this last point would require a knowledge which none of us possess, of the molecular or cellular basis of higher mental function.

* I wish to acknowledge a grant from the Medical Research Council, with additional help from the National Fund for Research into Crippling Diseases, and the Spastics Society. I especially thank my colleagues Dr. B. P. F. Adlard, Miss Jean Sands and Dr. J. L. Smart for their continuing help with this work.

20

With these reservations, however, it must be conceded that the effects on mental function described above bear some striking resemblances to the known effects of infantile malnutrition on the physical growth and development of the brain. It is a common finding in all the field studies that the period of life before 2 years of age is vulnerable to growth retardation in the sense that such retardation is not completely recoverable; whereas a similar retardation later in childhood is capable of much more complete catch-up.

THE VULNERABLE PERIOD

Experimental paediatric pathologists (4, 5, 6) using simple experimental designs and comparatively crude techniques, have already demonstrated that there is also a specific period of brain growth during which the organ is susceptible to growth restriction resulting in permanent physical deficit. One version of this idea relates vulnerability to that period of brain growth when cells are undergoing mitosis (6). Brain cells comprising any particular region undergo a once-and-for-all growth-hyperplasia (discounting pathological reactions) at an early stage of development, corresponding well with the timing of the observed period of clinical vulnerability (7). Restriction of general bodily growth at this time reduces the rate of brain cell mitosis in a manner which is not recoverable, even when optimum growth rates are subsequently restored (6).

However, when this general hypothesis is applied specifically to the brain, it tends to ignore that the two main cell types, neurons and glia, multiply at quite different times. Are both periods of mitosis vulnerable? Furthermore it may be wrong to assume that reduction of glial (or even neuronal) cell *number* is functionally significant (8). It seems much more likely that brain function is more dependent on a correct and orderly sequence of cellular migration and the formation of the appropriate histological micro-architecture. Of central importance to proper function is probably the growth of neuronal processes (axons and dendrites) and the proper establishment of their myriads of synaptic interconnections. Both of these aspects of brain growth *post-date* the achievement of neuronal cell number, although they do overlap with the period of glial multiplication known to pathologists as myelination gliosis (9). Indeed it may be significant that most of the known experimental work up to the present time which has produced permanent deficits of cell numbers by undernutrition during the vulnerable period, has imposed the experimental stress during the later period of *glial* mitosis, *after* adult neuronal numbers have been achieved, and the reported deficits in cell numbers must almost certainly refer to glial cells. Functional consequences have sometimes been observed, and it seems more likely that these may be the result of permanent reduction of post-mitotic neuronal development, rather than of restriction of glial cell number. Neurochemists and others could help to resolve this question with a quantitative assessment of the effects of vulnerable-period undernutrition on the ultimate extent of later neuronal growth.

Such speculation led some years ago (5) to a rather wider vulnerable period hypothesis, of which the cell multiplication theory mentioned above forms only an early part. This states in general terms that vulnerability of the brain is greatest during the transient period known as 'the brain growth spurt'. It is thus suggested that vulnerability may be directly related to the growth velocity of all the brain growth processes. This whole vulnerable period is broadly encompassed by the period of fastest accumulation of brain fresh weight, and includes post-mitotic neuronal growth as well as glial hyperplasia and myelination. It is also a time when many enzymes are being rapidly elaborated resulting in dramatic increases in their activity (10, 11), and so it raises the possibility that the developing enzymology of the brain may also be directly and permanently restricted at this time.

Much experimental evidence is being accumulated which relates the degree of vulnerability to the velocity of brain growth. In neurochemical terms all the evidence is crude, but at least it is sufficiently substantial to make a more sophisticated neurochemical approach worth while.

THE BRAIN GROWTH SPURT

If the whole growth spurt is a period of greatest vulnerability, it is first necessary to define its extent in quantitative and qualitative terms. The growth curve of whole brain wet weight has a sigmoid shape, and the brain growth spurt can be easily represented as a first order velocity curve (12). Figure 1 shows the velocity curves of brain growth in various species, from which it is clear that there is an important species difference in its timing in relation to birth. Maximum vulnerability in the guinea pig should be during foetal life, and so it can be shown to be. In the rat it is postnatal, whereas in humans it is perinatal. The characteristics of human brain growth velocity will be illustrated in more detail in a later figure (Fig. 2).

The principal events of whole brain growth are related to these velocity curves as follows. Neuronal cell division is complete to adult numbers before the growth spurt begins (13). Oligodendroglial multiplication, quantitatively much more important than neuronal multiplication, occupies the first half of the growth spurt. Lipid accumulation, in which myelination is prominently included, occupies the second half (12). Lipid accumulation occurs partly at the expense of water content, leading to a progressive dehydration of the tissue (14). The greatest contributor to growth in fresh weight, however, is probably growth in cell size, including the all-important special growth of

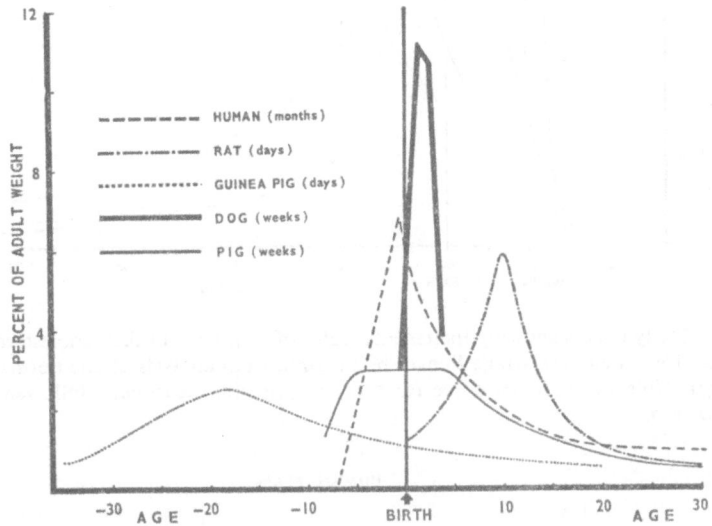

Fig. 1. Rate curves of brain growth in relation to birth in different species. Values are calculated at different time intervals for each species.

neuronal processes and their interconnections, and this occurs throughout the main growth spurt.

Most of these events can be quantitatively defined even in whole brain using the velocity curves of DNA (nuclear) and lipid accumulation. For these purposes the comparatively few tetraploid cells can be ignored, and the accumulation rates of many lipids inferred from the estimation of cholesterol, to which they bear a known temporal relation. The need to employ such crude descriptions is imposed by the extremely laborious nature and questionable validity of much quantitative histology, although it must be conceded that much topographical detail is lost. It is difficult to distinguish different cell types (but see fig. 5), and the migration of cells as well as the death of some of them which forms such a striking feature of brain development is unrepresented. It is therefore perhaps surprising that a recognisable developmental pattern emerges from analysing whole brain such as is seen in figure 2.

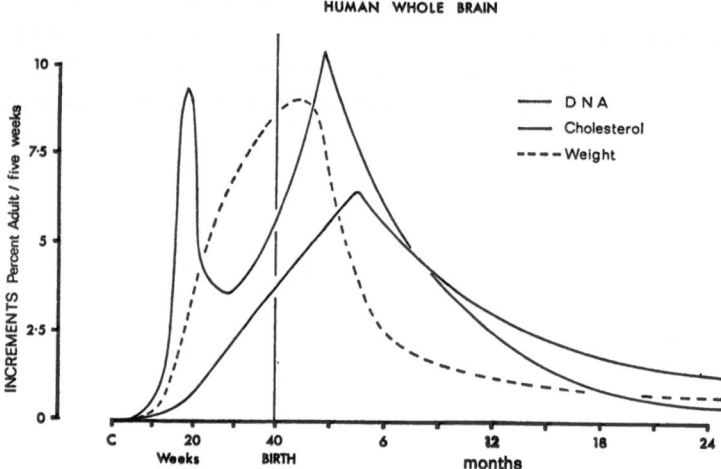

HUMAN WHOLE BRAIN

Fig. 2. Velocity curves showing incremental rates of DNA (two peaks), cholesterol (single peak) and fresh weight in whole human brain. Data from analysis of 200 normal human brains (7). Note the bimodel curve for DNA, representing neuroblast followed by glial multiplication.

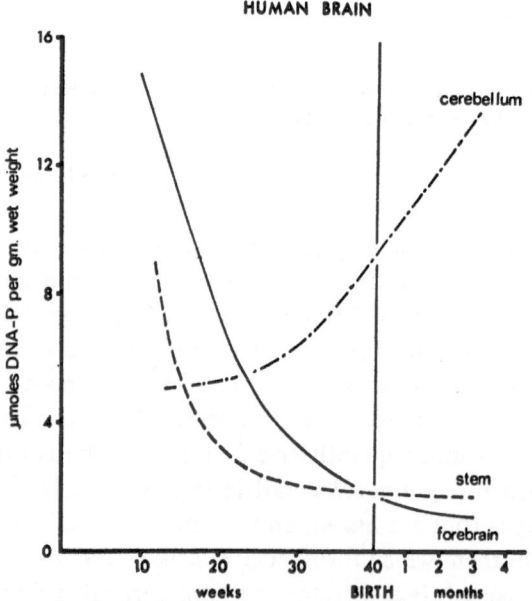

HUMAN BRAIN

Fig. 3. Changing concentration of DNA (per gram wet weight) in human forebrain, cerebellum and stem. Data from analysis of 200 human brains (7).

A little more meaning can be derived by dividing the brain into anatomical regions, but in a developing series this must be done according to anatomical landmarks and not by linear measurement. Thus the very different growth characteristics of the cerebellum can be distinguished from those of fore-brain and stem (15, 16). Unfortunately subdivisions into smaller regions makes it almost impossible to derive benefit from DNA estimations, since these are only of value when expressed as totals per whole region. Cellularity, or DNA concentration per unit volume or weight is more influenced in a developing series by changes in the denominator of the expression than by the DNA itself and is consequently almost impossible to interpret. Thus DNA concentration will fall in some regions as it rises in others with increasing age, even though cell division is occurring in both (Figs. 3 and 4). The meaning of the different ways of expressing analytical data has been discussed elsewhere (17).

TESTING THE VULNERABLE PERIOD HYPOTHESIS
It is not difficult to show that the brain is much more easily influenced during

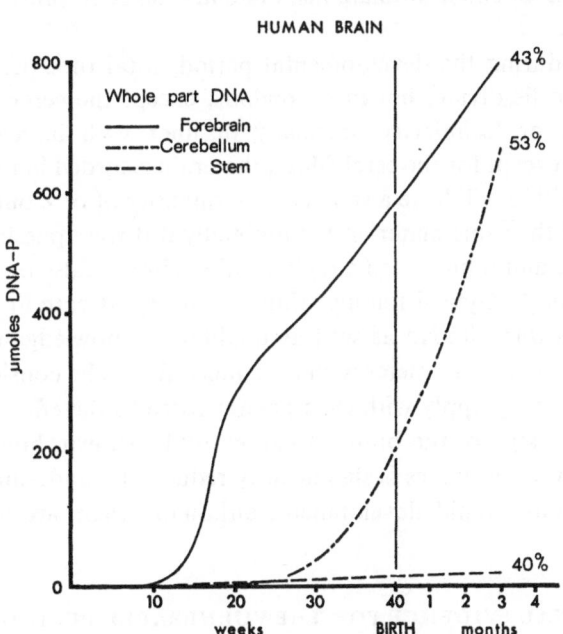

Fig. 4. Rising levels of whole part DNA in human forebrain, cerebellum and stem. Data form analysis of 200 normal human brains (7). Percentage figures denote percent of adult values achieved at 3 postnatal months.

the time of the brain growth spurt than either before or afterwards. Much of the early results is summarised elsewhere (5) and it may now be added that the progress of behavioural ontogeny is depressed just as are the other gravimetric and analytical parameters. The age at which important milestones of reflex and other behavioural growth occur in undernourished animals is significantly later than in normal controls (18).

Growth retardation in the physical parameters manifests itself in ways which can appear contradictory unless the normal direction of progress is taken into account. Thus although the undernourished brain weight is *less* than the controls during development, the *relative* brain weight, or the brain: body ratio is *higher* (5). This is *not* a brain sparing phenomenon as is so often assumed. It simply reflects that the brain weight increases with age before the body weight; and the brain: body ratio thus declines with increasing age. A simple growth retardation must therefore inevitably lead to a *higher* value for the brain: body ratio. Eventually, in the adult, this same brain (again contrary to earlier claims) can be shown to be relatively, as well as absolutely smaller (19). This new finding in rats compares well with the similar finding of small ultimate head circumference in previously underfed children (26).

Similarly, during the developmental period, total DNA per whole region increases as cells divide, but in all regions, except the cerebellum the DNA *concentration* or 'cellularity' normally declines with increasing age (see fig. 3). Thus, except for the cerebellum, the brain retarded in its development by undernutrition will have a smaller total quantity of DNA but a higher concentration of the same material. Undoubtedly if it were possible to examine much smaller and more specific regions other similar false paradoxes would be discovered. Analytical findings thus require great care in their interpretation, and a quantitative as well as qualitative knowledge of the normal movements of each parameter with time must always be considered.

This caveat may apply with even greater force to the effects on the developing enzymology of the brain. It can easily be shown, however, that the activity of several enzymes is significantly reduced by undernutrition only at the time of most rapid development, although others are apparently unaffected (10).

EXPERIMENTAL EVIDENCE FOR THE VULNERABLE PERIOD HYPOTHESIS
Interesting as it may be to study the contemporaneous effects of undernutrition on the developing brain, it is presumably much more important to examine those long-term results which persist in spite of nutritional rehabili-

tation after the vulnerable period. It may be argued that temporary retardation of developmental processes is of little permanent significance if it can be reversed. However this raises completely uninvestigated aspects of the problem. Educationalists are well aware of the permanent effects on a child's prowess of even temporary restrictions of progress which allow him to get cumulatively behind his fellows. In the same sense the orderly sequence of morphological and neurochemical development of the brain may be sensitive to such retardation, leading to an accumulating lag or deficit.

At present probably the most significant research is that which attempts to detect deficits or differences in adults who were undernourished at the time of the vulnerable period. Accounts of these will be found elsewhere and will only be summarised here (17).

Perhaps the most important positive finding refers as much to the whole body as to the brain. This is the finding that if whole body growth retardation is imposed at the time of the brain growth spurt, neither the whole body nor the brain are able to undergo complete recovery on restoration of a normal diet (5). The relevant period is in the last half of pregnancy in the guinea pig or the first three postnatal weeks in the rat. (It is interesting that guinea-pig birth weight can be reduced by as much as forty percent by maternal undernutrition, contrary to the old, outworn hypothesis of perfect foetal parasitism. Growth restriction is not related to the foetal or postnatal condition, but to the stage of development of a species at those particular times.)

Having imposed permanent stunting in this way, the *adult* brains will show the following permanent deficits:

1. Small size. This will be somewhat smaller than is appropriate for the body weight (19).
2. Deficits in total numbers of cells which may spuriously appear to parallel the reduction in weight (5). The cell deficit is not uniform throughout the brain but is largely concentrated in the cerebellum.
3. A *selective* cell deficit in the cerebellum compared with the remaining brain. This is probably related to the faster rate of growth and hence greater vulnerability of the cerebellum (15, 20).
4. A reduced concentration (per gram fresh weight) of myelin lipids (5, 21).
5. It has been very recently shown that acetylcholinesterase activity in rehabilitated animals is increased (22).

As has been already stressed, there is no evidence that any of these deficits are of functional significance. The idea that they may be mentally deleterious is mere hypothesis.

SIGNIFICANCE FOR HUMAN CHILDREN

It is quite clear that similar findings can never be experimentally demonstrated in human children, although a few analyses of the brains of malnourished children have already shown all the deficiencies mentioned above (23).

Assuming that the animal findings which can be extrapolated from one species to another can also be extrapolated to the human, it now becomes important to define the timing and duration of the human brain growth spurt.

Preliminary results from about two hundred human brains, ranging from ten gestational weeks to six postnatal years (7) suggest the following conclusions:

1. The human brain growth spurt begins at the end of the second trimester, and ends at between eighteen months and two years of postnatal life. This is significantly later (24) than the previous estimate of five postnatal months (25).

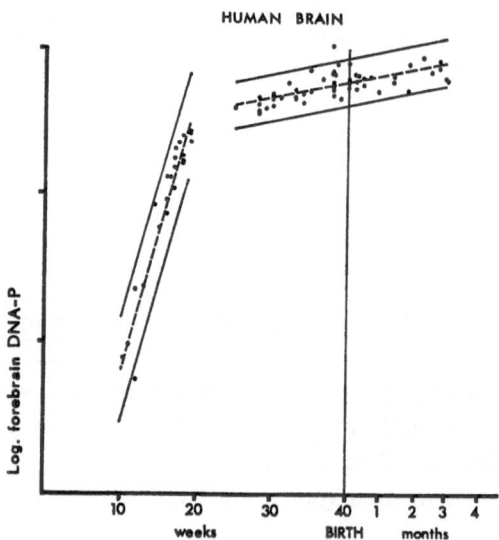

Fig. 5. Two phases of human forebrain DNA multiplication. The data has been analysed in two groups, from 0-22 gestational weeks and from 25 gestational weeks to 3 postnatal months. Two exponentials are shown, representing neuroblast followed by glial multiplication (7). (Broken lines are calculated regression lines, solid lines are 95% confidence limits.)

2. Human brain composition is about half-way towards the adult state by about three postnatal months (see fig. 4).

3. The differences between cerebellar growth and that of the remaining brain are the same as those previously shown in animals, and could perhaps lead to a similar differential vulnerability of the human cerebellum to growth retardation (see figs. 3 and 4).

4. There is a period between fifteen and twenty-five weeks of gestation when human neuroblasts complete their mitoses, before the commencement of glial multiplication. In this regard also the human brain resembles the animal in its growth sequence (see fig. 5).

CONCLUSIONS

Experimental studies of the long-term effects of undernutrition on the developing brain have shown results which emphasise the paramount importance of the *timing* of the undernutrition in relation to the brain 'growth spurt'. In humans this period is an extensive one, occupying the last half to one third of gestation and the first eighteen months to two years of postnatal life. This implies that permanent physical deficits in the brain could result from foetal growth retardation in the later months of pregnancy, and it underlines the importance of good postnatal growth in the prematurely born. Furthermore the first two years of postnatal life probably present a further hazard to the developing brain if malnutrition or any other growth-retarding influence is allowed to persist. Alternatively the postnatal period may also present an opportunity in our own species for compensatory brain growth, provided good nutrition or the correction of other deleterious influences is diligently pursued at this early stage. These remarks are based on the double assumption *a.* that the changes which can be permanently produced in developing animal brain are functionally significant; and *b.* that they can be extrapolated to man by carefully matching comparable stages of brain growth, especially the complex of interrelated events known collectively as the brain 'growth spurt'.

REFERENCES

1. Cravioto, J., Delicard, E. R., Mental performance in school age children – Findings after recovery from early severe malnutrition. *Amer. J. Dis. Child.* 120, 404 (1970).
2. Cravioto, J., Birch, H. G., de Licardie, E. R., & Rosales, L., The ecology of infant weight gain in a preindustrial society. *Acta Paediat. Scand.* 56, 71 (1967).
3. Scrimshaw, N. S. & Gordon, J. E. (eds.), *Malnutrition, learning and behaviour*, Boston 1968.

4. Dobbing, J., The effect of undernutrition on myelination in the central nervous system. *Biol. Neonat.* 9, 132 (1966).
5. Dobbing, J., Vulnerable periods in developing brain. In: Davison, A. N. & Dobbing, J. (eds.)., *Applied neurochemistry*, Oxford 1968.
6. Winick, M. & Noble, A., Cellular response in rats during malnutrition at various ages. *J. Nutr.* 89, 300 (1966).
7. Dobbing, J. & Sands, J., (in preparation).
8. Dobbing, J., Undernutrition and the developing brain: the relevance of animal models to the human problem. *Amer. J. Dis. Child.* 120, 411 (1970).
9. Rorke, L. B. & Riggs, H. E., *Myelination of the brain in the newborn.* Toronto 1969.
10. Adlard, B. P. F. & Dobbing, J., Vulnerability of developing brain: III. Development of four enzymes in the brains of normal and undernourished rats. *Brain Res.* 28, 97 (1971).
11. Chase, H. P., Dorsey, J. & McKhann, G. M., The effect of malnutrition on synthesis of a myelin lipid. *Pediatrics* 40, 551 (1967).
12. Davison, A. N. & Dobbing, J., The developing brain. In: Davison, A. N. & Dobbing, J. (eds.)., *Applied neurochemistry*, Oxford 1968.
13. Flexner, L. B., Enzymatic and functional patterns of the developing mammalian brain. In: Waelsch, H. (ed.), *Biochemistry of the developing nervous system.* New York 1955.
14. Dobbing, J. & Sands, J., Growth and development of the brain and spinal cord of the guinea pig. *Brain Res.* 71, 115 (1970).
15. Dickerson, J. W. T. & Dobbing, J., Some peculiarities of cerebellar growth. *Proc. Roy. Soc. Med.* 59, 1088 (1966).
16. Dickerson, J. W. T. & Dobbing, J., Prenatal and postnatal growth and development of the central nervous system of the pig. *Proc. Roy. Soc. B.* 166, 384 (1967).
17. Dobbing, J., Undernutrition and the developing brain. In: Himwich, W. A. (ed.), *Developmental neurobiology.* Springfield (Ill.) 1970.
18. Smart, J. L. & Dobbing, J., Vulnerability of developing brain: II. Effects of early nutritional deprivation on reflex ontogeny and development of behaviour in the rat. *Brain Res.* 28, 85 (1971).
19. Dobbing, J. & Sands, J., *Biol. Neonat.* (in press) (1971).
20. Chase, H. P., Lindsley, W. F. B. & O'Brien, D., Undernutrition and cerebellar development. *Nature* 221, 554 (1969).
21. Culley, W. J. & Lineberger, R. D., Effect of undernutrition on the size and composition of the rat brain. *J. Nutr.* 96, 375 (1968).
22. Adlard, B. P. F. & Dobbing, J., Elevated acetylcholinesterase activity in adult rat brain after undernutrition in early life. *Brain Res.* 30, 198 (1971).
23. Winick, M. & Rosso, P., The effect of severe early malnutrition on cellular growth of human brain. *Pediat. Res.* 3, 181 (1969).
24. Dobbing, J. & Sands, J., Timing of neuroblast multiplication in developing human brain. *Nature* 226, 639 (1970).
25. Winick, M., Changes in nucleic acid and protein content of the human brain during growth. *Pediat. Res.* 2, 352 (1968).
26. Stoch, M. B. & Smythe, P. M., The effect of undernutrition during infancy on subsequent brain growth and intellectual development. *S. Afr. Med. J.* 41, 1027 (1967).

DISCUSSION

Van der Werff ten Bosch: You have shown a slide comparing the growth rates of the brains of various species. For some species, such as the rat, the curve was very steep, whereas that of the pig was very flat and broad. It seems to me that this difference demonstrates one of the disadvantages of a cross-sectional study, because the shape of such curves largely depends upon the degree of variance there is between different individuals: if they all undergo a change in growth rate at the same time you get a steep curve, if this change is spread over a long period of time, some starting earlier, others starting late, you get a very flat curve. Now I was wondering if you could improve on these curves if, instead of plotting them simply against age, you would somehow allow for differences in body-weight, for example.

Dobbing: I think there are two points which I can answer you. You are perfectly correct about your observations, I think, about this particular disadvantage of the cross-sectional study. However, on that particular diagram I was going too quickly to elaborate on the point. In that particular diagram in which you had to plot the very different life-spans of humans and rats, the time-scale was very seriously and artificially treated. I played concertinas with the time-scales in each case to hammer them into the same graph. All I wanted to show on that particular graph was the relation of the timing of the peak in both. The playing concertinas with the time-scale also made nonsense of both the rates of growth and the shape of the curve. The pig one may not be flat. I don't know how you draw curves which are truly comparable between one species and another. The shapes of those curves were not comparable, and could not be from the way they were drawn. All it showed was the difference of timing of the velocity peak in relation to growth. Your second and last point is really a very interesting one, whether you would get less variance if you used body weight on the base line than if you used age. Or if you took it into account. The answer is yes. The answer also is, though, that in an experimental series, provided you take the trouble

31

to standardize litter-sizes in rats and go through a lot of other trouble to produce a 'standard' product, you will find that the variance in body-weight is really quite small. It only becomes large if you don't take steps to regulate the litter-size. In those cases where there is variation, if you don't take steps, and you get a lot of 12 day old rats for example of all different sizes, then it works out that the brain-parameters are more closely related to the body-weight than they are to age.

Van der Werff ten Bosch: How about prenatal animals?

Dobbing: In the case of prenatal animals there are a number of different sizes of litter particularly in the guinea-pig. It has not been our experience from the variances which I think I showed, that this has made a great deal of difference to the brain-parameters. There is a difference in body-weight but one of my comments this morning was to the effect that the difference in brain-weight appears to be buffered out from the difference in body-weight. But it has to be taken into account.

Polman: I should like to ask you a question. Does oxygen-tension have an influence on the development of DNA in brain tissue and has the air-pressure something to do with it?

Dobbing: The smart answer to that is that it is open to anyone to make this discovery. Because it only needs to be experimented with. It would be a comparatively simple thing, at least in these crude terms, to investigate. Presumably the effects on both intra-uterine and extra-uterine growth of living in the mile-high city of Denver, Colorado, are well-known and presumably these have something to do with the effects of the factors you mention on general somatic growth. What precisely their effect is on DNA synthesis, I have not any idea. But what I suspect is that environmental factors such as oxygen-tension and atmospheric pressure will in some global way affect growth rather than in a specific way. This is of course quite different from the concept of anoxia or hypoxia producing a focal pattern of lesions. This is quite another matter. We are speaking of a brain growth pattern. Have you anything to add to that Elsie?

Widdowson: I have nothing to add to that. It is an interesting fact that the average weight of babies at birth is lower at high altitude than it is at sea-level (J. A. Lichty, R. Y. Ting, P. D. Burns & E. Dyar (1957). *Am. J. Diseases*

Children 93, 666). As far as I know, no studies have been made on the brain, but only on the size of the whole body.

Freedman: Do you have any information on atmospheric differences in development of brain DNA-levels or cell number?

Dobbing: No we have not any information on that. Here again, however crude may be the technique of estimating cell-numbers in this way, it is a remarkably sensitive technique if all you want to know is what is the total number of cells there. It would be amenable to an investigation of that particular point where the one cerebral hemisphere is different from another. But we have not done it.

Steendijk: I have been listening very carefully and I have never heard Dr Dobbing use the word abnormal. You said that your small rats were lively and active, even more active than the big ones, and that they were not under-fed while the big ones were not over-fed. What is normal? Can you in fact say that undernourishment creates abnormal, sick animals, or are they just different? And what would you consider normal?

Dobbing: We are in the realm of philosophy, are we not? It is not a thing that we can really talk about. As Miss Widdowson said, she and I and many others of us don't regard, I think, certainly the fast growing rats, as abnormal. But assuming that you believe that the normal range merges with the abnormal, and I think in this field until there is evidence to the contrary we must, what we are trying to do with our experiments was to give ourselves the acid test. If we could produce permanent changes with such a comparatively mild restriction at this time, this seemed to us to make it useful then to go on and do others things. So we deliberately made it difficult. I would not like to argue about what is normal and what is not normal.

Steendijk: What I am referring to is the trouble we are having nowadays in trying to find out whether children which were undernourished at an early age and are later found to have lower IQ's, will ultimately catch-up in mental development. No one knows accurately as yet whether this different brain development is conducive to a lower or slower mental development.

Dobbing: This is my third lecture to-day, whereas Miss Widdowson had only one! In very brief summary: is it not the case that we know quite certainly that there is an association between severe undernutrition before the age of 18 months and ultimate (I mean by ultimate at the age of 10 years) deficits of various kinds in behaviour? The problem, and this is the one you have expressed, is: has this anything whatever to do with the nutritional effect on the physical growth of the brain?

I think all of us in the field and certainly those who are working in under-developed and underpriviliged communities, with the actual children, are well aware of the 5246 other factors and the immense capacity, at least in our own species, to compensate post-natally for even quite severe and gross physical deficits. Prof. N. Butler was divulging to us the other day some features of their analysis of a peri-natal mortality survey which is still in course of preparation, from which it clearly emerges that there were a very large number of different factors, the algebraic sum of which ends up with your result: that you can have some quite negative factors, detrimental factors, cancelled out by postnatal positive ones. But if you have poor social class, if you have large family-size, if you have a mother who has smoked heavily during the last part of the pregnancy or during the whole of the pregnancy, and if you add all of these negative, detrimental factors, then you don't just end up with a slightly lower point on the IQ-scale. You end up with an alarming proportion of mentally retarded children. But cancel any of those out, it is the algebraic sum that matters. I think that is what you are driving at.

Visser: I am very glad that you stress the fact that small-for-date babies should get a lot of calories and should be treated at neutral temperature and so on, at optimal environmental conditions. I like to add another piece of clinical information from the studies of my colleague Dr. Van Gils. We have premature infants, just prematurely born infants, who are not small-for-date. When you look for head circumference, they have normal head circumference, which means it is between the percentiles. And if treated well, head circumference grows just along the percentile. So a prematurely born infant, born at 32 weeks of pregnancy, grows for 8 weeks (until the 40th week) right along the percentile; it has no catch-up growth as far as head circumference is concerned. Which is a great difference from the group of infants showed this afternoon, which did show catch-up.

Dobbing: I think it is also very interesting to introduce another comment about the questions that have not been answered. Miss Widdowson did not mention that you can reduce the birth-weight of a guinea-pig by 40 or 50%

by underfeeding the mother. It is not that the foetus is a parasite which is being spared. It is not the fact of rats or ourselves being foetal when our mothers are underfed during pregnancy, which saved us. It is the stage of development we as a species are at as a foetus. If you take a species like the guinea-pig that is at its vulnerable stage in intra-uterine life, you can produce enormous deficits in the birth-weight. It is almost as if the deficit you can produce and even its lasting effect in *body-weight,* is related to the timing of the *brain* growth spurt. And this could support the idea of Dr. Tanner and Dr. Marshall, that somewhere in the brain there may be the organization of all this. Unfortunately for their idea, decapitated foetal rabbits grow remarkably normally.

Widdowson: In considering these small rats, and other species undernourished early in life I think we have got to differentiate between the effects of immaturity and effects of undernutrition. In both the runt-pigs that I talked about and in the small rats at 3 weeks, the small animal is less mature than the larger animal of the same age. On the other hand it is considerably more mature than a well-nourished animal of the same size, so that it is in many ways more mature than it ought to be for its body size. When we come to our severely undernourished pigs, we have got much greater changes, and these animals have reverted in some ways to the composition of an animal younger than they were when the undernutrition began. For example the muscle has more water in it than the muscle of a new-born pig.

Dobbing: Yes. I think the most dramatic thing about effects of undernutrition on the brain, which has been the first thing to be noticed for all the time it has ever been studied, which is about a century now, is the sparing. What one cannot assess is the degree of importance of the extent to which it has been affected; and it could just be that in concentrating on the sparing, which is the obvious and most dramatic thing, we may have neglected the possibility that the degree of affection is the most important. But this is only guessing.

Van Gils: The effect of the impairment of growth of the cerebellum in the last part of gestation, or the effect of the impairment of myelinization, has this anything to do with the hyperirritability you see in small-for-date infants?

Dobbing: I don't know and neither does anyone else. And I don't know whether it may be to do even with clumsiness in children, which is a fashionable subject to be thinking about. What I do know is that these quite mildly treated rats, who turn out to have deficits concentrated in the cerebellum, are very bad if you make them do quite outlandish things for a rat, like making them walk along a pair of thin rods, or making them run around the rim of a large beaker for a food-reward. This is a stupid thing to ask a rat to do of course, but push it to that extent and even in those mildly under-fed ones of the large litters you can detect deficits of performance, which may well be related to that cerebellum deficit. Now human pathologists don't measure the relationship in babies between, say, cerebellum-weight and the rest of the brain, do they? It would be very nice if some of them began to. It is just possible. I don't see any reason at all why, if it can happen to the cerebellum of the guinea-pig and of the rat and of the pig, and so on, why it should not happen in the human too. But we just have not looked.

Slob: I would like to ask one question. I have never seen in all those graphs what the sex is of the animals. Are you only working with males?

Dobbing: This is one of the things I should have said. We have only worked with males. The reason for it is, that, as Prof. McCance and Dr. Widdowson have shown in many different species, including birds (hens and cockerels), when it comes to catch-up potential following growth retardation at this time, the females of the species are much better at catching-up than the males. Now our only reason in this preliminary work in selecting males and only looking at males is, we wanted to give ourselves the best chance of producing the difference. In an experimental procedure this is quite fair to do. You deliberately set up your experiment to produce conditions you want to investigate. It does not necessarily reflect on the truth of life. But it is an attempt to isolate. And it is true of hens, is it not, Elsie, as well as pigs and rats and so on. They catch-up much better.

Widdowson: Yes, females do catch-up better than males, and then there is the interesting fact that males normally finish up with bigger brains than females. Why is this?

Dobbing: I know why this is! You can have it both ways, but the male human brain is on the average 100 g heavier than the female and this is presumably a factor related to lean body mass. The females, if you like, are working more efficiently, expressed by weight of brain.

De Groot: What you and Dr. Widdowson have demonstrated is the very strong protective capacity of the brain against malnutrition at the cost of other organs. It is quite remarkable that the growth and chemistry of the brain is so little disturbed by malnutrition. I think there must be a special positive factor which protects the brain. Perhaps, for example, there is a special nutritive substance which can only be metabolized by the growing brain. Do you have any suggestion?

Dobbing: Yes, I have lots of suggestions. We are not short of suggestions. We are just short of facts. I think Miss Widdowson's idea is, and I am sure that she would agree with this, a newish one and one of very many. As a chemical pathologist, thinking in terms of mild disorders of general pathology, I have always tended to think that we should not be thinking whether carts come before horses or horses before carts. During the development of vascularity in the developing brain it is not that the brain is developing because the vessels come in, or even perhaps that the vessels are coming in because there is the metabolic requirement there to pull them. But this is organized, I would have thought, at a much higher level of the hierarchy, both being in fact results of a higher order. You know one can talk, and perhaps the bar is the best place afterwards to talk in these terms. For it means absolutely nothing without some evidence.

Akiyama: I believe there is always a problem of comparing the data from animal experiments to the human in terms of undernutrition, but I think there must be some data on the effects of maternal malnutrition in some of the war-time studies.

Dobbing: Indeed. There is a paper which I was looking at, dating from 1905, somewhere in the States, where human mothers were deliberately underfed, not to see what was the effect on the foetus. It was the fashion in those days, and few of us can remember it, I suppose, it was the fashion to reduce foetal weight in cases of suspected disproportion by obstretricians, and the mothers were very severely starved. And they got deficits and this is all well documented, if you delve far enough back in the ancient literature. They got deficits of the order of 12-15%. Now here in Holland, of course, you had perhaps one of the most severe war-time episodes of undernutrition in your occupied population. There are a couple of studies, which are quoted still and very rightly so and very commonly quoted. But what gets quoted is the degree of brain sparing. If you look into the original papers from Holland about this the thing to realize is that undernutrition first of all affects fertility, and you are looking at the ones which were actually born, which are obviously the product of a fertile conception. And the second thing is that if you look at the actual figures they too show a deficit of 12-15% and it is written off as not significant. Well, of course it may not be significant. How do we know what is significant? All I am suggesting, and I think the rest of us are suggesting, is that quite mild growth retardations at the time when the brain is growing fastest, can produce ultimate deficits in the brain. And therefore a straight numerical assessment of significance is not of a very useful order.

Levine: We keep talking about sparing and indeed there is sparing in one strict sense, but there is another sense of sparing we don't know about. And that is, although we may be sparing some of the physiological changes, we don't know how that brain is responding to inputs at that time, which may be one of the most critical questions of all. Here you have a developing brain, and there have been a number of very interesting series of relationships between rates of development and adaptive significance in terms of the length of the infantile period, in order for more input, for greater cortical development to occur. Now in essence you measure only what is happening to that animal in terms of the chemical changes in the brain. But how is it responding to a variety of inputs which may go on? That may be one of the more critical questions to ask in terms of what is being spared and what is not being spared. A deficit may really exist as a function of how this animal is responding to its environment.

Dobbing: Clearly I would only respond with a plea to you, Dr. Levine, and others like you who really are the people who know about these things behaviourally, that here is in your own terms 'an open field'. I do seriously think that it is no good our regretting that we have got to do this in rats. We are not going to be able to do it in humans, it is far too complex a situation. You can't do it experimentally in humans anyway. So let us accept that we have got to do it in rats, and let us recruit you and others like you and try to seduce you into doing this job for us. I know you have other things which you are interested in too. That is the plea I would leave you with.

EFFECTS OF EARLY MALNUTRITION ON GENERAL DEVELOPMENT IN ANIMALS

E. M. WIDDOWSON

The theme of this course is the normal and abnormal development of the central nervous system. It is important, however, not to think of the brain in isolation. It forms part of the body, and if the young child or animal is malnourished all parts suffer, but – and this is the important thing – they do not all suffer to the same extent. Some organs develop sooner than others, and the effect of malnutrition may vary from one organ to another, depending on the stage of development each of them has reached when the malnutrition is imposed.

I am going to compare the growth in size and the increase in the number of the cells in 5 organs, and the brain is one of them, first during normal development in the well-nourished animal, second during periods of malnutrition early in development, and third during rehabilitation. I shall speak only about the effects of undernutrition – too little of all food – and not of specific dietary deficiencies. I shall illustrate my points by reference to the rat and the pig and, where possible, show when and how the general principles apply also to man.

All mammalian species go through a similar sequence of developmental events between conception and maturity, but birth takes place at different stages in them. The rat is born in a very immature state, before its development has gone very far. Its eyes and ears are closed, it has no hair and it is completely helpless. The pig is much more mature at birth. It can walk about, and in fact has to do so in order to find its food. The human baby is in some ways more and in other ways less mature than the newborn pig. It cannot move about as the pig can, but on the other hand it has already got considerable amounts of fat in its body, which the pig does not acquire until after birth.

Some animals are much nearer the adult size than others when they are born, but this is not necessarily a sign of greater maturity. Table I shows the weights of the newborn rat, pig and human baby compared with the weights of the adults. Although the newborn rat is so much less mature than the newborn pig, its weight is a greater proportion of that of the adult, and this is important in two ways. Thus undernutrition after birth can delay the normal course of development of, say the brain, of the rat much more than that of the pig because it is less highly developed at birth but it is possible to make a much greater impression on the somatic growth of the pig than it is on that of the rat because the newborn pig is so small compared with the adult. Figure 1 shows the growth of the three species the rat, the pig and man during the first year after birth, all related to a weight of unity at birth. The human baby merely trebles its weight, the rat multiplies its birth weight 70 times and the pig 180 times. It is clearly possible theoretically to retard the growth of a pig after birth more than that of a rat, and of both species far more than the human child is ever likely to be retarded.

Table 1. Weight at birth compared with weight of adult.

	Rat	Pig	Man
Weight at birth g	5	1,500	3,500
Weight of adult g	350	300,000	70,000
Weight at birth as % adult weight	1.4	0.5	5

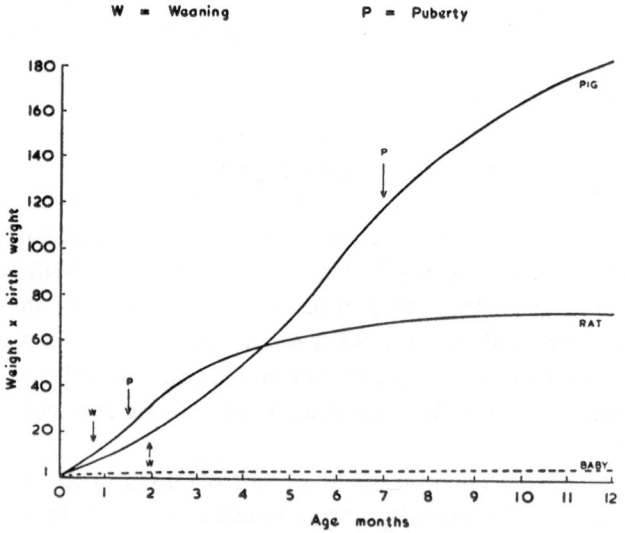

Fig. 1. Gain in weight of the pig and rat during the first year after birth compared with growth of the human baby. Birth weight = 1.

Table 2 shows the weights of the organs of the three species at birth compared with weights in the adult. The values for the whole body are given again for comparison. The brain is nearest to its adult weight and the muscle is the farthest away. Figure 2 shows the changes in weights of the organs of the rat after birth; the values are all expressed as a percentage of the weights at 18 weeks, by which time the rat is fully mature. The rat's brain goes on growing more rapidly after birth than the other organs and it reaches its mature weight first; the skeletal muscle and liver remain behind and are the last to reach mature size.

The different parts of the body not only grow in size at different rates, but

Table 2. Weights of organs at birth as a percentage of the adult weight.

	Rat	Pig	Man
Whole body	1.4	0.5	5
Brain	10.2	30	25
Liver	1.6	4.5	6
Kidneys	1.8	5.2	8
Heart	3.1	4.6	7
Muscles	0.2	0.4	4

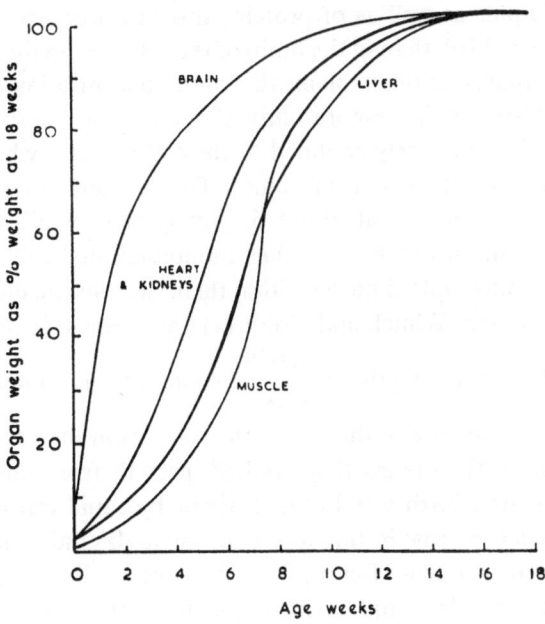

Fig. 2. Weights of organs of rat as percent of weight at 18 weeks.

they also move towards chemical maturity at different speeds. One of the characteristics of chemical development is a decrease in the percentage of water and an increase in the percentage of solids, of which the most important quantitatively in most organs is protein. Table 3 shows the concentration of protein in the organs of the rat and pig at birth expressed as a

Table 3. Concentration at birth of protein in organs and tissues and of cholesterol in brain, expressed as a percentage of the adult value.

	Rat	Pig
Brain	80	77
Liver	76	80
Kidneys	69	78
Heart	79	86
Muscles	57	67
Cholesterol in brain	28	43

percentage of the adult value. The heart is nearest its adult composition in this respect and the muscle the farthest behind. The brain is in a special position because it has 3 major components, water, protein and lipids. The later stages of development are associated with a large increase in the concentration of lipids as well as of protein; this has proceeded farther in the brain of the pig at birth than in the brain of the rat because the former is more mature at this time, and this explains the lower concentration of protein in it.

Protein synthesis is the responsibility of the nucleic acids. Desoxynucleic acid, DNA, is almost entirely confined to the cell nucleus, where it is an important constituent of the chromosomes. The amount of DNA in a diploid nucleus is rather constant at about 6.2 picograms so if we measure the amount of DNA in an organ which has mononucleated cells, and which is known to have only diploid nuclei within them, we can calculate the number of cells in that organ. Winick and Noble (1) have done this systematically in the rat, and they have used the $\frac{\text{protein}}{\text{DNA}}$ ratio, or the amount of protein per nucleus, as a measure of the size of the cell. From their results they concluded that in all the organs they studied, growth from the embryo until about 15 days after birth was brought about by rapid cell division. Some organs continued to grow in this way until 40-50 days after birth, in others cell division slowed down after 15 days, but eventually it ceased in all the organs except the spleen and thymus, and from then on growth was due entirely to increase in size of each cell.

At a particular time after conception, 15 days for the heart, at about the time of birth for the brain, and about 14 days after birth for the kidney, the protein per nucleus in each organ began to increase rapidly, indicating that cell division was now being accompanied by an increase in the size of the cells. Finally, this too came to an end, and at this point growth of the organ ceased. Not only do organs start to grow at different ages after conception but, as we have already seen, they also cease to grow at their own appointed time.

The first effect of undernutrition, whether before birth or afterwards, is to hinder growth. All parts of the body are not retarded equally, and the brain is always in a very favoured position when food is short. We have made studies on rats and pigs, and have found that the same general principles apply to both species, and to undernutrition before and after birth.

STUDIES ON RATS

Since the rat is so very immature when it is born it can be undernourished after birth at a stage of development which other species pass through before birth. The device for undernourishing was first described by Kennedy (2) and developed by Widdowson and McCance (3). Two litters born on the same day are mixed, and 3 young rats returned to one mother to suckle and all the remainder, 15-20 are given to the other. Those in the group of 3 get

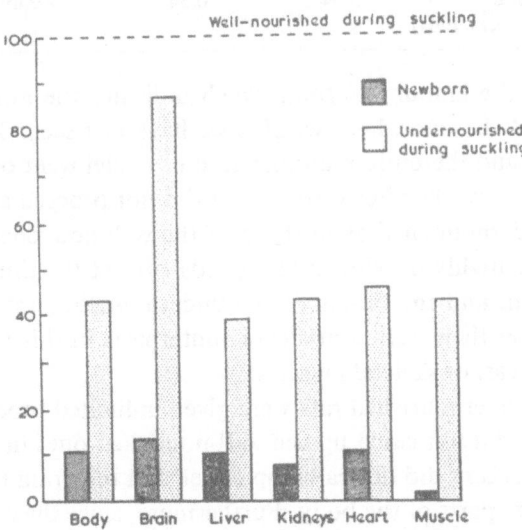

Fig. 3. Weights of organs of newborn rats and of rats undernourished for 3 weeks after birth expressed as a percentage of those of well-nourished 3 week old animals.

more milk and grow more rapidly than the others and at 3 weeks of age they weigh 2-3 times as much. Figure 3 shows that the undernourished animals suckled in a large group have smaller organs. The weights of the body and of the organs of the small animals are expressed as a percentage of those of the large ones, and the values for the newborn rat, also expressed as a percentage of the values for a well-nourished 3 week old animal, are given. Growth of the organs of the well-nourished animal during the first 3 weeks after birth is indicated by the difference between the newborn and 100, and growth of the undernourished by the difference between the height of the two blocks. It is clear once again that the brain is a little further on in size than any other organ at birth, and that undernutrition has considerably less effect on the growth of the brain than on other parts of the body.

Table 4. Total DNA in organs of rats.

	Newborn	3 weeks	
		Undernourished	Well-nourished
Body weight g	5.2	21	49
DNA mg			
Brain	0.59	1.6	2.2
Liver	0.73	2.8	5.5
Kidneys	0.29	1.4	3.0
Heart	0.14	0.25	0.51
Muscles (Gastrocnemius)	0.04	0.34	0.69

Table 4 shows the amount of DNA, which indicates the number of nuclei, in the organs of the rats whose weights we have just seen. The amounts of DNA increased, and therefore multiplication of nuclei went on, in all the organs during the 3 weeks after birth, but it did not proceed so far in the organs of the undernourished as in those of the well-nourished animals. The brain was more highly developed as regards DNA at the time of birth than any other organ, and the brains of the undernourished rats 3 weeks after birth were nearer their well-nourished counterparts in this respect than the liver, kidneys, heart or skeletal muscles.

When these undernourished rats were given unlimited food from weaning at 3 weeks they did not catch up the well-nourished ones in weight; table 5 shows that the organs did not catch up either, but the brain more nearly did so than the other parts of the body. Furthermore, since the concentration of DNA was the same whether the organ was large or small there was less DNA in the organs of the animals that were undernourished. Winick and Noble

(4) explained this by suggesting that if the cells of an organ are still dividing rapidly when the animal is undernourished, and cell multiplication is sufficiently delayed or has stopped, the full number of cells may not be reached even when the animal is rehabilitated and hence the organ will be small. If undernutrition is imposed later, after the full number of cells has already been achieved, then it will only prevent the cells growing in size, and this can be made good when plentiful food is supplied.

Table 5. Weights of organs of rats 15 weeks old, all well-nourished from weaning at 3 weeks.

	Undernourished first 3 weeks	Well-nourished first 3 weeks
Body g	310	372
Brain g	1.60	1.76
Liver g	14.4	16.5
Kidneys g	2.11	2.45
Heart g	0.81	0.99
Muscles g (Gastrocnemius)	3.71	4.20

STUDIES ON PIGS

We have studied pigs undernourished at two stages of their growing period, before birth and during the first year afterwards. In large litters of pigs there is sometimes one – the runt – that weighs only one half or one third as much as the rest of the litter at birth. This is because the blastocyst became implanted at an unfortunate site in the uterus, where the blood supply was particularly poor for, since blood provides the foetus with all its nourishment, the foetus becomes undernourished if the flow rate is too low. We do not know how early in gestation the undernutrition began to make itself felt, and to compare the runt with a well grown animal of the same size I have selected for this purpose well grown foetuses from other litters at about the 90th day after service, which is three-quarters of the way through gestation. I have also compared it with its well grown littermate, born along with it at term.

Figure 4 shows the mean weights of the organs of the 'runt' pigs expressed, as in the case of the rats, as a percentage of those of their large littermates, and the weights of the organs in well grown foetuses of the same size are also shown. The brain at once arrests our attention. It was nearer its full term weight than any other organ in the foetus, and the mean weight of the runts' brains was 80% of their large littermates, whereas those of the liver and muscle were less than 30%. These last two organs in fact weighed less than those of the foetus, and table 6 shows that the muscle contained less DNA. Nuclear division in the muscles of the runts must have begun to be delayed at some age well before the 90th day of gestation.

Some of these runt pigs and their large littermates are now growing to maturity. The runts are not going to catch up their large littermates in weight. None have yet been killed at maturity so I can say nothing about the size of their organs or the amounts of DNA in them.

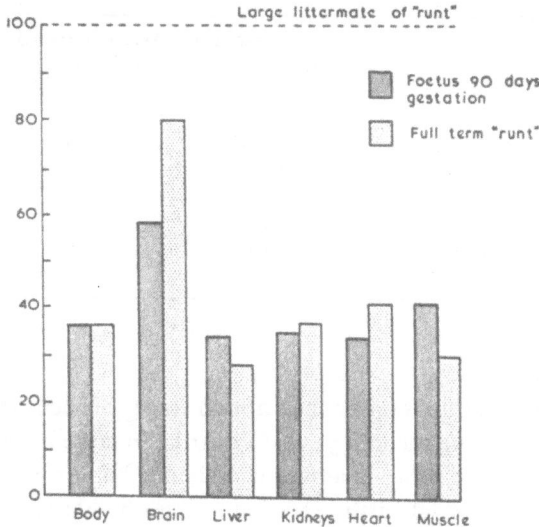

Fig. 4. Weights of organs of foetal and 'runt' pigs born at term expressed as a percentage of those of large littermates of the runts.

Table 6. Total DNA in organs of foetal and newborn pigs.

	Foetus	'Runt'	Large littermate of runt
Body weight g	576	578	1586
DNA mg			
Brain	26	35	48
Liver	34	43	102
Kidneys	29	38	66
Heart	16	30	46
Muscles (Quadriceps)	22	16	31

We have also undernourished pigs after birth. We have given them so little food that they weigh only 5-6 kilograms when they are a year old and their well-nourished littermates weigh 170 kilograms (5). This enables us to compare in the same species the effects of undernutrition before birth with that of severe undernutrition afterwards. We start the deprivation when the pigs are about 10 days old and weigh 3-4 kg. We give them just enough food to enable them to grow very very slowly during the year, and figure 5 shows

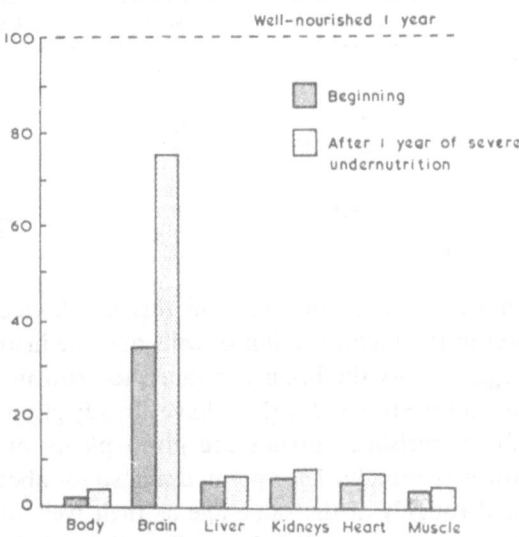

Fig. 5. Weights of organs of pigs at the beginning and end of a year of severe undernutrition expressed as a percentage of those of well-nourished littermates.

the weights of their organs expressed as a percentage of those of the well-nourished littermates one year old. The starting point is the 10 day old pig, and the weights of its organs are expressed in the same way. Some parts of the body have barely changed in weight during this time, but the brain once again has gone on growing, and has more than doubled its weight, largely because it has been depositing protein and lipids. It weighs 80% of the weight of the brain of the littermate, although the whole body weighs only 3%.

Table 7 shows the amount of DNA in the brain and anterior tibialis muscles of these three kinds of pigs. There has been an increase in DNA in the brain during the year of undernutrition, but the increase is small, and no more relatively than the increase in DNA in the skeletal muscle. The effect of the undernutrition has been much more severe on the muscle, however, because at this stage of development the increase in DNA should be so much greater. Neither brain nor muscle had its full quota of DNA at 10 days of age when the undernutrition began, and the effects of undernutrition after birth were similar qualitatively to the effects before birth. The degree of deprivation

Table 7. Weight and total DNA of brain and anterior tibialis muscles of undernourished and well-nourished pigs.

	Well-nourished 10 days	Undernourished 1 year	Well-nourished 1 year
Body weight kg	3.3	5.6	170
Brain			
Weight g	38	83	111
DNA mg	48	54	76
Muscles			
Weight g	9.3	10.7	250
DNA mg	6.2	7.5	98

after birth was much greater, however, and this is reflected in the much greater retardation in the multiplication of cells and the increase in weight of most of the organs. Only the brain continued to grow in weight to any appreciable extent and the reason for this I have already given you.

When these undernourished animals are given plenty of food they at once begin to grow very rapidly. They go on doing so for about 2 years, but then they stop, and roughly at the same age as their well-nourished litter-mates stop, so that they become slightly smaller adults. Table 8 shows the weights of the organs of pigs 3½ years old, the one group undernourished till they were a year old and then rehabilitated, the others well-nourished throughout. By this time all the pigs had stopped growing. All the organs were smaller in the previously undernourished animals, just as they were in the rats rehabilitated after being undernourished for the first 3 weeks after

Table 8. Weights of organs of pigs 3½ years old, all well-nourished from 1 year.

	Undernourished first year	Well-nourished first year
Body kg	240	290
Brain g	121	140
Liver g	1940	2950
Kidneys g	428	580
Heart g	577	736
Muscles g (Anterior Tibialis)	530	656

birth. Complete recovery was not possible, even of the brain, and no organ contained as much DNA as the corresponding organ of the well-nourished animal. There was a big increase in DNA in all organs, however, and that is perhaps more striking than the fact that nuclear division stopped a little too soon.

Why both rats and pigs undernourished early in life stop growing before they have reached full size is a question we cannot answer. Although cell division had been held up almost completely for a year in some of the organs of the undernourished pigs, it started up again when plentiful food was supplied and the amount of DNA almost, but not quite, reached its full quota.

Skeletal development, like the development of the soft tissues, can be hindered by undernutrition before or soon after birth. The bone development of the 3 week old rats that had been undernourished since birth was behind that of well grown animals of the same age (6), and the runt pigs had smaller bones and fewer ossification centres than their larger littermates. The bones of these animals that are undernourished during the early part of their lives never grow as long as those that grew well in the early stages (7). Closure of the epiphyses is not the explanation for the rat's epiphyses never close, and those of the pig are said not to close till $3\frac{1}{2}$-4 years, long after the bones have ceased to grow in length. If the bones do not grow as long it is difficult to see how the skeletal muscles can do so, and it makes one wonder how much the growth of the brain is limited by the smaller skull. We may have too look to the skeleton for the explanation of why previously undernourished animals and their organs never grow to full size.

REFERENCES

1. Winick, M. & Noble, A., Quantitative changes in DNA, RNA, and protein during prenatal and postnatal growth in the rat. *Devl Biol.* 12, 451 (1965).
2. Kennedy, G. C., The development with age of hypothalamic restraint upon the appetite of the rat. *J. Endocr.* 16, 9 (1957).
3. Widdowson, E. M. & McCance, R. A., Some effects of accelerating growth. I. General somatic development. *Proc. R. Soc. B.* 152, 188 (1960).
4. Winick, M. & Noble, A., Cellular response in rats during malnutrition at various ages. *J. Nutr.* 89, 300 (1966).
5. McCance, R. A. & Widdowson, E. M., Nutrition and growth. *Proc. R. Soc. B.* 156, 326 (1962).
6. Dickerson, J. W. T. & Widdowson, E. M., Some effects of accelerating growth. II. Skeletal development. *Proc. R. Soc. B.* 152, 207 (1960).
7. Lister, D. & McCance, R. A., Severe undernutrition in growing animals. 17. The ultimate results of rehabilitation. Pigs. *Br. J. Nutr.* 21, 787 (1967).

DISCUSSION

Van der Werff ten Bosch: There is a question that I have wanted to ask you for a long time. When you talk about catch-up in the undernourished rats, which have been undernourished for the first three weeks of life, you compare them to the what you call well-nourished animals. Would it be fair to say that you are really seeing an effect of overnutrition in some animals and that it is perhaps illegitimate to compare the growth of the other animals to these 'overfed' animals.

Widdowson: This is a nice point. I would like to suggest that the big ones are not overnourished, but that they are well nourished, and the rats that have been suckled in litters of eight are perhaps a little undernourished. They provide an intermediate group. They grow faster than those suckled in very large groups, but more slowly than those suckled in groups of three.

Van der Werff ten Bosch: That's why I was wondering. One might argue the point whether normal growth is optimal growth.

Widdowson: What is optimal growth? If you are not satisfying full growth potential by suckling in litters of eight can you really consider those animals perfectly nourished? I don't know. This is a debatable point.

Freedman: As I understand it, the skeletal growth is inhibited at puberty by testosterone production. And I am wondering if one might be able to experimentally postpone the introduction of high titers of testosterone for a while to enable these runts to try and catch-up.

Widdowson: I've been discussing this with Dr. Steendijk and he has told me about a nice trick to stop the skeleton growing. I mean to try this and when I've done it we should be able to be more certain about the role of the skeleton in controlling the growth of the soft tissues.

Ader: Dr. Widdowson, as you probably know, if you rear rats in litters of three, litters of eight, twelve or fifteen, there are also very large differences in the interaction between the mother and the litter; that is, behaviour towards the litter is quite different. I like to ask, first, to what extent and in what organs do you think this might have contributed to part of the differences; secondly, do you know of any behavioural deficits in either the rats or the pigs; and, thirdly, do you have any data on the longevity of these animals?

Widdowson: I'll start with the last question first. We made studies on longevity of these animals some years ago (Widdowson, E. M. and Kennedy, G. C., *Proc. Roy. Soc. B.* 156, 96, 1962) and what we found was that the death-rate among the slow growing ones was much higher than among the fast growing ones in the first year. Many more of them got respiratory infections. If you take the death rate from the end of the first year onwards, there was no difference between the mortality rates, but if you consider it from the beginning then the mortality was greater and earlier in the slow growing ones. I personally don't think that the interaction of the mother with the young makes any difference. I don't know whether Dr. Van der Werff ten Bosch would be prepared to say something about this.

Van der Werff ten Bosch: Mr. Slob and some other of my collaborators are at the moment studying the effect of malnutrition brought about in a different way: by having litters of eight, half of which remain with their mother for 24 hours a day, while the other half spend 12 hours with the lactating mother and the other 12 hours with the foster mother, which does not produce milk.

Slob: What we try to do is to keep the number of animals constant and also the control animals within one litter will always be with the same number of litter mates with their own mother.

Widdowson: Can you tell us what you have found?

Slob: Well, the first thing we did is try and find out if it is possible to deprive suckling animals for 12 hours of their milk supply, and it works fine. The resulting big differences in weight and length are of the same orders as you have found. We plan to carry out behavioural tests in adulthood.

Ader: I would like to hear very much more about this study. We have some

recent data that indicate that there is a 24 hour rhythm in maternal behaviour
in the rat (Ader, R. and Grota, L. J., *Animal Behaviour* 18, 144, 1970;
Grota, L. J. and Ader, R., *Animal Behaviour* 17, 722, 1969). Therefore, if you
want to have a mother with a litter for only 12 hours a day it is likely to be
very critical which 12 hours those are in relation to the light-dark cycle and
how much time the mother spends with them and nurses them.

Slob: We have a day-group and a night-group. So some animals are food-
deprived during the day when it's light, from 9 A. M. till 9 P.M. (we have a
12-12 hours light-dark schedule) and the other group is deprived during the
other 12 hour period, from 9 P.M. till 9 A.M. From the preliminary data we
have, there does not seem to be any difference between these two groups.

POSTNATAL GROWTH AND DEVELOPMENT IN SMALL-FOR-DATE BABIES

J. F. VAN GILS

Until recently, all newborns with a birth weight lower than 2500 grams were defined as premature regardless of the gestational age, as proposed by the First World Health Assembly in 1948. The effect of this classification was that all newborns with a low birth weight were grouped together, so that infants with a low birth weight due to short gestation were compared with infants having a low birth weight due to intra-uterine growth retardation. Several authors pointed out the differences between these two kinds of infants: divergence in external appearance resulting from foetal malnutrition during the last weeks of gestation, in organ weight, as pointed out by Gruenwald (1, 2, 3, 4) or in oxygen consumption per kilogram body weight. Both groups have their own specific problems in postnatal life, which can influence the results of follow-up studies.

Unanimity has not been reached concerning the definition of intra-uterine growth retardation. This is partly a consequence of ethnic and geographical differences in birth weight, which influence in particular the shape of the intra-uterine weight curve. The American Academy of Pediatrics (5) cites as an example of a useful standard the Colorado Intra-uterine Growth Graph (6), and defines 'small for gestational age' as a birth weight below the 10th percentile. Gruenwald defines chronic foetal distress as a birth weight below two standard deviations of the mean for the relevant gestational age.

In our department we use the intra-uterine growth curves for weight, length, and head circumference given by Usher and McLean (7). The 10th percentile in the weight curve of the Denver studies is the same as 2 S.D. below the mean in the so-called Montreal curve. Birth weight below the 2 S.D. is defined as intra-uterine growth retardation.

There is equally little unanimity about the nomenclature, as can be judged from the variety of terms in use: chronic foetal distress (1), intra-uterine growth retardation (10), dismaturity (11), pseudo-prematurity (12), light-for-dates (13), small-for-dates (14). We shall use the expression small-for-

53

date to describe the result of a pathological process during intra-uterine life, namely intra-uterine growth retardation. It is not my intention to discuss here the various causes of intra-uterine growth retardation. The main cause of this developmental disturbance is a decreased flow of nutrients and oxygen through the placental membrane from the mother to the child. Maternal causes are in the first place hypertension irrespective of development during pregnancy or other chronic maternal diseases, undernutrition of the mother, smoking during pregnancy, use of certain drugs, and environmental influences such as living in low oxygen tension surroundings. Placental causes include gross macroscopic aberrations such as partial solutio placentae, infarction or haemangioma, or only microscopically visible aberrations such as circulatory disturbances or degenerative changes in the villi (1).

A relative placental insufficiency can originate in twin pregnancy (18, 19). An otherwise normal placenta can be functionally inadequate for optimal growth in twin pregnancy after the 31st week, mainly at the cost of one of the twins. In triplet pregnancy this relative insufficiency occurs even sooner. Foetal causes of intra-uterine growth retardation can be genetic in nature or caused by intra-uterine infections such as rubella, cytomegalic inclusion disease, or listeriosis.

The question is now, what are the consequences of intrauterine malnutrition for the developing foetus? Much information about the consequences of malnutrition for the ultimate growth of the whole body as well as of different organs has been gathered from animal experiments, particularly in rats and pigs. Without detracting from the merits of the work of several other authors, I would like to refer here to the important publications of Wigglesworth (15-17), Widdowson and McCance (20-23), Dobbing et al. (24-27), Winick et al. (28-31), and Zamenhof (32). These authors describe the effect of malnutrition on body composition and in particular on the cellular growth of the brain. In addition, I would like to mention the publication by Barnes (33) on the influence of malnutrition on the functional development of the brain of rats and pigs.

The interesting experiments of Widdowson and Dobbing are reported in this monograph, and I shall therefore not review these experiments, although they form the basis of our own work. With respect to the experimental work on animals, the following facts are the most important.

In organ growth in general, and with reference to the present subject in the development of the brain in particular, three phases can be distinguished (31):

I.   cell multiplication, distinguished by a proportional increase in weight and in the DNA and protein contents;
II. cell multiplication and cell volume increase, distinguished by an increase of DNA and a disproportional increase in weight and protein content;
III. cell volume increase without cell multiplication, distinguished by the absence of DNA increase while weight and protein content increase.

Myelination of the brain, i.e. the deposition of several lipids, takes place under the influence of oligodendroglia cells and is always preceded by multiplication of these cells. Malnutrition during the phase of cell multiplication impairs this process. If malnutrition persists beyond the phase of cell multiplication, this impairment is irreversible. If malnutrition is restricted to only some part of the cell multiplication phase, then after the resumption of normal nutrition we find a restoration of the normal number of cells by 'catch-up' growth. If, however, malnutrition takes place during the phase of cell volume increase, it will only cause impairment of cell volume, reflected in a decreased protein-to-DNA ratio. There is no alteration in the number of cells, and this process is fully reversible.

Of all the organs, the development of the brain is the most rapid, and its ultimate growth the first to be completed. In man there is a linear increase in brain DNA during intra-uterine life that decelerates after birth and stops at about 6 months postpartum (28). Further increase of brain weight is influenced by increase of cell volume and by myelination.

It may be assumed that in man malnutrition during the phase of active cell multiplication causes the same impairment of brain growth as in animals, the effect being dependent upon the length and severity of the malnutrition in relation to the phase of cell multiplication. Malnutrition can take place in either the intra- or extra-uterine period and worst of all in both periods, in which case it results in a 60 per cent reduction of the total number of brain cells, as has been shown in young rats (28).

Winick (30) investigated the brains of nine children whose death occurred during the first year of life due to severe malnutrition. All these children showed a severe reduction of head circumference, corresponding to a reduction of brain weight as compared with that of normal children of the same age. Total DNA, protein, and RNA were reduced proportionally to the reduction in brain weight. However, in three cases the DNA content was even lower, i.e. only 40 per cent of the normal DNA content. These three children had a birth weight of less than 2000 grams. It was not known whether these children had been born prematurely or as small-for-dates. In either event, however, these three cases illustrate the more extreme effect of malnutrition during early life, as had already been showed in the doubly-deprived rats. No data have yet been published concerning the myelination of the brains of these children.

More information is available about the late effects of malnutrition on the functional development of the brain. The literature on this subject can be divided in two groups, one dealing with the effect of malnutrition during the first year of life and the other with the effect of malnutrition during intra-uterine life, consisting of studies on the intellectual development of small-for-dates. The results pertaining to these groups show a striking divergence. In the first group such authors as Stoch and Smythe (34, 35), Cabak and Najdanvic (36), and recently Chase and Martin (37), found a significantly lower IQ in the malnourished group, as well as decreased weight and length and, what is more, a reduced head circumference persisting years after the period of malnutrition. On the other hand, representatives of the follow-up studies on small-for-date infants do not always report the same effect. Babson (38) did not find a significantly lower IQ or head circumference in the under-nourished group, but did find a persisting impairment of growth expressed in weight and length (40). Yet the same author found a significant difference in growth and mental development between twins of dissimilar size (39). Drillien (41) points out the effect of social class expressed in the results of studies done in small-for-dates. At the age of 10-12 years in children of middle class and superior working class parents there was no difference in IQ between those with a birth weight below the 10th percentile as compared to those above the 25th percentile. There was, however, a difference between the two groups originating from poor workingclass parents. As has already been said, the ultimate effect of malnutrition on brain development is dependent on the duration of malnutrition in relation to the growth phase of the brain as a whole or some part of it. Recovery of normal nutrition before the end of cell multiplication can give catch-up growth of the impaired cell multiplication. This perhaps partly explains the difference between the group of long-term malnutrition during the first year of life and that of the relatively short period of malnutrition for small-for-dates. If a catch-up growth of the brain mass indeed takes place after restoration of a normal diet, this phenomenon must be observable in measurement of head circumference (29).

In our neonatal ward we investigated this phenomenon in small-for-date infants. The group under study consisted of 35 girls and 17 boys. In fig. 1

these children are arranged according to gestational age. The mothers' height is shown at the top. In fig. 2 the same children are arranged according to birth weight combined in groups of 250 grams; the mothers' height is

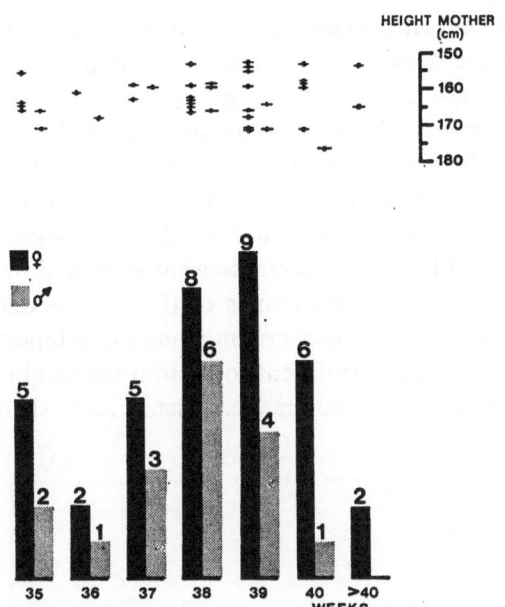

Fig. 1. Distribution of the length of gestation of 54 small-for-date babies.

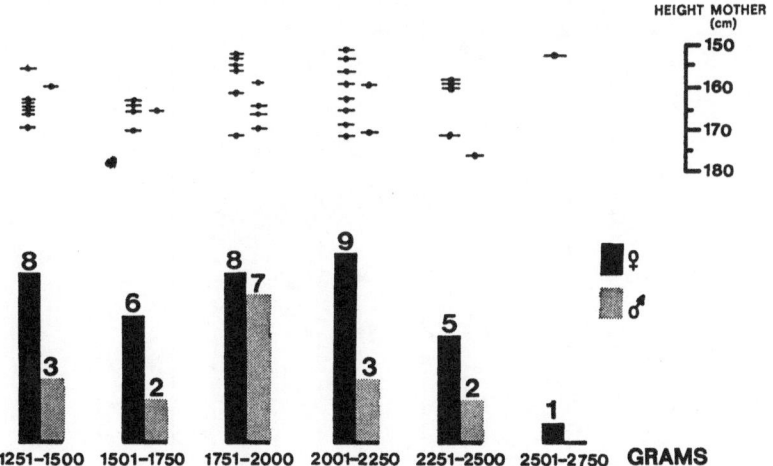

Fig. 2. Distribution of birthweight of 54 small-for-date babies.

shown as before. These children have in common a birth weight of 2 S.D. or more below the mean for the appropriate gestational age. Small-for-dates with gross congenital malformations were not included, and those forming the smaller child of twin pregnancies were analysed separately.

All infants were treated in the same way, the purpose being on the one hand to give a large amount of calories and on the other to have the least possible loss of calories by heat production. After the 8th day of life these infants receive a formula of humanized milk providing per kilogram: 200 ml water, 140 kilo calories, and 3 grams of protein. During both the clinical observation and the regular check-ups at the out-patient department, the length, weight, and head circumference were measured by the same person. Double skin thickness and the course of the bone development were also measured. An investigation concerning mental development is in progress. The available space is not sufficient to go into the results of these different kinds of anthropometric measurements in detail, and I shall confine myself to

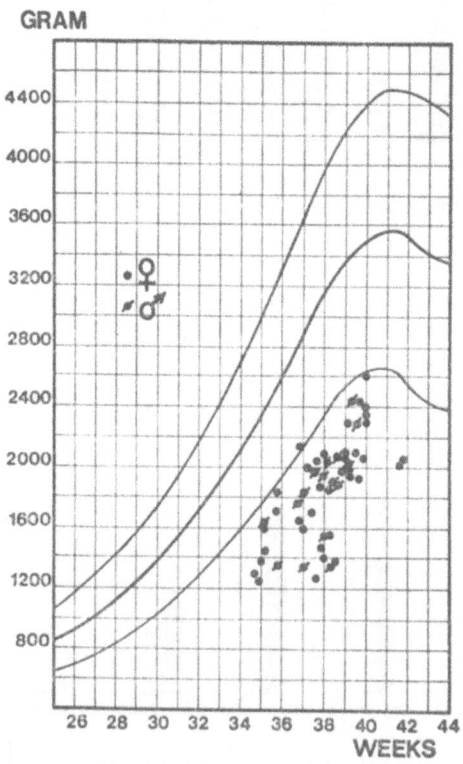

Fig. 3. Birthweight of 54 small-for-date babies; 37 girls, 17 boys.

showing some striking facts observed in this series. Foetal malnutrition impairs not only the development of body weight, which is shown in fig. 3, but also of the length and the brain expressed in the cranial circumference (Figs. 3, 4, 5).

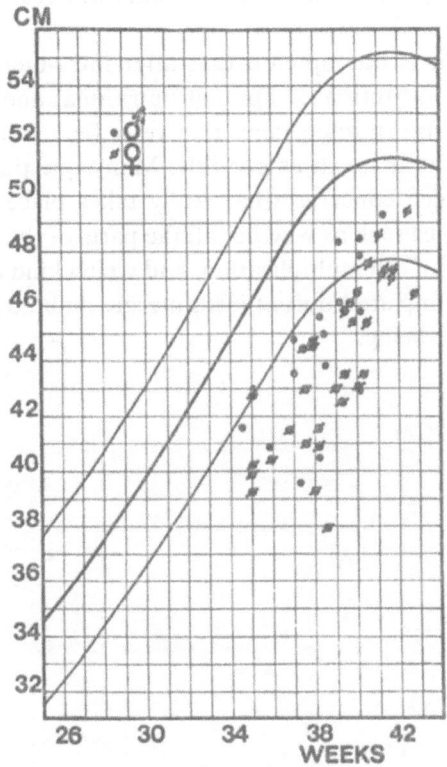

Fig. 4. Birth length of 54 small-for-date babies; 37 girls, 17 boys.

During the first month of life there was a striking increase in head circumference, apparently leading to a fully normal value. This striking catch-up growth was not observed to the same degree in the length and weight. Figs. 6 and 7 show the growth patterns of 4 boys and 4 girls born before the 38th week of gestation, and 4 boys and 4 girls born after the 38th week of gestation. All these children were small-for-date infants. To determine whether the normal head circumference is achieved, we compared the growth of twins of dissimilar size. As can be seen from figs. 8 and 9, there is a very rapid increase in the head circumference of the smaller child, until the value of the other child has been reached. Comparison of the growth rate of the head circumference of small-for-dates with that of normal infants shows an even more striking difference (see figs. 10 and 11). For several reasons, a double-blind investigation was not possible, nor do we have at our disposal a well-documented group of small-for-date infants not reared according the described method.

Nevertheless, it is our opinion that after intra-uterine malnutrition the earliest possible institution of optimal nutritional and environmental conditions is of the utmost importance to reverse the effects of malnutrition on brain development as much as possible. Many questions remain, the most important of which concerns what really takes place in the brain during recovery. Questions such as whether all the parts of the brain can recuperate after impairment of cell multiplication, and which kind of cells in which part of the brain are impaired during intra-uterine malnutrition, remain unanswered for the time being.

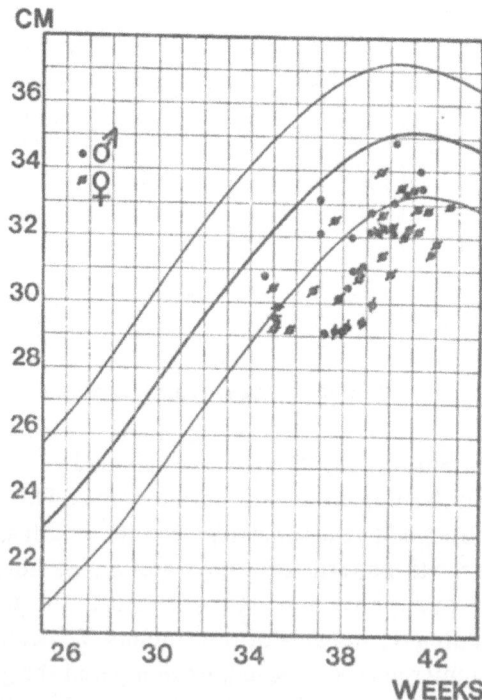

Fig. 5. Birth head circumference of 54 small-for-date babies; 37 girls, 17 boys.

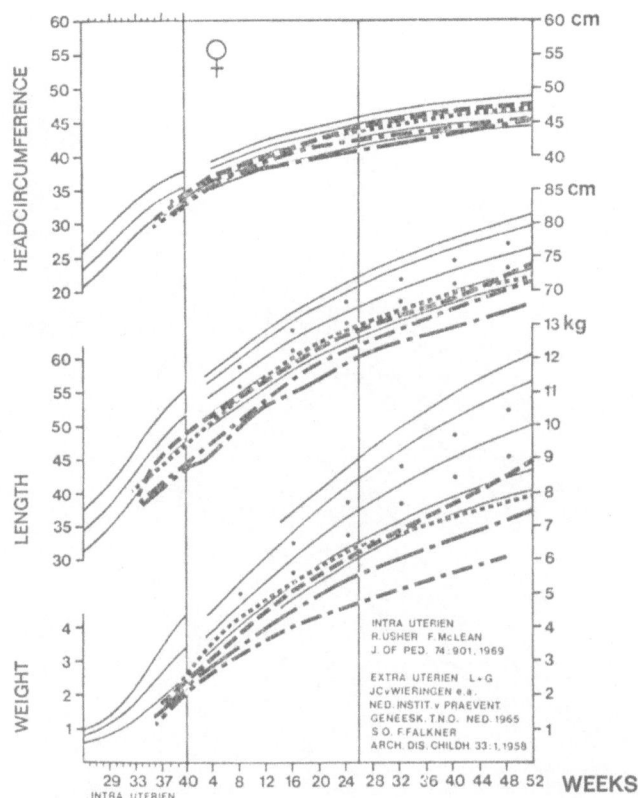

Fig. 6A. Example of postnatal growth of 4 small-for-date girls, born after 35-36 weeks of gestation.

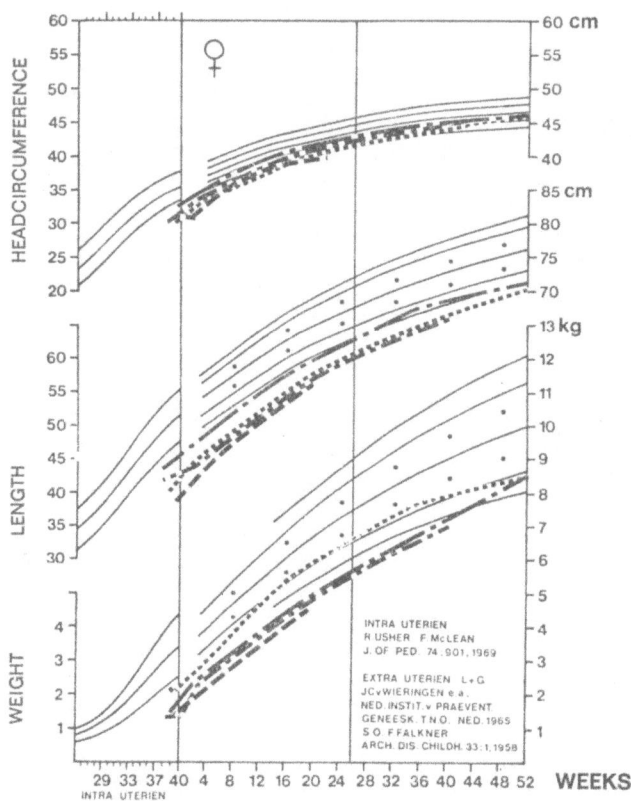

Fig. 6B. Example of postnatal growth of 4 small-for-date girls, born after 38-39 weeks of gestation.

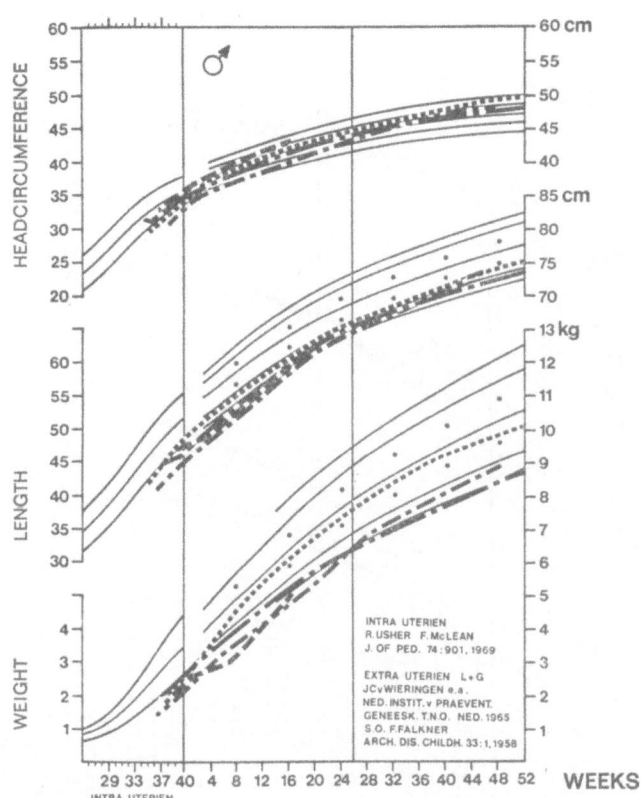

Fig. 7A. Example of postnatal growth of 4 small-for-date boys, born after 35-36 weeks of gestation.

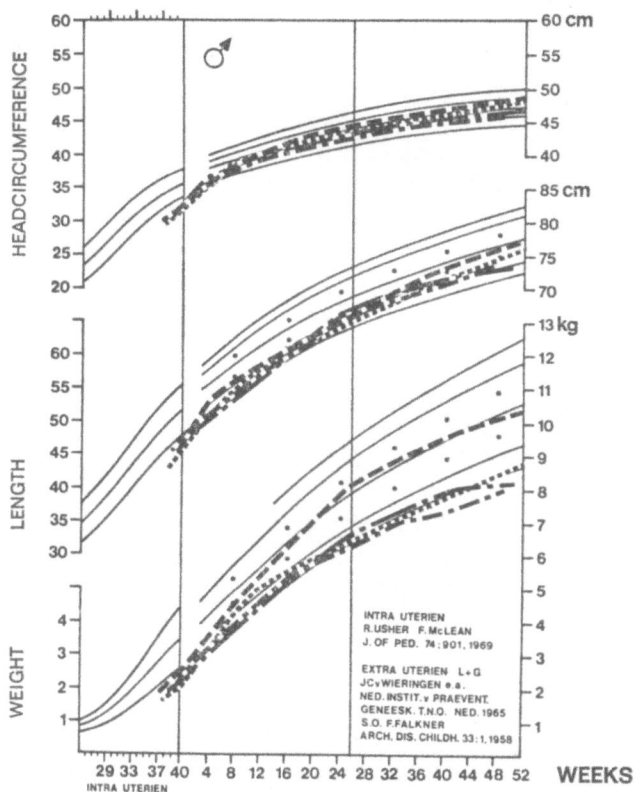

Fig. 7B. Example of postnatal growth of 4 small-for-date boys, born after 38-39 weeks of gestation.

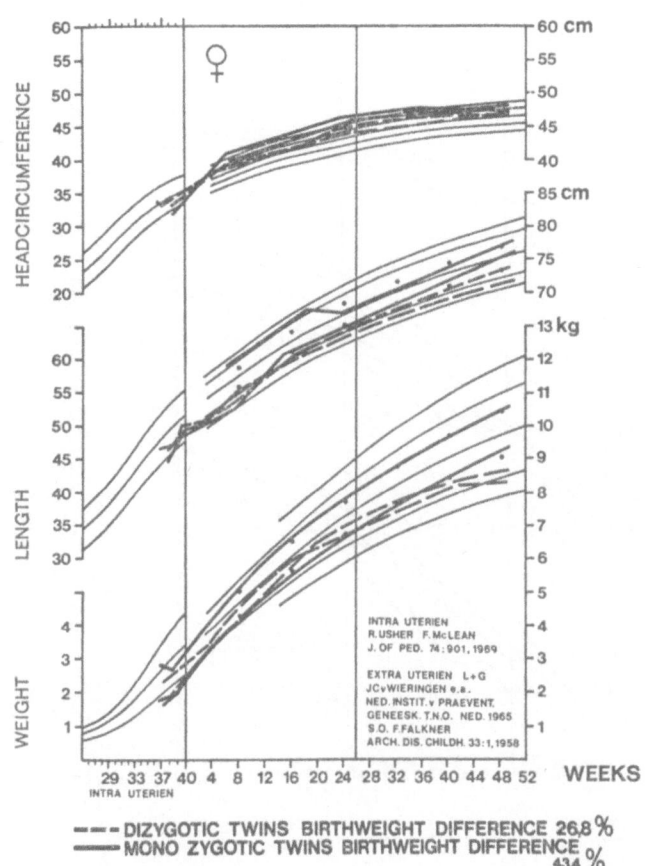

Fig. 8. Example of postnatal growth of one pair of dizygotic and one pair of monozygotic twin girls of dissimilar size at birth.

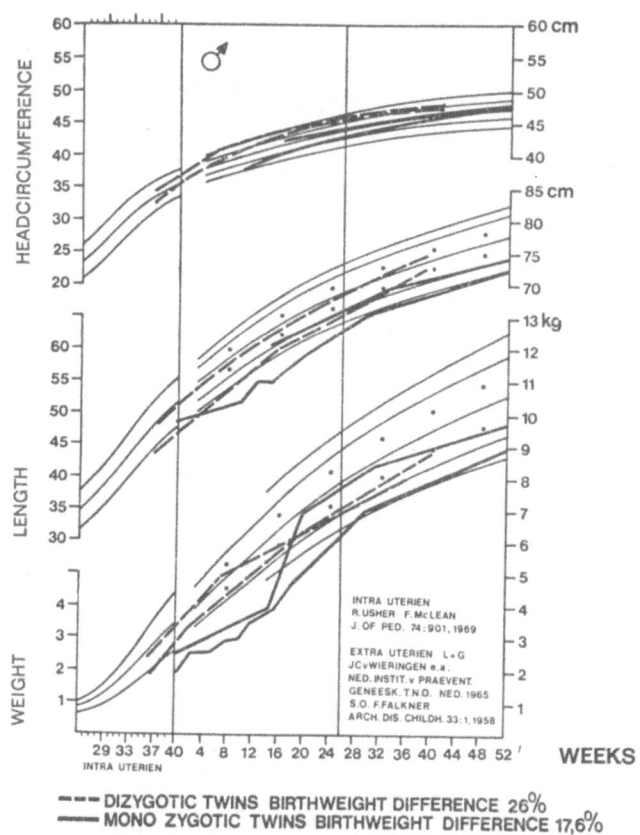

Fig. 9. Example of postnatal growth of one pair of dizygotic and one pair of monozygotic twin boys of dissimilar size at birth.

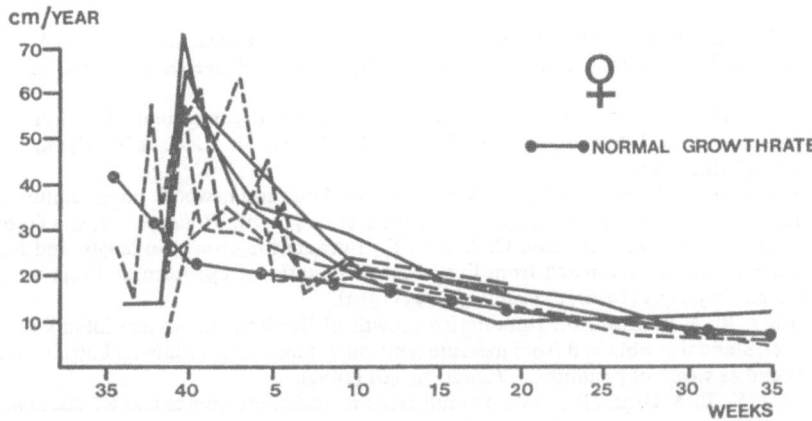

Fig. 10. Postnatal growthrate of the largest occipitofrontal head circumference in seven small-for-date girls.

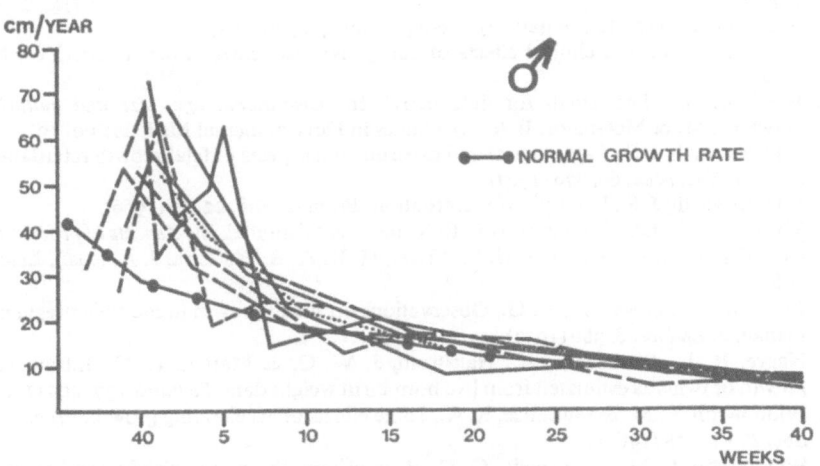

Fig. 11. Postnatal growthrate of the largest occipitofrontal head circumference in eight small-for-date boys.

REFERENCES

1. Gruenwald, P., Chronic fetal distress and placental insufficiency. *Biol. Neonat.* 5, 215 (1963).
2. Gruenwald, P., Growth of the human fetus. *Am J. Obst. Gynec.* 94, 1112 (1966).
3. Gruenwald, P., Infants of low birth weight among 5000 deliveries. *Pediatrics* 34, 157 (1964).
4. Gruenwald, P., Growth pattern of the normal and the deprived fetus. In: *Aspects of praematurity and dysmaturity.* Jonxis, J. H. P., Visser, H. K. A. & Troelstra, J. A. (eds.), Leiden 1968.
5. American Academy of Pediatrics, Committee on fetus and newborn nomenclature for duration of gestation, birthweight and intra-uterine growth. *Pediatrics* 39, 935 (1967).
6. Lubchenco, L. O., Hansman, C. & Boy, E., Intrauterine growth in length and head circumference as estimated from live births at gestational age from 26 to 42 weeks. *Pediatrics* 37, 403 (1966); *J. Pediat.* 32, 793 (1963).
7. Usher, R. & McLean, F., Intrauterine growth of live-born Caucasian infants at sea level: standards obtained from measurements in 7 dimensions of infants born between 25 and 44 weeks of gestation. *J. Pediat.* 74, 901 (1969).
8. Scott, K. E. & Usher, R., Fetal malnutrition: its incidence, causes and effects. *Am. J. Obst. Gynec.* 94, 951 (1966).
9. McLean, F. & Usher, R., Measurements of live born fetal malnutrition infants compared with similar gestation and with similar birth weight normal controls. *Biol. Neonat.* 16, 215 (1970).
10. Warkany, J., Monroe, B. & Sutherland B., Intrauterine growth retardation. *Am. J. Dis. Childh.* 102, 127 (1961).
11. Sjöstedt, D., Engleson, G. & Rooth, G., Dysmaturity. *Arch. Dis. Childh.* 33, 123 (1968).
12. Soderling, B., Pseudo-prematurity. *Acta Paediat.* 42, 520 (1953).
13. Neligan, G. A., The clinical effects of being 'light for dates'. *Proc. R. Med.* 60, 877 (1967).
14. Dawkins, M., The 'small for date baby'. In: *Gestational age, size and maturity.* Dawkins, M. & McGregor, B. (eds.). Clinics in Developmental Medicine no. 19.
15. Wigglesworth, J. S., Pathological and experimental aspects of fetal growth retardation. *Proc. R. Soc. Med.* 60, 879 (1967).
16. Wigglesworth, J. S., Fetal growth retardation. *Br. med. Bull.* 22, 13 (1966).
17. Wigglesworth, J. S., Dysmaturity in the experimental animal. In: *Aspects of praematurity and dysmaturity.* Jonxis, J. H. P., Visser, H. K. A. & Troelstra, J. A. (eds.), Leiden 1968.
18. McKeown, T. & Record, R. G., Observations on foetal growth in multiple pregnancy in man. *J. Endocr.* 8, 386 (1952).
19. Naeye, R. L., Benirschke, K., Hagstrom, J. W. C. & Marcus, C. C., Intrauterine growth of twins as estimated from live born birth weight data. *Pediatrics* 37, 409 (1966).
20. Widdowson, E. M. & McCance, R. A., Some effects of accelerating growth. *Proc. Roy. Soc. B.* 52, 188 (1960).
21. Widdowson, E. M. & Kennedy, G. C., Rate of growth, mature weight and life-span. *Proc. Roy. Soc. B.* 156, 96 (1962).
22. Widdowson, E. M. & McCance R. A., The effects of finite periods of undernutrition at different ages on the composition and subsequent development of the rat. *Proc. Roy. Soc. B.* 158, 329 (1963).
23. Widdowson, E. M., Harmony of growth. *Lancet* 901 (1970).
24. Davison, A. N. & Dobbing J., Myelination as a vulnerable period in brain development. *Br. med. Bull.* 22, 40 (1966).

25. Dobbing, J., Effects of experimental undernutrition on development of the nervous system. In: *Malnutrition, learning and behavior*, Scrimshaw, N. S. & Gordon, J. E. (eds.), Cambridge (Mass.) 1968.
26. Dickerson, J. W. T. & Dobbing, J., Prenatal and postnatal growth and development of the central nervous system of the pig. *Proc. Roy. Soc. B.* 166, 384 (1967).
27. Dickerson, J. W. T. & Dobbing, J., The effect of undernutrition on the postnatal development of the brain and cord in pigs. *Proc. Roy. Soc. B.* 166, 396 (1967).
28. Winick, M., Malnutrition and brain development. *J. Pediat.* 74, 667 (1969).
29. Winick, M. & Rosso, P., Head circumference and cellular growth of brain. *J. Pediat.* 74, 774 (1969).
30. Winick, M. & Rosso, P., The effect of severe malnutrition on cellular growth of the human brain. *Pediatric Research* 3, 181 (1969).
31. Winick, M. & Noble, A., Quantitative changes in DNA, RNA and protein during prenatal and postnatal growth in the rat. *Dev. Biol.* 12, 451 (1965).
32. Zamenhof, S., Van Marthens, E. & Margolis, F., DNA (cell number) and protein in neonatal brain: alteration by maternal dietary protein restriction. *Science* 19, 322 (1968).
33. Barnes, R. H., Moore, A. U., Reid, I. M. & Pond, W. G., Effects of food deprivation on behavioral patterns. In: *Malnutrition, learning and behavior*, Scrimshaw, N. S. & Gordon, J. E. (eds.), Cambridge (Mass.) 1968.
34. Stoch, M. B. & Smythe, P. M., Does undernutrition during infancy inhibit growth and subsequent intellectual development? *Arch. Dis. Childh.* 38, 546 (1963).
35. Stoch, M. B. & Smythe, P. M., Undernutrition during infancy and subsequent brain growth and intellectual development. In: *Malnutrition, learning and behavior*, Scrimshaw, N. S. & Gordon, J. E. (eds.), Cambridge (Mass.) 1968.
36. Cabak, V. & Majdanvic, R., Effect of undernutrition in early life on physical and mental development. *Arch. Dis. Childh.* 40, 532 (1965).
37. Chase, H. P. & Martin, H. P., Undernutrition and child development. *New Eng. J. Med.* 282, 933 (1970).
38. Babson, S. G. & Kangas, J., Preschool intelligence of undersized term infants. *Am. J. Dis. Child.* 117, 553 (1969).
39. Babson, S. G., Kangas, J., Young, N. & Bramhall, J. L., Growth and development of twins of dissimilar size at birth. *Pediatrics* 33, 327 (1964).
40. Babson, S. G., Growth of low-birth-weight infants. *J. Pediat.* 77, 11 (1970).
41. Drillien, C. M., The small-for-date infant: etiology and prognosis. *Pediatric Clinics of North America*, 17, 9 (1970).

DISCUSSION

Freedman: I was wondering how you explain the recovery in head circumference and the lack in recovery in length and weight.

Van Gils: I think I cannot do so. I only know from animal experiments that the same has been seen there, especially in pig studies. There seems to be a brain-sparing effect, and after recovery it is observed that the brain has a relative priority for recuperation over body length. I do not know, however, if the difference in length of the monozygotic twins will persist because they have a much longer time to recuperate. We shall have to wait to see whether there is a difference after puberty.

Freedman: I have seen curves presented by Tanner in which identical twins retain about the same disparity in height and weight through eighteen years of age.

Casaer: I would like to ask you if you further subgrouped your infants that were small-for-date?

Van Gils: No, we did not. But I agree with you that this is the next step, because dysmature babies do not constitute a homogeneous group; they form a very heterogeneous group. Some of them are small-for-dates, because of a very long period of undernutrition, and others are small-for-dates due to a relatively short period of undernutrition, and that is the difference found when you differentiate between the two groups.

Steendijk: May I ask if you would elaborate on the method of measuring the growth rates of headcircumference? You express this in cm/year. Of course, you must have used a multiplication factor, because you measured far more often than twice a year. How often, in fact, did you measure, and did you smoothe the curves or use the actual measuring points?

Van Gils: No, we did not smoothe, but we tried to measure the infants at regular intervals. That was not always possible. What we want is to measure them every week, but that is not always possible for technical reasons. If the children are in a serious condition we cannot measure them, of course. On the other hand, in the out-patient department we took measurements every two months for the first half year: fourteen days after leaving the clinic and then every two months. During the second half year every three months. And after that every half year.

Steendijk: I am not concerned about the larger infants. I am concerned about the very beginning, when they show this catch-up. And I wonder whether I would not rather have smoothed the curves. From my own experiments I find that errors in measurements are quite likely to occur in these young children, and I would rather have a lot of points, then smoothe, and calculate growth rates from the smoothed curve. This is a question of method that may be important in this respect.

Van Gils: Yes, it is very difficult to measure these infants accurately. It is very easy to make mistakes by using bad measuring tapes. Sometimes there are two peaks and I think that this is caused by such errors.

Marshall: I think it is always a difficult problem to know how to relate a possible error in measurement to the amount of increase that is taking place. First, one must discover as exactly as possible what the extent of one's error is by doing a reliability test, with repeated measurement on the same individuals on the same day. And then one has two possibilities. If the error is small in relation to the amount of increase taking place, it can for many purposes be ignored depending on what the object of the exercise is. Failing this, it is usually desirable to do some kind of smoothing or curve fitting, the complexity of which again will vary according to the circumstances. I think your curves in fact came out reasonably smooth most of the time.

Van der Werff ten Bosch: Your main conclusion, I find, is that you get a greater catch-up in the brain or in head circumference than in length and weight measurements. I think you draw this conclusion from the fact that the change in percentile position of one measurement (head circumference) was greater than the change in percentile position of other measurements (length and weight). Have you any information on what happens in normal children? I think it is a mistake to assume that a child with a length percentile of, let's say 5, will usually also have its weight on the 5th percentile. In other words, the correlation between percentiles of different measurements, I would have thought, may not be very high at all. What happens if you follow children of normal birth weight? Do you find that there is a marked correlation between the percentile positions of the different measurements? Because this is really what you draw your conclusions from: the absence of such a state of affair in these children, and I wonder whether this supposition is correct for normal children.

Van Gils: I don't know, because we see relatively few normal children.

Visser: Not much is known on this subject. There are not many normal children who have a head circumference on the 10th percentile and the height and weight on the 10th percentile as well. But what is important, I think, is the growth rate curve. I think that normal children follow a normal growth rate curve for weight and height and head circumference with respect to the position of the percentiles. And so I think that the conclusion that there is an increased catch-up in the growth rate curve for head circumference as compared with the increase in growth rate in weight and length is a valid one.

Roebers: Do you have an explanation for the fact that there is such a great difference in number between the boys and the girls you had in your investigation?

Van Gils: We wondered ourselves, but I think the only explanation is that there is a difference between the intra-uterine growth curves of boys and girls. There must be more, another explanation, but this difference has been observed by others too, and they did not have an explanation either.

Roebers: Brain damage caused by birth is in general more frequent in boys than in girls.

Van Gils: Is it? I don't know.

Freedman: Perhaps someone should bring up the obvious fact that boys are genetically different from girls. And there should really be two different norms for what is small-for-date. Just as there should be different norms for what is small-for-date for an African population and a Dutch population, for example. It is well known, for example, that small-for-date girls have a better prognosis than small-for-date boys.

Barth: Dr. Van Gils, I presume that you have been using head circumference as an index of brain mass in your study. I have had my hesitations about this method, especially when one is comparing not simple spheres but skulls which may be a bit distorted from specimen to specimen. I am thinking especially about prematures with their hypotonia and secondary bilateral skull flattening. And I think that perhaps this may have some influence. Actually, I would suggest that if you wish to make a measurement of intracranial mass you could use the radiological method of taking X-rays from two directions and apply the formula developed for computing intracranial mass from these radiograms.

Van Gils: There have been two publications concerning brain mass and head circumference. One was a radiological study, as you suggested, and the results showed a positive correlation between skull content and head circumference. The other study was done by Winick in infants whose death had been due to an accident or poisoning. A positive correlation was found between head circumference and brain weight.

ON THE STRUCTURE, DEVELOPMENT, AND CONNECTIONS OF THE LIMBIC SYSTEM

J. ARIËNS KAPPERS

In 1878, Broca (1) first used the term *grand lobe limbique* for at least part of the limbic system with which we are concerned in this paper. Broca thus anticipated the demonstration of the close functional relationship between such very different structural elements as the cingulate gyrus and the hippocampus. He chose the term *limbique* because his *lobe limbique* lies like a ring or limbus around the brain stem, forming, as it were, a transitional zone between it and the neocortex. Actually, Broca's *lobe limbique* included the parahippocampal gyrus, the isthmus region, the cingulate gyrus, and the parolfactory area (Fig. 1). More specifically, the limbic lobe includes the hippocampal formation and the dentate gyrus as well. These structures form what is presently called the rhinencephalon in the broad sense.

Broca considered his *grand lobe limbique* to be *la partie brutale de l'encéphale*, being functionally opposed and in man subordinated to the neocortical part of the brain, his *partie intelligente de l'encéphale*. This suggests that, at that time, the opinion prevailed that strictly separate divisions of the brain regulate the 'lower' and the 'higher' drives and motivations of mankind and that, clearly, man should aim at a complete neocortical control of his 'lower passions', localized in the *grand lobe limbique*. It is now known, however, that there is a strong functional interrelationship between the rhinencephalon in its broader sense, many other parts of the brain, and the neocortex, leading to the integrated activity of these different divisions of the brain.

For a long time Broca's brilliant insight was more or less forgotten. The parts of the brain he distinguished as one system were originally generally considered to be exclusively related to the sense of smell. Comparative neuroanatomical investigations finally showed, however, that microsmatic and even anosmatic mammals demonstrate a similarly well-developed 'rhinencephalic area' which proved to be very constant during phylogenetic development. Consequently, it became evident that this system cannot be exclusively related to olfaction.

On the basis of the well-developed fibrous connections between the cingulate gyrus, the anterior thalamic nuclei, the hippocampus, and the mamillary bodies, Papez (2) suggested that the system probably acts as a neural correlate of the functional mechanism for emotional expression, being involved in the shaping of emotional behaviour. After Broca, Papez was one

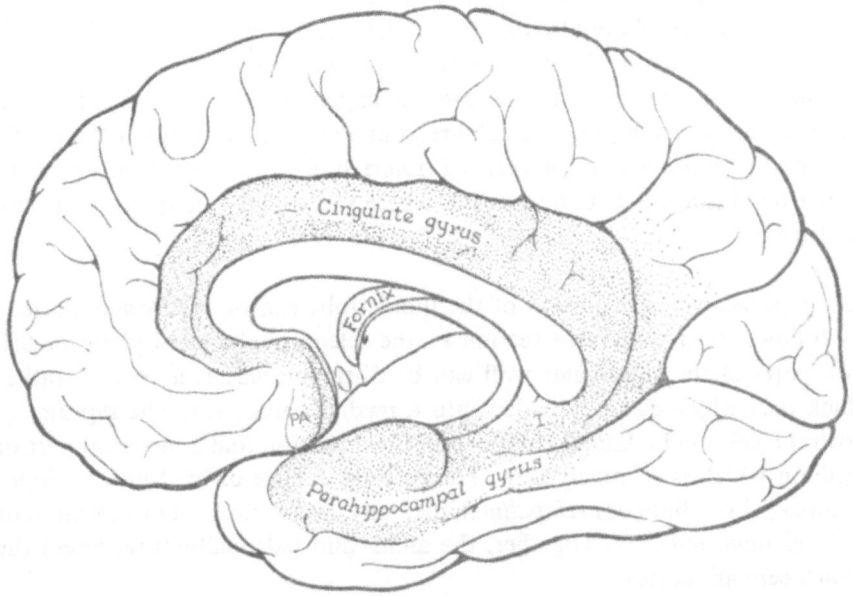

Fig. 1. Medial aspect of the right cerebral hemisphere. Shading indicates the *lobe limbique* as defined by Broca. This lobe encircles the upper brain stem. I: isthmus region; PA: parolfactory area. (Fig. 20-8 from reference no. 6).

of the first to regard the limbic lobe as the morphological substrate of affective and emotional life. This author also stressed the presence of many neural connections of this lobe with the hypothalamus as well as with different parts of the neocortex.

In 1949 and subsequent years, basing himself mainly on electrophysiological investigations, McLean (3) showed once again the great value of the conception 'limbic system', which has also been called 'the visceral brain'. As defined by McLean, the limbic system comprises the limbic lobe as well as associated nuclei and nuclear regions such as the amygdaloid complex, the septal nuclei, the hypothalamus, the epithalamus, the anterior thalamic nuclei, and parts of the basal ganglia including the fibre systems connecting these parts.

It has since been demonstrated that the limbic system indeed has a great many afferent and efferent fibrous connections, not only with the neocortex but also with centres in the brain stem, especially with the midbrain reticular formation, part of which has even been included in the limbic system by Nauta (4). It should, moreover, be stressed that the output of this system is not only of a neural but also of a hormonal nature by virtue of the hypothalamic magnocellular and parvocellular neurosecretory nuclei.

Due to space restrictions, the present paper offers only a very reduced account of the development, structure, and neural connections of the limbic system. For more details the reader is referred, for instance, to the extensive paper by Gastaut and Lammers (5), where most of the pertinent literature is also cited.

The *phylogenetic development* of the limbic lobe can be briefly summarized as follows. In a transverse section of the telencephalic hemisphere of fish two parts of the ventricular wall can be distinguished: 1. a ventral, rather thick part which can be divided into a medial component, the septum, at rostral levels, and a lateral component, the striatum; and 2. a dorsal part or pallium which is relatively thin. The pallium can be divided into a hippocampal primordium or *archipallium*, medially, and a piriform primordium or *paleopallium*, laterally. Together, the archi- and paleopallium represent the rhinencephalic cortex.

In amphibians a neopallial primordium can be distinguished which is situated between the paleopallium and the archipallium. In reptiles the neopallial part of the cortex is still small. It lies between the archipallium or hippocampal primordium medially and the piriform lobe or paleopallium laterally. From the ventral striatal division of the hemispheric wall, an area olfactiva develops.

In aplacental mammals such as Monotremata and Marsupialia, a strong development of the neopallium, i.e. of the neocortex, occurs. This neocortex, occupying the entire dorsal and even part of the medial and lateral components of the ventricular wall, presses the archipallium or hippocampal primordium to the medial aspect of the hemisphere and the paleopallium or piriform lobe in a lateral and even a ventral direction. The anlage of the hippocampus now starts to invaginate into the ventricular lumen, leading to the formation of the Ammon's horn and of a hippocampal sulcus at the medial aspect of the hemisphere (Fig. 2).

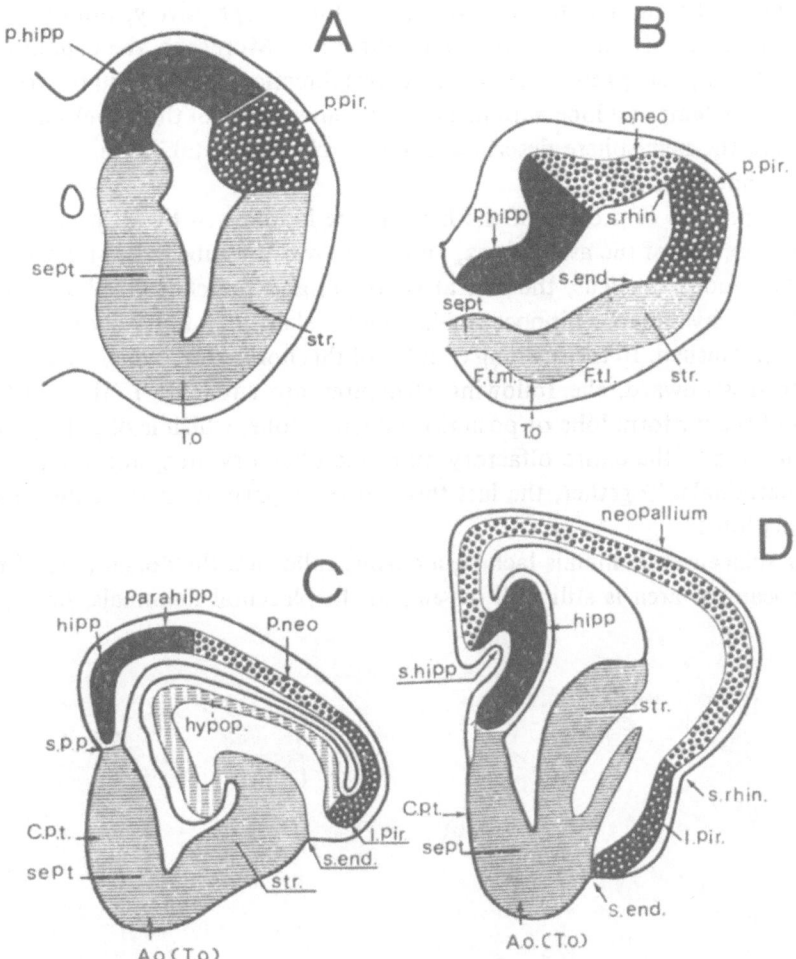

Fig. 2. Phylogenetic development of the wall of the cerebral hemisphere as seen in transverse sections. A: fish; B: lungfish and amphibians; C: reptiles; D: aplacental mammals. A.o.: area olfactoria; C.p.t.: corpus paraterminale; hipp.: hippocampus; hypop.: hypopallium; parahipp.: area parahippocampi; l. pir.: lobus piriformis; p. hipp.: primordium hippocampi; p.neo.: primordium neopallii; p.pir.: primordium piriforme; sept: septum; s.end.: sulcus endorhinalis; s.hipp.: sulcus hippocampi; s.p.p.: sulcus parolfactoria posterior; s.rhin.: sulcus rhinalis; str.: striatal anlage; T.o.: tuberculum olfactorium. (Fig. 2 from reference no. 5).

In placental mammals the neocortex develops progressively, not only in a transverse but also in a rostro-caudal direction. Moreover, the caudal part of the hemisphere grows in a ventro-rostral direction, resulting in the formation of the temporal lobe with its pole. In consequence of this developmental process, the hemisphere describes a semi-circle, finally taking the form of a horse-shoe or limbus.

This process of growth of the hemisphere is followed by all parts of the neocortex and of the archicortex, and, moreover, by subcortical nuclei such as the caudate nucleus, the lateral ventricle, and the choroid plexus. This explains why a limbus hippocampi having the shape of a horse-shoe can now be distinguished. In the opening or hilus of this horse-shoe, which is directed ventro-rostralward, the following structures are situated: 1. the anterior part of the piriform lobe or posterior olfactory lobe, which is of paleopallial origin, and 2. the entire olfactory bulb, the olfactory area, and the corpus paraterminale. Together, the last three of these parts form the anterior olfactory lobe.

In aplacental mammals lacking a corpus callosum, the dorsal part of the hippocampal area is still well developed. In placental mammals, however,

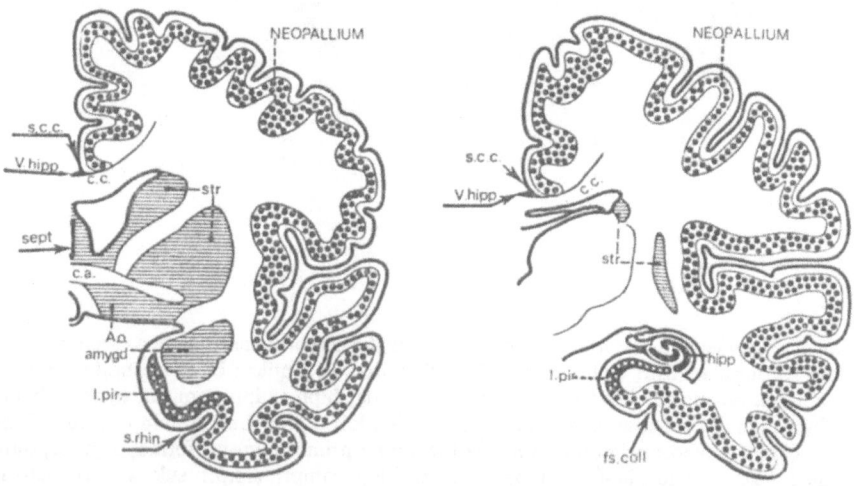

Fig. 3. Diagrams of transverse sections of the human cerebral hemisphere. On the left, at a rostral level; on the right, at a more caudal level. amygd: amygdaloid nuclear complex; A.o.: area olfactoria; c.a.: commissura anterior; c.c.: corpus callosum; fs. coll: fissura collateralis; hipp: hippocampus; l. pir.: lobus piriformis; s.c.c.: sulcus corporis callosi; s. rhin.: sulcus rhinalis; str: striatum; v. hipp: vestigial remnant of the hippocampus. (Part of Fig. 3 from reference no. 5).

this largest of the neocortical telencephalic commissural systems develops progressively. In this way, the part of the hippocampus situated dorsal to the strongly developing corpus callosum is flattened and reduced to a thin band, the indusium griseum. The postcommissural and temporal parts of the hippocampic limbus are, however, left intact.

Due to the enormous development of the neocortex, the paleopallium shifts from a ventrolateral to a basal position. In man it is even situated at the medioventral side of the temporal lobe of the hemisphere.

In aquatic anosmatic mammals, such as Pinnipedia and Cetacea, seals and whales, the olfactory apparatus in its strict sense is absent. However, the hippocampus with its fornix, the amygdaloid nuclear complex with its terminal stria, and the entorhinal cortex, which is part of the piriform lobe, do persist. This indicates that these parts have a greater functional significance than just an olfactory one.

The amygdaloid nuclei develop from the primitive striatum, that is from the lateral component of the ventral or basal part of the hemisphere wall, and, according to some authors, also from the neighbouring part of the paleopallial piriform lobe.

In placental mammals the piriform or posterior olfactory lobe shifts to a position next to the hippocampus due to the enormous development of the neocortex. This is why the piriform lobe is now called the parahippocampal gyrus (Fig. 3).

After this outline of the *phylogenetic development* of some of the more important parts of the limbic lobe, its *ontogenetic development* in man will be briefly dealt with.

During the third and fourth months of embryonic development, a regional differentiation can be observed at the ventral side of the caudal part of the frontal lobe and the ventral aspect of the temporal lobe. An olfactory vesicle, of earlier origin, is still present, now showing a short pedicle. This structure is subsequently transformed into the olfactory bulb and the olfactory peduncle, after which the caudal part of the peduncle forms the olfactory trigone (Fig. 4).

Caudal to the anlage of this trigone and partly also somewhat laterally, the following structures can now be distinguished: 1. the frontal prepiriform area, somewhat later represented by the lateral olfactory gyrus merging caudalward with the tip of the temporal lobe and, more laterally, with the subinsular area; 2. the olfactory area, medial to the prepiriform area, which differentiates into an area perforata anterior and the anlage of the olfactory tubercle; and 3. the medial olfactory gyrus.

The basal surface of the temporal lobe shows, in a rostro-caudal direction, the development of a temporal prepiriform area and of the paleopallial piriform lobe which differentiates into: *a.* a periamygdaloid area, covering the anlage of the amygdala, *b.* the so-called entorhinal area, and *c.* the presubicular area.

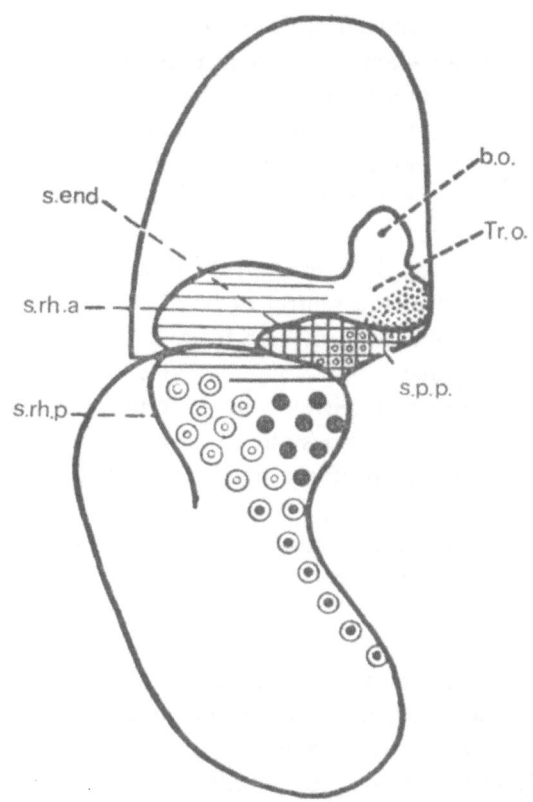

Fig. 4. Basal aspect of the frontal and temporal lobes of the cerebral hemisphere in a human embryo aged 4 months. Small black dots: gyrus olfactorius medialis; horizontal hatching: area prepiriformis frontalis and area prepiriformis temporalis, respectively; double hatching: area olfactoria; double hatching with small circles: anlage of tuberculum olfactorium; double hatching with large circles: anlage of gyrus diagonalis; black dots: area periamygdaloidea; concentric circles: area endorhinalis; circles containing black dots: area presubicularis. Most of the blank part of the basal aspect of the temporal lobe belongs to the area piriformis. b.o.: bulbus olfactorius; s.end: sulcus endorhinalis; s.p.p.: sulcus parolfactoria posterior; s.rh.a. and s.rh.p.: sulcus rhinalis anterior and posterior, respectively; Tr.o.: tractus olfactorius. (Part of Fig. 7 from reference no. 5).

At the medial aspect of the embryonic hemisphere the following structures can now be observed: 1. the hippocampal area forming a limbus, and 2. quite rostrally, the corpus paraterminale. The developing corpus callosum, growing in a caudal direction, divides the rostral part of the primordium hippocampi into the supracallosal indusium griseum and, quite rostrally, ventral to the genu of the corpus callosum, the infracallosal dorsal part of the septal area.

The corpus paraterminale gives rise to the following structures: 1. the subcallosal gyrus at the surface of the medial aspect of the hemisphere, and, deeper, 2. three nuclear masses, a ventral one, the nucleus accumbens septi, and two dorsal ones, the medial and lateral septal nuclei.

After the fourth month of embryonic development, virtually only the temporal piriform lobe, with its three divisions as mentioned, and the retrocommissural part of the hippocampal limbus with the dentate gyrus and the hippocampus, develop and differentiate to a considerable extent. In man the fornix, which contains most of the efferent and afferent fibres of the hippocampus, also develops rather early.

Concerning the *histogenesis* of these different parts, the following brief remarks may be made. In the neopallial area a peripherally situated cortical layer of neurones develops exclusively. This part of the cortex develops into the six-layered isocortex or homogeneous cortex. In the archipallium and the paleopallium, however, atypical cortices develop. This atypical cortex is also termed allocortex or heterogeneous cortex.

On the medial aspect of the hemisphere, archipallial cortex or archicortex develops in the entire area of the primordium hippocampi or hippocampal area. From early histogenesis on, the matrix layer is rather thin here, the intermediate nuclear layer is not very dense, and initially an outer nuclear or cortical layer of neurones is altogether lacking. In the fourth month a not very dense and not very well circumscribed outer nuclear layer develops. Locally, the structure of the archicortex differs according to its different parts.

During its development, the original paleopallium shows a thickening of the matrix layer and of the mantle layer, which form the intraventricular foldings of the eminentia ganglionaris and of the septum, respectively. At the periphery of this paleocortex a very incomplete cortical layer of neurones is formed. The paleocortex has also been termed semicortex.

In addition, a periallocortex archipallialis and a periallocortex paleopallialis have been distinguished. The archipallial periallocortex develops bordering on the archicortex dorsally forming the cingulate gyrus, the cortex of which is also termed mesocortex. Here, the outer cortical cell layer is very thin and, moreover, double. The cyto-architectonic pattern of the paleopallial perialloxortex is still less characteristic. It forms a transition to the neo-cortical pattern. This type of periallocortex is situated in the most ventral part of the insula and borders on the prepiriform and periamygdaloid paleocortices.

The main part of the amygdaloid nuclear complex originates from the caudoventral part of the eminentia ganglionaris, the primitive striatum or archistriatum. The rostrodorsal part of this eminence gives rise to the corpus striatum, that is the caudatum, putamen, and pallidum, and to the nucleus accumbens septi. The rest of the amygdaloid complex may originate from neighbouring parts of the cortex.

These phylogenetic and ontogenetic data indicate that olfaction is not the primary function of the rhinencephalon in its broader sense. The olfactory lobe may be absent, as is normally the case in aquatic mammals or abnor-

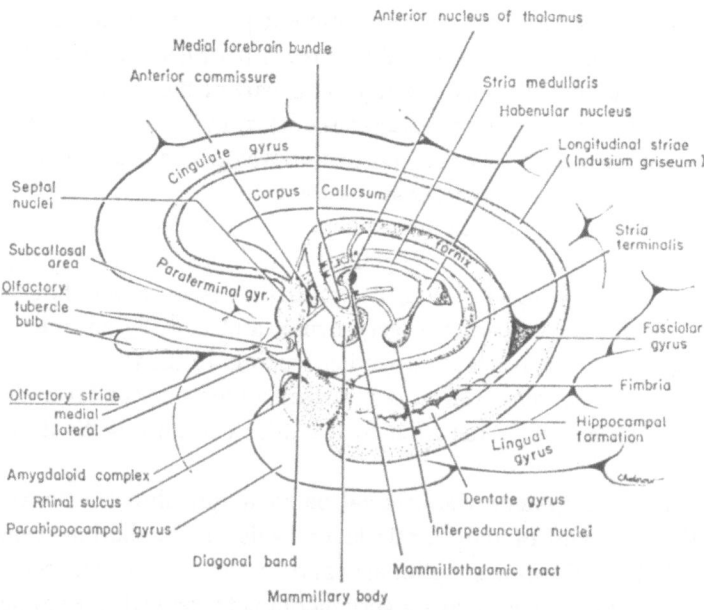

Fig. 5. Semi-schematic drawing of the rhinencephalon, the limbic lobe, and some centres and tracts functionally involved in the limbic system in its broader sense, as seen in the medial aspect of the right cerebral hemisphere in man. (Fig. 20-3 from reference no. 6).

mally in monsters, without any obvious alteration in the development of the rest of the rhinencephalon. It is also striking that the hippocampo-mamillo-thalamo-cingulate gyrus system is very strongly developed in microsmatic man. The same holds for the piriform lobe and the amygdala. From this it follows that especially the limbic part of the rhinencephalon must have important extra-olfactory functions.

In the adult brain the rhinencephalon, including the rhinencephalic cortex in the strict sense and the limbic lobe, shows the following divisions: (1) the olfactory lobes or the pars basalis rhinencephali, and (2) the pars limbica rhinencephali. The former consists of the anterior and posterior olfactory lobes, each of which shows several subdivisions, the latter comprises the hippocampal limbus, the medullary limbus with its fimbria and fornix, and the choroid plexus. All of these divisions with their several parts are illustrated in fig. 5.

We will now deal briefly with the *afferent and efferent neural connections of the rhinencephalon*. Their number is extremely large and only a few can be mentioned here.

In the posterior olfactory lobe, the entorhinal area forms the greater part of the parahippocampal gyrus. It is a secondary olfactory integration centre showing, moreover, afferent and efferent connections with many other parts of the brain. The other parts of the parahippocampal gyrus, i.e. the prepiriform and the periamygdaloid cortices, can be regarded as direct olfactory projection areas receiving impulses from the lateral olfactory stria.

The parts mentioned are the specific olfactory projection areas. Their function is to analyse the incoming olfactory stimuli.

Besides these, non-specific olfactory pathways and centres can be distinguished. They serve for the integration of olfactory stimuli reaching these centres along multisynaptic pathways with sensory stimuli of a different nature. Such centres are: the septum, the amygdala, the hippocampus, the cingulum, the habenula, the midbrain reticular formation, etc. These non-specific olfactory pathways and centres are involved in somatic as well as in visceral emotional behaviour. Many of them receive afferents from the specific olfactory areas.

The *hippocampus* is a very important part of the limbic system, being an integration centre for sensory impulses of various origin. The hippocampus shows afferent connections with the prepiriform and periamygdaloid areas and with the area entorhinalis. It also receives visual and tactile impulses along fibre systems of which only the bundles running from the neocortical visual association areas to the hippocampus are well-established neuro-anatomically. Gustatory stimuli reach the hippocampus either directly or indirectly via the entorhinal area. In addition, it receives afferent fibres from the septum via the fornix. The fornix is also the most important efferent pathway of the hippocampus. It contains more than two million fibres. In addition, efferent fibres from the hippocampus reach the area entorhinalis.

The fornix contains the following fibre systems: fibres originating in the cornu Ammonis and running to the septum and further to the preoptic area together with septo-hypothalamic fibres; fibres running along the same pathway to the anterior and lateral hypothalamic areas; fibres from the septum to the cornu Ammonis; septo-temporal as well as temporo-septal fibres; fibres running to the mesencephalic tegmentum coursing via the supramamillary decussation and the mamillary peduncles; and fibres originating in the cornu Ammonis and running to the medial mamillary nucleus.

Some of the fibres running to the latter nucleus are, however, of a different origin, that is they come from septal nuclei, the parolfactory area, the cingulate gyrus, and from several areas of the neocortex. The strong development of the fornix in man is, indeed, due to its neocortical components.

The anterior nuclei of the dorsal thalamus have a double connection with the cornu Ammonis, that is along a circuitous route via the fornix, the mamillary body, and the mamillo-thalamic tract, as well as directly via the fornix.

In view of its probable connections with the intralaminar nuclei of the dorsal thalamus and its discharge to neocortical areas, the hippocampus is also involved in non-hypothalamic diencephalic as well as in neocortical telencephalic functions. It may well be, moreover, that via the thalamus hippocampal activity is correlated with the multisynaptic ascending system in the brain stem.

On the hippocampus, a motor pattern can be distinguished (Fig. 6). The pathways along which this activity is conveyed are not yet well known. It can be still evoked after bilateral lesions of the fornix, but not after lesion of the alveus along which most of the efferent hippocampal fibres run before entering the fornix.

The function of the hippocampus and of the parahippocampal gyrus is closely related to that of the amygdala and of the neocortex of the temporal pole, because these areas are so closely connected. Often, they are involved in the same lesion because of their close topographical relationship.

The hippocampus being also a centre of motor activity, it is evident that scar tissue may cause epileptogenic foci. From areas activated in this way, secondary foci may arise in the temporal pole, causing the so-called temporal epilepsy. Sometimes, patients with this kind of epilepsy show bilateral sclerosis of the hippocampus.

The hippocampus is also involved in recent memory. Loss of recent memory occurs in patients having extensive lesions of both hippocampi but also in patients showing lesions of the orbital parts of the frontal lobe, that is in the area where the uncinate fascicle ends. This association bundle connects the uncus, the parahippocampal gyrus, and the neighbouring temporal areas with the orbital surface of the frontal lobe.

According to Papez (2), the hippocampus is the regulator of hypothalamic centres involved in emotional behaviour. This agrees with the observations in patients with bilateral hippocampal lesions. Papez' circuit runs as follows: hippocampus → fornix → mamillarybody → thalamus → cingulate gyrus and back to the hippocampus. It is now certain that this circuit is only one of many involved in emotional behaviour and expression.

The *cingulate gyrus* is also a very important part of the limbic system. Its principal afferent connection is by way of thalamo-cortical fibres originating in the anterior nucleus complex of the dorsal thalamus, in particular in

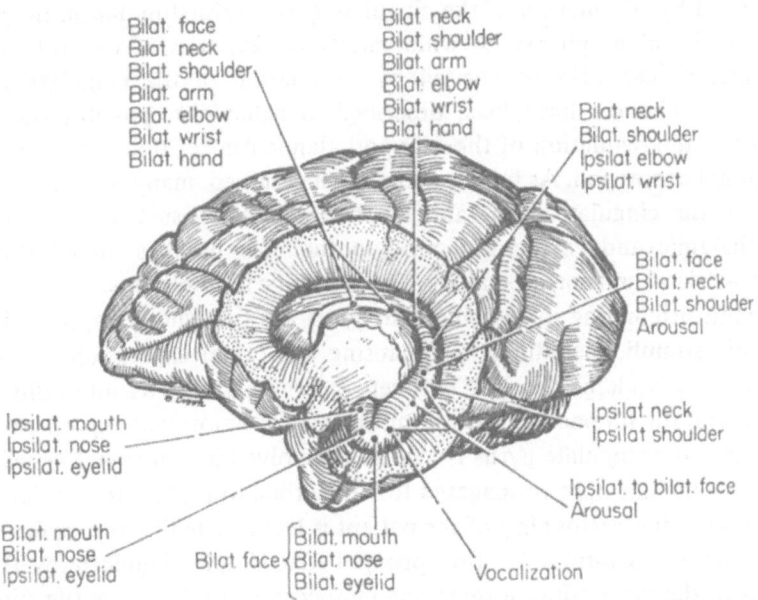

Fig. 6. Drawing showing the hippocampus and fornix in the macaque brain. The pattern of movements on stimulation of various points is indicated, as is also the area from which arousal was obtained. (Fig. 1 from C. L. Votaw, *J. comp. Neurol.* 112, 353 (1959).

the anteroventral nucleus, and projecting on all parts of the large cingulate gyrus. The impulses reaching the gyrus in this way result, via the mamillary-thalamic tract, from an integration, in the hypothalamus, of ascending gustatory stimuli, descending olfactory stimuli, stimuli from the hippocampus and the parahippocampal gyrus, and stimuli from the septum reaching the mamillary body via the septomamillary fibres. Besides a great many thalamo-cortical afferents, the cingulate gyrus also receives an input from many neocortical areas.

Efferent fibres originating in this gyrus run to many neighbouring neocortical areas, to the septum, the caudate nucleus, and the globus pallidus, to thalamic nuclei, to the anterior, posterior, and lateral hypothalamic areas, and, finally, to the midbrain tegmentum.

A very important long association bundle running through the cingulate gyrus is the cingulum. Its fibres establish connections between parts of the limbic system and many neocortical areas such as the motor areas 4, 6, and 8 in the frontal lobe, and the visual association areas 18 and 19 in the occipital lobe.

Interestingly, motor activity associated with striated musculature can be elicited by stimulation of the cingulate gyrus. Overstimulation may even cause Jacksonian epilepsy. A wide variety of activities of visceral smooth musculature can also be elicited by stimulation of the cingulate gyrus. Moreover, changes have been described in behaviour, possibly due to a change in the regulation of those hypothalamic centres that are involved in emotional expression. As has already been mentioned, many connections run between the cingulate gyrus and the hypothalamus, such as the cortico-hypothalamic and cortico-thalamo-hypothalamic bundles, in addition to cortico-striatal and cortico-pallido-hypothalamic fibre systems.

Stimuli originating in the cingulate gyrus are thought to suppress hypothalamic stimuli, including those causing emotional expression. An equilibrium is considered to exist between the cingulate gyrus inhibiting such stimuli and the hippocampus evoking stimuli for emotional expression.

Because the cingulate gyrus is evidently involved in emotional behaviour, cingulectomy has been propagated for some time to replace frontal leucotomy, because the personality of the patient is less affected by the former than by the latter operation. It also appeared that simple cingulotomy, that is cutting of the gyrus without removing mesocortex, is effective in the elimination of fear and pain that are refractive to drug treatment. Changes in personality do not occur.

Sufficient space is not available to deal with another very important centre of the limbic system, the *amygdaloid nuclear complex*. It must suffice to mention that its nuclei receive, among other things, fibres from secondary and tertiary olfactory centres, the most important efferent fibre bundle being the stria terminalis via which many efferent impulses reach the hypothalamic centres.

Lastly, we shall deal with *the connections of the limbic lobe with the diencephalon and the brain stem*. These connections are formed by two main large pathways: the hypothalamic and the epithalamic. The hypothalamic pathway is the most important of the two. It comprises: 1. the olfacto-hypothalamic fascicle, and 2. the septo-hypothalamic fascicle, and their continuation to the midbrain tegmentum. The olfacto-hypothalamic fascicle originates in the basal olfactory centres, the septo-hypothalamic fascicle in the nuclei of the septal area. The fascicles run ventral to the anterior commissure to enter the preoptic area of the hypothalamus, where they are joined by fibres originating in the amygdala, the cingulate gyrus, the hippocampus, the parahippocampal gyrus, the orbital neocortex, and the neocortex of the temporal pole. The large fascicle formed in this way is the medial forebrain bundle, which courses in the lateral hypothalamic area and reaches the midbrain tegmentum. Here, most fibres end in the reticular formation.

In the lateral hypothalamic area the medial forebrain bundle is joined by the anterior and posterior hypothalamo-tegmental fascicles originating, respectively, in the lateral preoptic area and the anterior hypothalamic nucleus, and in the posterior hypothalamic area and the ventromedial hypothalamic nucleus. Both tracts end in the deep tegmental nucleus of the midbrain. A dorsal hypothalamic tegmental tract is also distinguished by some authors (Fig. 7).

Fibres running from the hypothalamus to the midbrain tegmentum and vice-versa also course in a third system, the more or less diffusely spread periventricular fibre system. Its descending fibres originate in the entire hypothalamic area, the preoptic and ventromedial nuclei excepted. In the midbrain, fibres of this system join the dorsal longitudinal fascicle of Schütz. Some of the fibres of this bundle run to the nuclei of the superior collicles and to the parasympathetic oculomotor nucleus of Edinger. Other descending fibres distribute to all tegmental nuclei present in the central grey substance of the midbrain, some running even farther caudalward to end in the medulla oblongata on the salivatory nuclei, the dorsal vagus nucleus, the nucleus ambiguus, and other motor nuclei of cranial nerves. In this way impulses set up in the hypothalamus can reach centres in the midbrain and, from there, centres in the lower brain stem either directly or indirectly via multisynaptic tegmento-bulbar pathways. Motor centres in the cord, somatomotor as well as visceromotor, can also receive impulses by these systems.

In addition, two tracts run from the mamillary bodies to the midbrain tegmentum: 1. the mamillo-tegmental tract and 2. the mamillo-peduncular tract. The fibres of the former tract (Fig. 8) end directly in the dorsal tegmental nucleus from which the impulses are relayed to parasympathetic

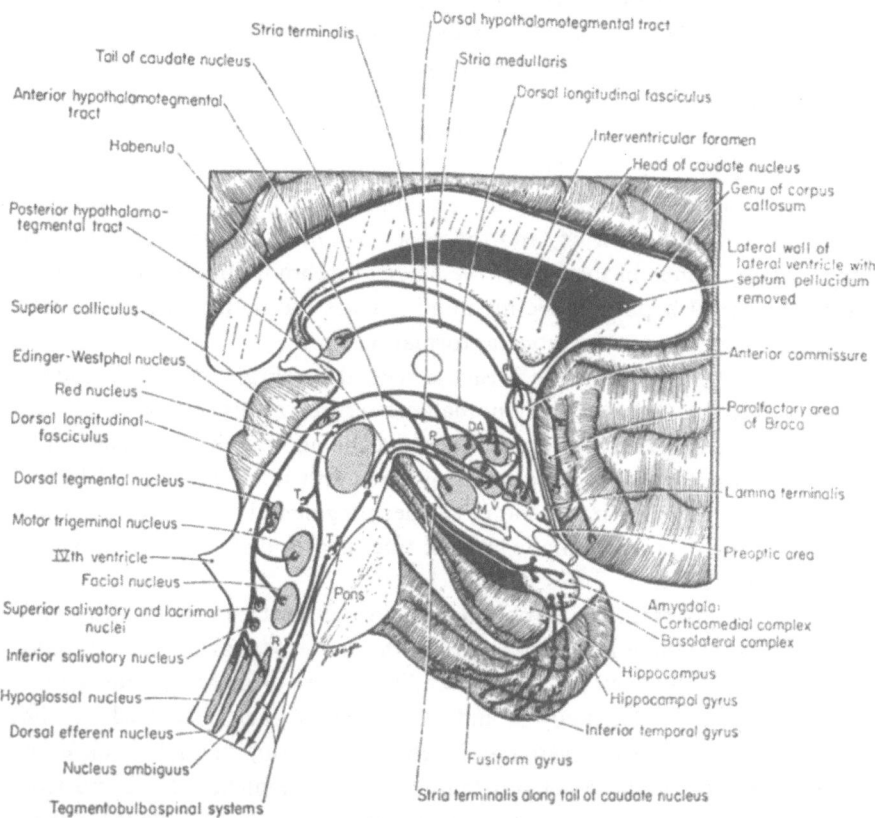

Fig. 7. Schematic drawing illustrating some of the discharge pathways of the hypothalamus to the midbrain tegmentum and to motor nuclei in the medulla oblongata. A: anterior hypothalamic area; D: dorsomedial hypothalamic nucleus; DA: dorsal hypothalamic area; M: mamillary body; P: posterior hypothalamic area; R: reticular grey; T: tegmental grey; V: ventromedial hypothalamic nucleus. (Fig. 224 from Crosby, Humphrey and Lauer: *Correlative anatomy of the nervous system*, New York 1962).

nuclei and motor nuclei of cranial nerves. Impulses coursing by way of the mamillo-peduncular tract reach the dorsal tegmental nucleus via the inter-peduncular nucleus. Along the latter tract, tegmental ascending stimuli reach the mamillary nuclei where they are confronted with stimuli from such parts of the limbic system as the septum and the fornix.

The second large pathway along which impulses from the limbic system can reach the midbrain tegmentum and the lower brain stem is the epitha-lamic one. Its main components are the stria medullaris thalami, the medial

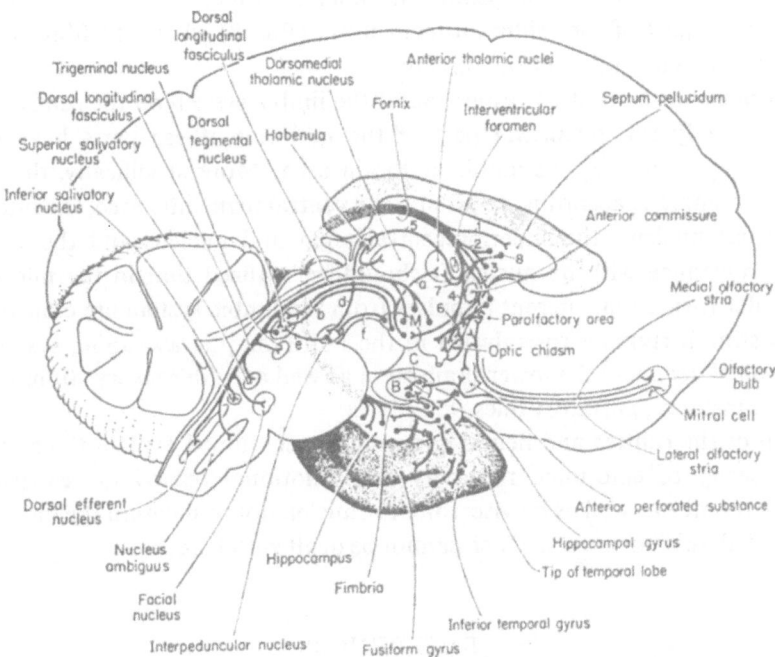

Fig. 8. Diagram illustrating some of the connections of the rhinencephalon in the strict sense and of the limbic system more generally. B: basolateral amygdaloid nuclear group; C: corticomedial amygdaloid nuclear group; M: mamillary body; a: mamillothalamic tract; b: mamillotegmental tract; c: habenulodiencephalic tract; d: habenulopeduncular tract; e: pedunculotegmental tract; f: mamillo (inter)peduncular tract; 1: hippocamposep-tal fibres; 2: septohippocampal fibres; 3: precommissural fornix; 4: postcommissural fornix; 5: medial corticohabenular fibres; 6: septopreoptic and septohypothalamic fibres of the medial forebrain bundle; 7: fibres of the fornix and the septum to the anterior thalamic nucleus; 8: connections from the septum pellucidum to the thalamus (septotha-lamic fibres), to the habenula and the postcommissural fornix (septohabenular or olfacto-habenular and septohypothalamic or olfactohypothalamic fibres). (Fig. 299 from Crosby, Humphrey and Lauer: *Correlative anatomy of the nervous system*, New York 1962).

habenular nuclei, and the efferent connections of the latter to the midbrain (Figs. 7 and 8).

The stria medullaris is composed of fibres originating in such centres as the septum, the olfactory area, the amygdala, the hippocampus, and the parahippocampal gyrus. In the medullary stria these fibres run to the ipsilateral and contralateral medial habenular nucleus.

From the habenular medial nucleus, three tracts originate: 1. the habenulotectal tract, 2. the habenulo-tegmental tract, and 3. the habenulo-interpeduncular tract or Meynert's fasciculus retroflexus. The fibres of the last of these tracts end in the interpeduncular nucleus, which sends its fibres to the middorsal part of the midbrain tegmentum (Fig. 8) where the fibres of the habenulo-tegmental tract end directly.

Because of the profuse projection of the limbic system on the central grey and the adjacent tegmental part of the midbrain, these parts have been termed by Nauta (4) the limbic midbrain area. More specifically, this area would comprise, according to Nauta, the ventral tegmental area, the interpeduncular nucleus, the superior central tegmental nucleus and the central grey substance with its nuclei. It should be realized that in the midbrain reticular formation, efferent impulses from the limbic system are confronted with stimuli running rostralward in the multisynaptic ascending system in the spinal cord and the lower brain stem as well as with sensory stimuli such as, for instance, gustatory ones.

All of the centres and neural connections mentioned explain the extreme complexity of emotional reactivity and emotional behaviour realized by somatomotor as well as by visceromotor nuclei, not to mention the output of hypothalamic hormones, which cannot be dealt with here.

REFERENCES

1. Broca, P., Anatomie comparée des circonvolutions cérébrales: le grand lobe limbique et la scissure limbique dans la série des mammifères. *Revue d'Anthrop.* 2e sér., 1, 385 (1878).
2. Papez, J. W., A proposed mechanism of emotion. *Arch. Neurol. Psychiat.* 38, 725 (1937).
3. McLean, P. D., Psychosomatic disease and the 'visceral brain'. Recent developments bearing on the Papez theory of emotion. *Psychosom. Med.* 11, 338 (1949).
4. Nauta, W. J. H., Hippocampal projections and related neural pathways to the mid-brain in the cat. *Brain* 81, 319 (1958).
5. Gastaut, H. & Lammers, H. J., Anatomie du rhinencéphale. In Vol. I of: *Les grandes activités du rhinencéphale.* Alajouanine, (ed.), Paris 1960.
6. Truex, R. C. & Carpenter, M. B., *Human neuroanatomy.* Baltimore 1964.

DISCUSSION

De Groot: Is anything known about the vulnerability of this system compared with other systems in situations of stress, e.g. oxygen lack, extreme malnutrition or disorders of metabolism in early life?

Ariëns Kappers: I am sorry I can't give you any information on this point. It is, however, known that the vascularization of e.g. the hippocampus is rather poor. Therefore, if atherosclerosis develops in the brain, this is one of the first parts of the limbic system that will drop out. This might explain the loss of recent memory at older ages as it has been suggested that the hippocampus is involved in the storage of recent memory.

BEHAVIORAL ASSESSMENT IN INFANCY

D. G. FREEDMAN

D. G. FREEDMAN

LIMITATIONS IN PREDICTIVE VALUE OF INFANTS TESTS

All present-day scales of infant behavior beyond the newborn period appear to stem from Arnold Gesell's test developed in the 1920's. Gesell was, of course, a research pediatrician, and his major aim was to determine norms of development so that criteria for abnormal development might be established. To a certain extent this aim was achieved, and the Gesell test is indeed most useful in pointing-up and predicting defective development. (The recent review by Hoben Thomas (1) documents this point, and provides an excellent overview of the baby-testing field today.)

However, its predictive value to five years of age for the middle of the distribution is typically no higher than .50 (accounting for 25% of the variance), and this holds as well for the closely related Cattell and Bayley tests. In our own studies we obtained an average of ten Bayley Mental and Motor tests per infant (N = 34), given over the first year, and still obtained a correlation with the Stanford-Binet at 5 and/or 6 years of only .33 for the Mental Scale and .13 for the Motor Scale. Similarly, the Bayley Infant Behavior Profile in the first year yielded no relationship with scores on a five-year version of the same test. The reasons for such poor prediction from mental, motor and personality scores can be summarized as follows.

1. Motor items, in infancy, usually involve the whole body, e.g., rolling over, sitting, standing, walking. Motor items in tests beyond 3 years are completely inadequate in assessing whole-body coordination. A true motor test in older children would attempt to quantify such tasks as skipping rope, climbing a pole, throwing a ball, etc. There is no scale which does so.

2. The so-called 'mental' items in infancy are predominantly assessments of eye-hand coordination and over-all sensory alertness. However, beyond 5 years abstraction plays a progressively greater role in mental test items, and there is no logical reason to propose that sensory acuity is a forerunner of

the ability to engage in abstract thinking; in fact, nothing in infancy appears to predict this capacity well. There is one possible exception: in Bayley's own long term study, precocity of verbalizations in infant girls correlates with verbal I.Q. at age 26 at an astounding .86 (2). This does make some logical sense in that common neural centers are probably involved in early verbalizations and in later language usage. (For the sex-specific nature of these findings see page 214).

3. Although personality items given in infancy have also had poor predictive value, we all know from watching children grow up, that certain personality traits persist over time, often starting in early infancy. Such traits are different in each child and contribute to his total uniqueness. Clearly, standardized scales, by their very nature, cannot handle such unique material.

The only successful scientific demonstration of this fact, to my knowledge, is the work of Neilon, who had judges match personality descriptions of the same individuals independently written at 3 years and 17 years. Their matching was well above chance. We have been able to replicate this finding with excellent matching of descriptions at *6 months* and 10 years in a series of fraternal twins.

Here is an example, abstracted from descriptions of filmed behavior, of what such continuities consisted of:

Arturo and Felix, a fraternal pair of twins, showed striking dissimilarity in their thresholds to smiling, as early as 2 months of age. At that age, Arturo would smile, with his eyes closed, to the stroking of his cheek, a soft voice, or the tinkle of a bell. Felix rarely smiled, but by contrast was alert and usually observant. At 9 months, when confronted by a stranger, both seemed equally uncomfortable. Arturo, however, tried to smile, despite his fear, while Felix simply kept his eyes from meeting those of the stranger. At the $5\frac{1}{2}$ year follow-up, the persistence of these differences in interpersonal approach were striking. Although both boys were nervous, Felix exhibited only one full smile during the entire interview, while Arturo smiled constantly over the entire time. Such striking differences were never seen among our identicals, and we must conclude that different genotypes were ultimately responsible.

While many other points could be brought up about the limitations of infant tests, we will focus on only one more aspect, their essential *survey* nature; that is, no trait is probed in depth, the process of acquisition is of no concern, and only presence or absence of behavior is registered. This point will concern us for the remainder of this paper.

THE USE OF INFANT PERFORMANCE TO TEST HYPOTHESES

Thomas (1) has pointed out (much to my surprise) that my study with Barbara Keller on identical and fraternal twins is a lone example of a baby test used to test a theoretical question.

I can see why this is so, for baby tests are constructed to provide a wide ranging but superficial assessment of behavioral status. For our initial purposes this was fine, for we were interested in comparing identicals and fraternals in just such a general way. But if one wants to focus at a higher microscopic power, he will invariably have to develop his own assessment procedures, tailor made for the questions he is asking.

The work of Bower (3, 4, 5, 6, 7) is a good example. Bower, addressing himself to such classic problems of perception as phenomenal identity, size and shape constancy, slant perception, visual apperception of texture, and object permanence has shown, in a brilliant series of experiments, that infants exhibit these characteristics in early infancy. As a result of these studies there now seems little doubt that whatever learning is involved in the achievement of the perceptual constancies, it accrues around built-in abilities. In one experiment, for example, a projected *virtual* image of a soft, puffy ball was presented before the seated 7-week-old who had never before seen such an object. The infant was then observed to reach for the image with the fingers of both hands set appropriately to touch a soft round object of the projected size. A projected metal ball, by contrast, drew quite another set to the hands, clearly appropriate for the size and surface of a hard sphere. Also, when the projected ball was small, only one hand was reached out. In each case, the absence of the object, for it was a virtual image, elicited unmistakable surprise (7).

In another experiment, which can be called a demonstration of movement constancy, unpracticed 6 week old infants visually followed a target moving in a constant arc, and continued following the target after its disappearance behind a screen – so that the eyes met the target as it emerged on the other side of the screen (7). Very young infants (6 weeks old) are also capable of recognizing an object in its various aspects (shape constancy). For example, a rectangle when placed at an angle, impinges on the eyes as a trapezoid, but it is nevertheless distinguished from a true trapezoid and recognized as a rectangle. This was determined by conditioning headturning responses to the rectangle, and then noting when this conditioned behavior again occurred (3). These studies have enabled Bower (3) to conclude, as follows, concerning the belief that perception is caused by the momentary retinal image:

'What the experiments seem to show is that evolution has tuned the human perceptual system to register not the low-grade information in momentary retinal images but rather the high-fidelity information in sequences of images or in simultaneous complexes of images – the kind of information given by motion parallax and binocular parallax. Rather than being the most primitive kind of perceptual ability, it would seem, that ability to register the information in a retinal image may be a highly sophisticated attainment and may indeed have to be learned.'

To briefly mention some other examples of infant behavioral assessment procedures intimately tied to theory, Robert Fantz (8) developed an instrument which allows the experimenter to assess what a baby prefers to look at. Again, his study stems from the innate-acquired problem, and Fantz was attempting to replicate work with chicks which, he had found, peck prefer-

EXPERIMENT I STIMULI

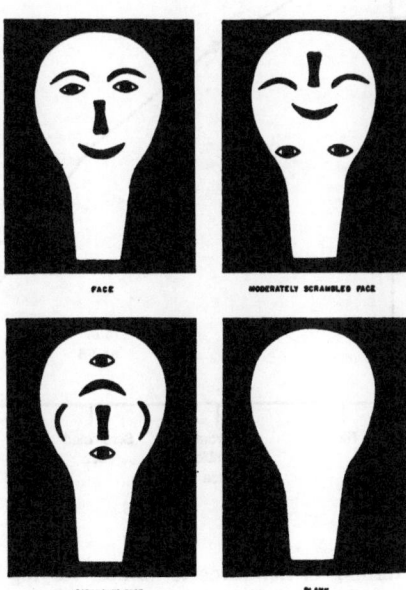

Fig. 2. Figures used in test.

entially from hatching at certain forms and colors. While the literature on
the infant apparatus developed by Fantz is now voluminous and somewhat
ambiguous, it appears that young infants prefer faces over most other
stimuli.

Inasmuch as conditioning might explain such results in older infants, my
own student, Carolyn Jirari, using yet another technique, was able to accom-
plish what those working with the Fantz apparatus could not; that is, she
was able to test visual preferences in a substantial number of *newborns*.

Newborns are much more attracted to a moving object than to one which
is still, so Jirari simply measured the degree of head-turning to a moving
stimulus. She held the infant in the lap and, with a large protractor behind its
head, measured the extent various stimuli were followed from midline to
either side (Fig. 1). There were three trials to either side, and the farthest ex-
cursions left and right were added to form the infant's score. As can be seen,
Jirari's results (Figs. 2, 2a, 3, 3a) support the aforementioned trend that a
face-like stimulus receives maximal attention. The next series of 6 figures
capture 12 seconds of filmed behavior of a crying newborn being cuddled in

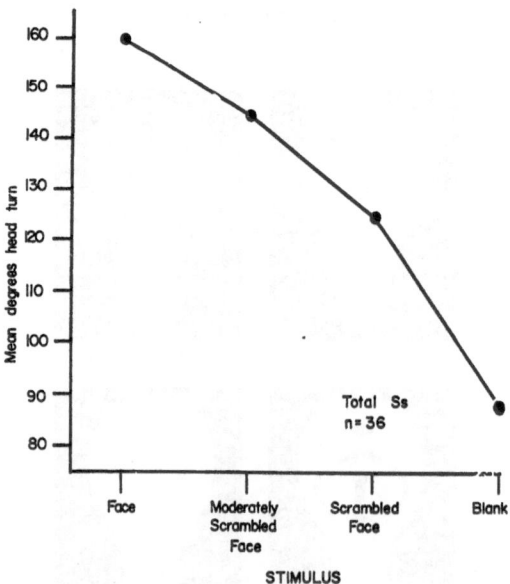

Fig. 2a. Averaged head turning in newborns to stimuli varying in degree of 'faceness'
(maximal score is 90° to each side or 180°). All the comparisons were significant (p. <. 005)
on the Wilcoxon matched-pair assigned-ranks test. From Jirari, 1970.

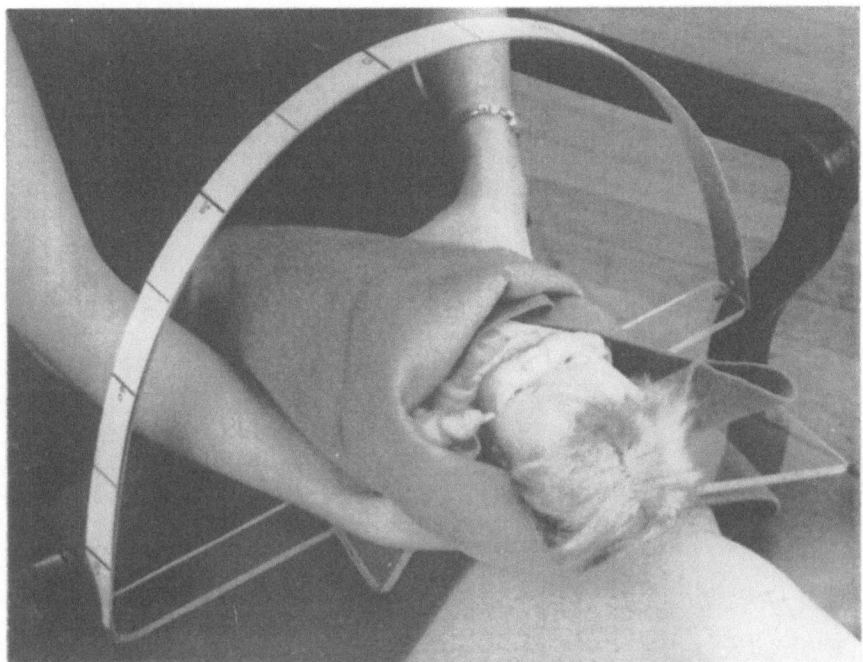

Fig. 1. Apparatus used in study of head turning demonstrated with a doll. In actual practice one of the experimenter's hands supported the baby's head at the junction of the neck and head, while the other hand held the stimulus in front of the baby's face.

Figs. 4-9. One day old girl is consoled in arms for the first time. She ceases crying almost immediately and looks to E's face. From motion-picture film covering approximately 12 seconds of action.

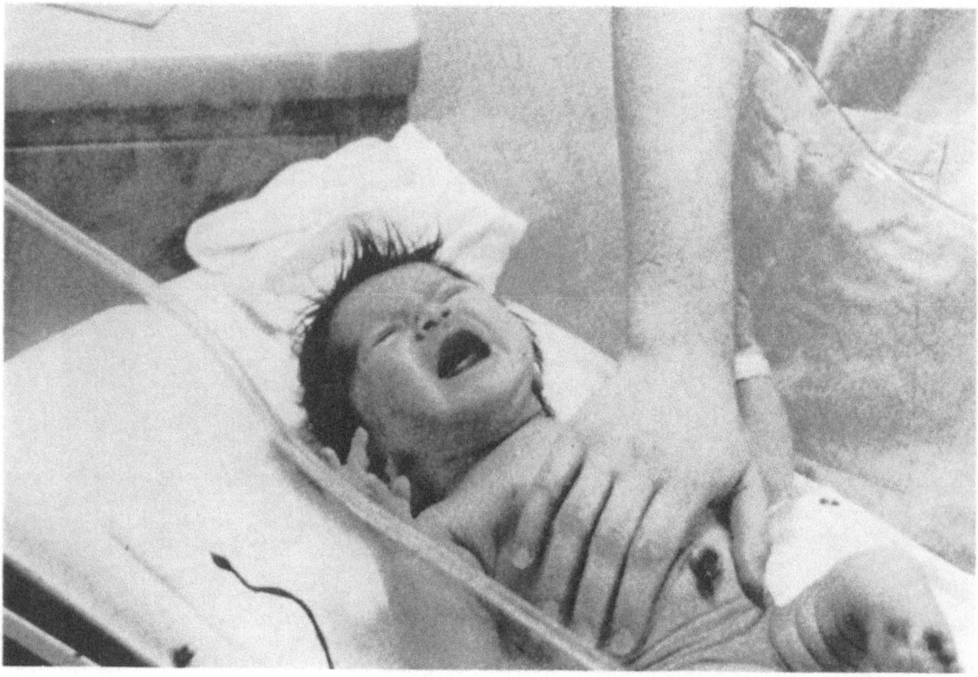

Fig. 4

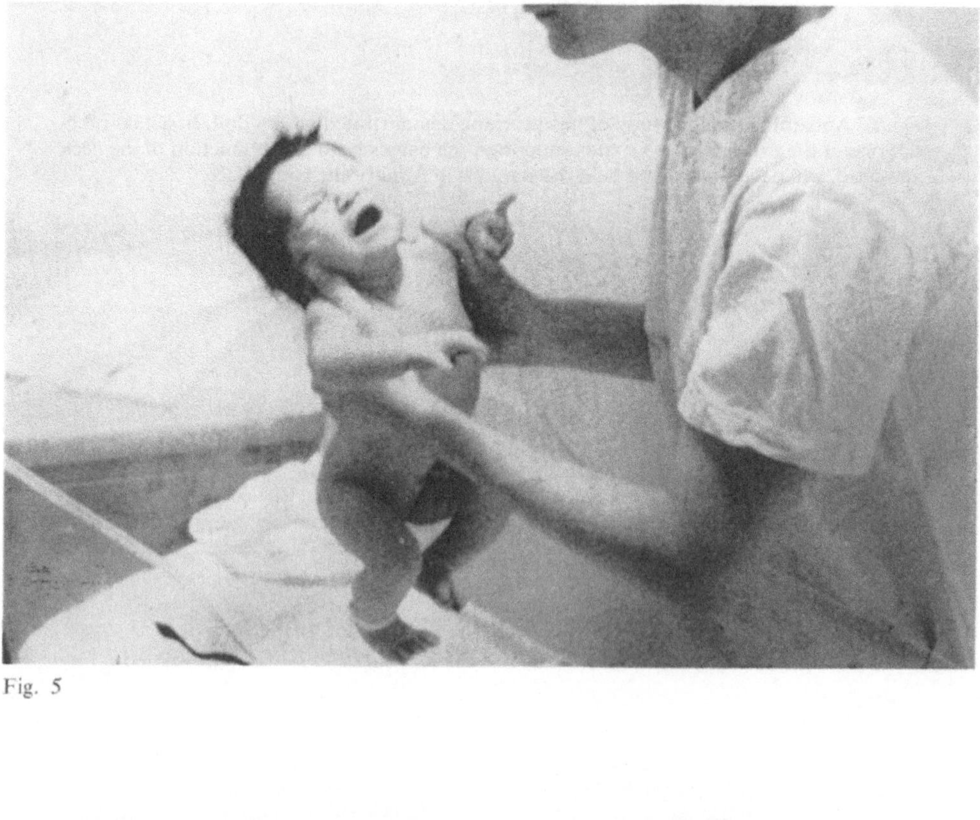

Fig. 5

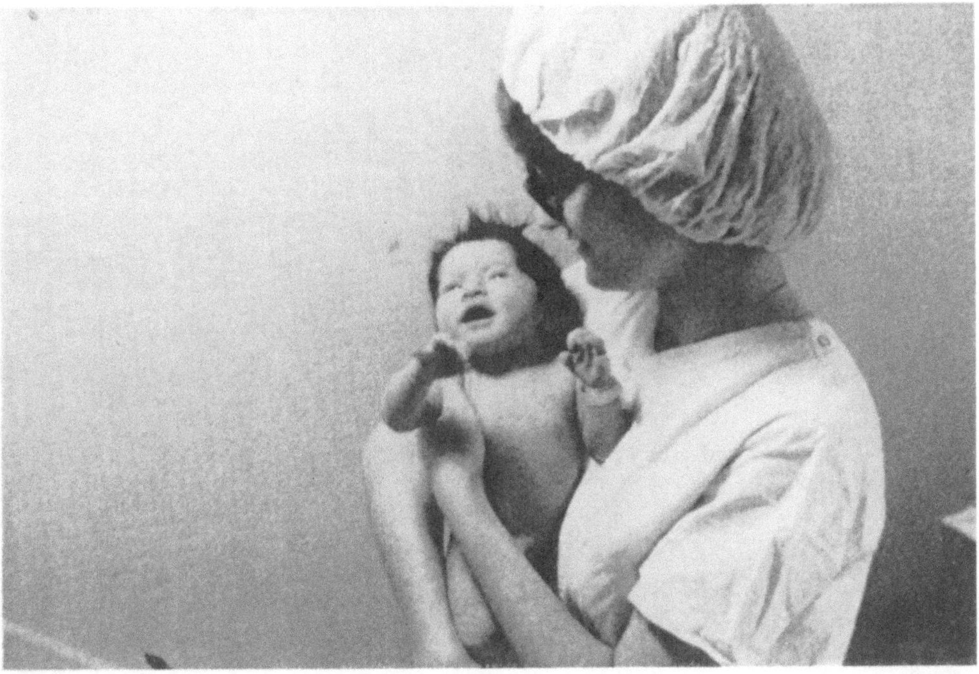

Fig. 6

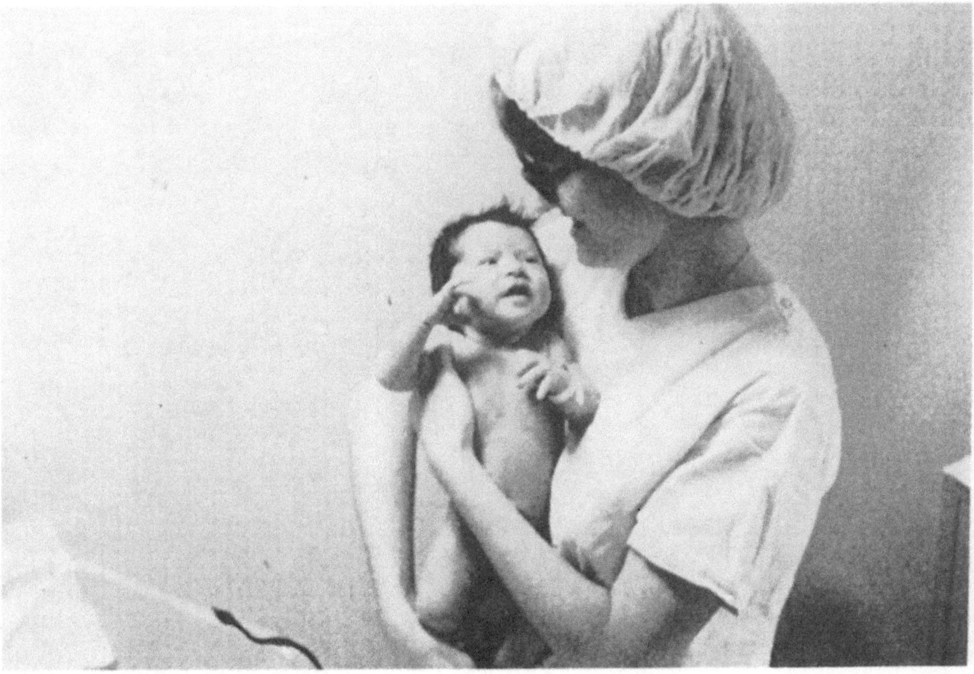

Fig. 7

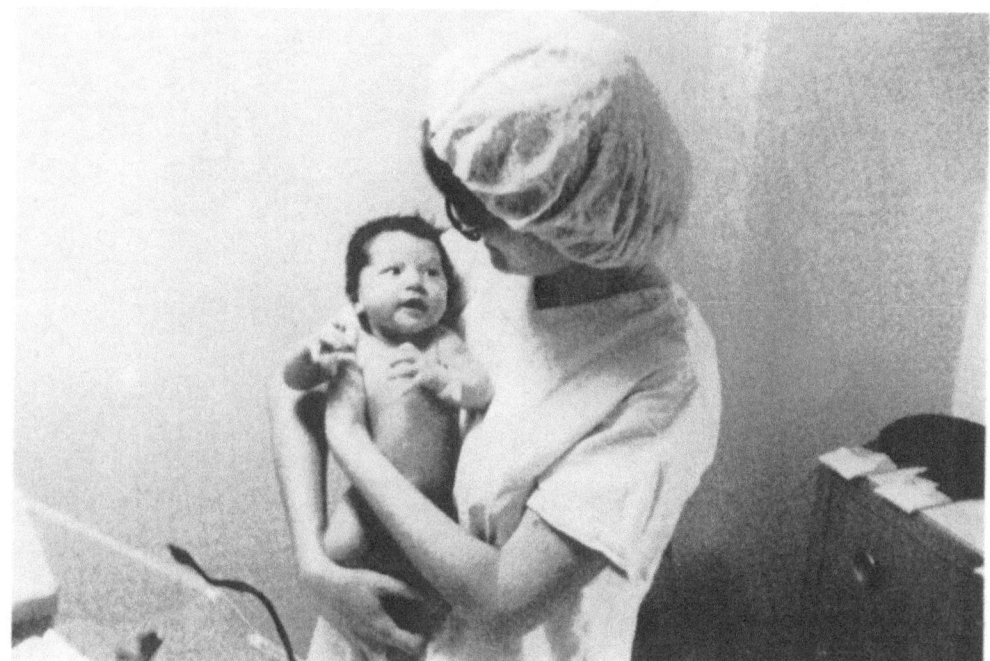

Fig. 8

Fig. 9

EXPERIMENT 4 STIMULI

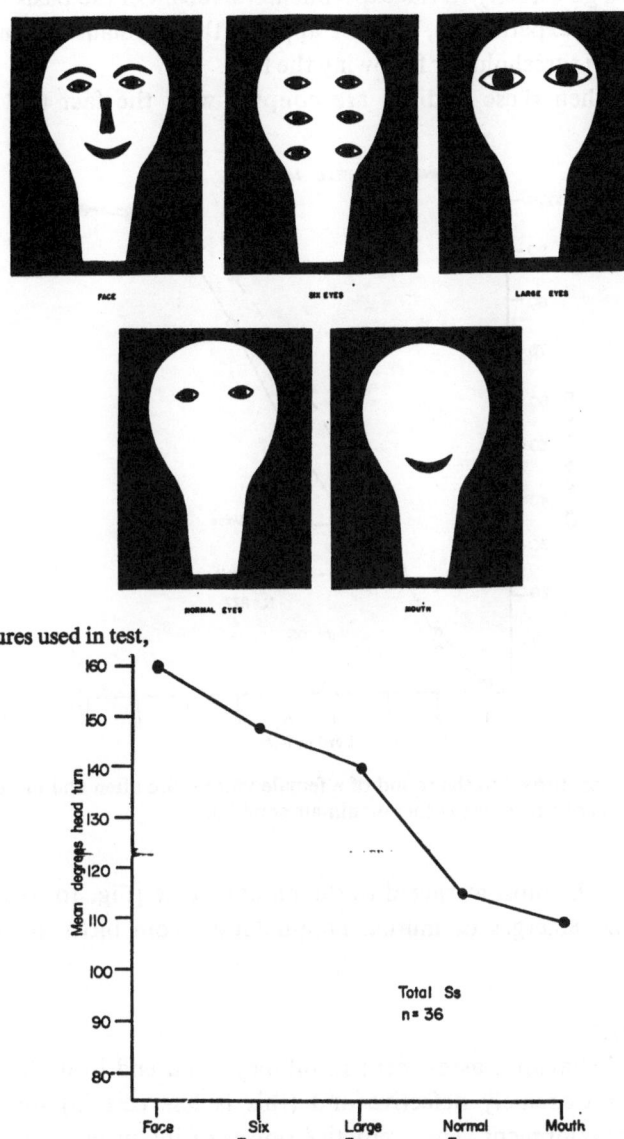

Fig. 3. Figures used in test,

Fig. 3a. Averaged head turning in newborns to schematic drawing of a face and face-parts. On the Wilcoxon test: Face > Six Eyes, p. <.01; Six Eyes > Normal Eyes (1 in schematic face), p <.005; Face > Large Eyes, p <.03; Large Eyes > Normal Eyes, p <.01; Six Eyes = Large Eyes and Normal Eyes = Mouth. From Jirari, 1970.

the arms for the first time. Note that crying stops almost immediately, and that the eyes go directly to the experimenter's face. On the basis of such observations and experiments, then, it appears that humans are indeed born with a lowered threshold for following the face.

Further, when these findings are coupled with the fact that newborns

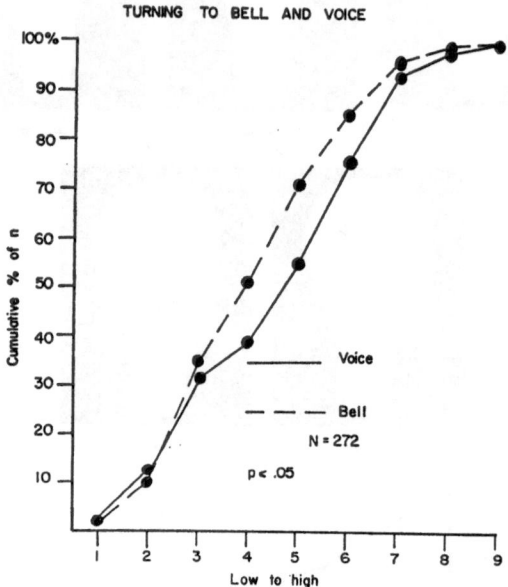

Fig. 10. Newborns turned to the sound of a female voice more often and more vigorously than to the sound of a bell (or to other inanimate sounds).

appear also to be most attracted to the human voice [Fig. 10; see also Hutt (9)], a picture emerges of mutual adaptedness, from birth, of infant and caretaker.

CONCLUSION

Mental and behavioral assessment in infancy is an end in itself only when screening for extremely defective and (this is less certain) for extremely precocious development. The predictive power of infant tests to later status is otherwise quite mediocre. While this undoubtedly could be improved by constructing more sensitive tests in both infancy and later childhood, new insights into the capacities of infants have arisen outside of the testing movement – from the work of scientists engaged in hypothesis-testing and theory construction. Out of such work new tests and assessment techniques have arisen, which have in turn served to encourage further behavioral investigations of infants.

REFERENCES

1. Thomas, H., Psychological assessment instruments for use with human infants. *Merrill-Palmer Quarterly of Behavior and Development* 16, 2 (1970).
2. Bayley, N., Behavioral correlates of mental growth: birth to thirty-six years. *Amer. Psychol.* 23, 1 (1958).
3. Bower, T. G. R., The visual world of infants. *Scient. Am.* 215, 80 (1966).
4. Bower, T. G. R., Slant perception and shape constancy in infants. *Science* 151, 832 (1966).
5. Bower, T. G. R., Phenomenal identity and form perception in an infant. *Perc. Psychophys.* 2, 74 (1967).
6. Bower, T. G. R., The development of object permanence: some studies of existence constancy. *Perc. Psychophys.* 2, 411 (1967).
7. Bower, T. G. R., Unpublished lecture, University of Chicago 1968.
8. Fantz, R. L., The origin of form perception. *Scient. Am.* 204, 459 (1961).
9. Hutt, S. J., Hutt, C., Lenard, H. G., Bernuth, H. V. & Muntjewerff, W. J., Auditory responsivity in the human neonate. *Nature* 218, 888 (1966).

DISCUSSION

Baum: I wonder if you or somebody else have tried some of these face-scrambling experiments in non-human primates.

Freedman: Nobody has tried the face-scrambling experiments but perhaps you know the experiment at Wisconsin by Sackett (1) in which isolated rhesus monkeys were able to choose the picture of another monkey they preferred by touching a lever. Monkeys under four months were greatly disturbed by the picture of a threatening monkey, although they had never seen this expression. On the other hand, pictures of other infants were most frequently sought and investigated.

Baum: But that is not quite analogous to what you were describing; in a sense that was a preference for a stimulus which aroused the monkey.

Freedman: Since we are on this topic, the work with the 'Fantz'-box is pertinent. The box is an apparatus the supine baby is slipped into; a visual stimulus is placed over the infant and you can see what he is looking at by peeping through a little hole and noting the reflection in his pupil. A baby's interest may be judged by the amount of time he spends looking at the stimulus. Vine (2) has recently summarized this voluminous literature and it appears that something that looks like a face is, in general, the preferred stimulus. However, these studies have been primarily with older infants since newborns tend not to look at a stationary stimulus. Thus, the advantage of using head-turning to a moving stimulus is that you can record a measurable response immediately after birth. As advice to inexperienced paediatricians, then, who wish to check a newborn's alertness, please don't use a torch although it may seem more scientific to do so. Instead, use your own face and talk to the baby, for the best stimulus that anyone has yet found is the vocalizing human face.

Marshall: This question has partly been answered, but in comforting the infant there appear to be several things involved: it is picked up, there is a face, there is possibly a voice. Is there any evidence as to the importance of the picking-up, cuddling aspect as distinct from the presence of the face and the baby being removed relative to it, which creates, in effect, a moving face. Is the picking-up and cuddling more for the benefit of the mother than the baby?

Freedman: No, we have taken all these steps in trying to quiet a baby, and the effect is cumulative. I believe my co-workers all agree, however, that the quickest way to quiet a newborn is to pick him up and walk with him, jostling him rhythmically. This works as well in the dark and without talking. Swaddling, too, is an effective way to console a crying newborn.

Levine: In most pictures there was no face. In effect, the face was covered with a mask and all that was seen was eyes, unless eyes are the only relevant character of a face that are important.

Freedman: It certainly appears that the eyes are the most important part of the face to newborns. There is an old study by Ahrens (3) in which he found a progressive trend. In the first weeks eyes alone were a sufficient target to attract an infant, but by the third month babies were not interested and did not smile unless a model of the full face was present. Eventually an actual smiling face was necessary to elicit a smile. With regard to newborns, then, it appears that a nose-mouth mask does not interfere with the baby's response. It sounds mysterious to non-evolutionists, but much data has now been accumulated which indicate that newborns preferentially respond to the stimuli which adults normally exhibit: human sounds, the human face, the universal tendency to pick-up and cuddle a baby. Not surprisingly, then, it appears that if one wanted to build a robot based on what babies best respond to, it would be a duplicate of ourselves.

Dobbing: I simply wanted to ask if you have any information about the various categories of babies of low birth-weight in this regard.

Freedman: I can't tell you how prematures compare with full term babies in their response to adult cues, but it does give me an opportunity to tell of a study with prematures undertaken by a student of mine, Louisa Powell. If one carries forward the logic that evolution has yielded beautifully coordinated systems between adult and infant, he must reject much of standard premature care. Consider a modern Isolette, and compare it with the uterine situation, where the premature baby should be: for one thing, there is always a bright light on, which seems to force the baby's eyes shut to ward it off. Secondly, prematures frequently startle themselves, for they now lie free and unswaddled, so that the new units seem a step backwards compared to the bundling practiced 20 years ago. Third, there is no movement in the environment and movement does appear to stimulate fetal development (4). To illustrate the potential importance of this last point, we placed prematures in a rocker developed by the Isolette Co. for apneic babies as phase one of these studies. The rocker was set at the gentle rate of 12 rocks per minute, and we began to see some interesting things. For one thing, the rocked infants gained weight at a somewhat faster rate. For another, they smiled more (eyes-closed smiling) while being rocked, and we have taken that to be a signal of increased well being, even as it is later in life (cf. 5). In Mrs Powell's study (phase two) mothers of prematures, instead of being separated from their babies for as much as 60 days, as might occur in the case of a very low-weight baby, have been permitted instead to help care for their infants on the premature ward. This work is now in progress, but we are convinced that the very act of touching the baby, let alone caring for it, will help create social bonds. The study will therefore involve a comparison, later in the first year, of these mother-infant pairs and a control group who had the more usual experience of prolonged early separation.

REFERENCES IN THE DISCUSSION

1. Sackett, G. P., Monkeys reared in isolation with pictures as visual input: evidence for an innate releasing mechanism. *Science* 154, 1468 (1966).
2. Vine, I., significance of facial-visual signals in human social development. In: *Expressive movement and nonverbal communication*. Vine, I. & Von Cranack, M. (eds.), New York 1971.
3. Ahrens, R., Beitrag zur Entwicklung des Physiognomie- und Mimikerkennens. *Z. Experim. Angew. Psychol.* 412, 599 (1954).
4. Gottlieb, G. & Kuo, F. Y., Development of behavior in the duck embryo. *J. Compar. Physiol. Psychol.* 58, 183 (1965).
5. Freedman, D. G., Smiling in blind infants and the issue of innate vs. acquired. *J. Child Psychol. Psychiat.* 5, 171 (1964).
6. Freedman, D. G. & Omark, D., Ethology, behavior genetics and education. In: *Cultural relevance in educational issues: a reader in anthropology and education*. Ianni, F. A. J. New York 1971.
7. Geber, M. & Dean, R. F. A., Precocious development in newborn African infants.

Readings in infancy and childhood. Brackbill & Thompson (eds.), New York 1966.
8. Kimura, D., Functional asymmetry the brain of in dichotic listening. *Cortex* 3, 163 (1957).
9. Montagu, M. A., *Prenatal influence*. Springfield (Ill.) 1962.

MANUAL TO ACCOMPANY CAMBRIDGE NEWBORN BEHAVIORAL AND NEUROLOGICAL SCALES*

T. B. BRAZELTON AND D. G. FREEDMAN

It should be made immediately clear that our goal in developing these scales has been to achieve a test which will distinguish differences among *normal* newborns, and the screening for pathology must be considered incidental to our interests here.

This manual is intended as a guide to objective scoring; it cannot replace an apprenticeship period under someone trained in these methods. In our experience excellent reliability is obtained between trainer and a reasonably talented trainee after testing and scoring approximately fifteen newborns together, usually over a period of ten days or so. (We are still in the process of gathering reliability data in an effort to pinpoint the most and the least valuable scales, and these figures will appear elsewhere.)

Despite this admonition, it is possible for researchers familiar with infants to use these scales without training, and to then develop reliability scores within their own group. Towards this end, most of the neurological items (elicited movements) are adequately described, as well as illustrated, in Prechtl and Beintema (1). Ideally, of course, all examiners should have a wealth of experience with a spectrum of normal infants against which they can establish norms for scoring the subject.

The test should take from 25 to 35 minutes. Since many of the scores are summary assessments, it is preferable that they be recorded after the test is complete. However, as it will be seen, some items may be immediately scored. It is recommended that when there is doubt about a performance, perhaps because states of receptiveness are constantly changing, that the item be repeated until doubt is eliminated (or at least alleviated). For reasons such as this, some babies simply take longer to test.

The examiner (E) should not be bound to the order in which items appear

* Our thanks to Dr John S. Robey, M. D., Joan Durfee, B. A., Joan Kuchner, M. A., and Nina Freedman, R. N., who helped in the development of these scales. The senior author is now preparing a modification of this test.

here. As a suggestive guide, the items are grouped on the last page according to convenience of administration.

There is evidence that newborns do not perform in a stable fashion on certain neurological items until 4 days of age (2) and that they tend to be relatively discoordinated for 48 hours after delivery, particularly if the mother has had systemic drugs. Thus it is advised that the scales will probably yield more stable scores with older neonates. However, while careful studies still need to be done, we have seen babies who have yielded quite stable performances starting at a few hours of age.

CONDITIONS OF EXAMINATION

The infant should be examined under relaxed conditions, for example in a private room adjacent to the nursery; in our experience a relaxed examiner is as important as a receptive baby. There should be some control over lighting, since many infants engage actively in shutting out bright lights, and thus are un-receptive to visual stimulation. The same logic holds for auditory stimulation.

Many infants attend better in the lap with head well up, and they should be given this opportunity. Similarly, some attend better when bundled than with limbs free, particularly highly irritable infants; propping the bassinet at about 30 degrees is yet another means of maximizing alertness.

An exam should ideally take place in the intermediate periods between feedings, not too soon after the last feeding (when the baby may be groggily asleep) or within an hour before the next feeding (when he may be unreachable as soon as he is aroused, because of hunger). However, even when babies are examined with such optimal timing, some will nevertheless show all the indications of being hungry. For such babies it is very helpful to have a bottle of sugar-water available. Pacifiers, on the other hand, while sometimes useful, tend to interfere with optimal performance because babies may then concentrate on sucking to the exclusion of everything else.

STATE

'State of consciousness' or 'state' is one of the most important variables in any observation period. All of the infant's reactions are state-related, and must be interpreted within the context of the presenting state of consciousness.

State depends on physiological variables such as hunger, nutrition, degree of hydration, time within the wake-sleep cycle, etc. The pattern of states as well

as the movement from one state to another appear to be important characteristics of infants in the neonatal period, and this kind of evaluation may be
the best predictor of the infant's receptivity and ability to respond to stimuli
in a cognitive sense. The criteria for delineating the states listed below are
drawn from our experience and that of others who have worked with newborns.

SLEEP STATES

S-1   Deep sleep with no spontaneous activity other than a few mild
        startles at regular intervals; external stimuli do not seem to penetrate
        and no behavioral response may be noted for long periods. This
        state may be induced as a homeostatic response to repeated, distur-
        bing stimulation.

S-2   Sleeps with little spontaneous activity except startles or startle
        equivalents; at quite regular intervals, external stimuli produce
        startles with some delay; suppressions of startles are rapid.

S-3   Light sleep with eyes closed; low activity level with random move-
        ments and mild spontaneous startles; responsive to internal and
        external stimuli with startle equivalents, often with a resulting
        change of state.

AWAKE STATES

A-1   Eyes generally open; semi-dozing; activity level low with inter-
        spersed mild startles from time to time; reactive to sensory stimuli,
        but delay in response often seen; state change after stimulation fre-
        quently noted.

A-2   Eyes open; considerable motor activity with thrusting movements of
        extremities; intermittent crying; few spontaneous startles; reactive
        to external stimulation with increase in startles or motor activity,
        but discreet reactions difficult to distinguish because of general high
        activity level.

A-3   Alert bright look; seems to focus attention on source of stimulation,
        e.g., pacifier, face or moving object, voice or bell; tends to shut out
        competing stimuli.

Crying Intense crying activity which is difficult to break through with stimu-
        lation.

INITIAL STATE

In the two minutes before stimulation is begun, an assessment of the infant's initial state is made by observing his spontaneous behavior, respirations (as observed by the movement of the gown or covering sheet), eye movements, startles, and responses to concurrent spontaneous events (sounds, vibrations, etc.) in the environment. The infant should be left covered or dressed as he is found in the Nursery to assess initial state. After he is disturbed, and undressed, he will be in an entirely different state of receptiveness.

PREDOMINANT STATE(S)

At the end of the examination period, the examiner should record the two or, at the most, three states within which the infant performed. Since the most important influence on the baby's scores will be his available states, it is important to have an idea of the range, as well as the kinds, of states used by him during the exam. For purposes of analysis, however, the examiner should also underline the one circled state which most nearly predominated during the exam.

Additional note: As conceptualized here, the states which the infant utilizes are ranged along a continuum from deep sleep to awake and very alert. It is implied that, as the infant moves from the S_1 to the A_3 state, he becomes progressively more 'alert', more receptive to stimulation. Intense crying would, thus, seem to represent a state qualitatively different from those on the sleep-wake continuum. It is unlikely that the infant will be asleep when very distressed, and, yet, he certainly is neither alert nor responsive to stimulation. Thus, very intense crying is listed as a separate 'state' and may be scored alone (not in conjunction with another state) if it persists and predominates.

I. GENERAL TONUS   (9 point scale)

This scale is designed to give a summary impression, after completion of the examination of the tone of the infant's musculature. Factors such as resistence to movement of the limbs, and adjustment to being held and handled are important indices of tonus. It is therefore imperative that the examiner handle as well as observe the infant to score this scale. Reactions relevant to other scales on the test will contribute toward an assessment of tonus: e.g., defensive movements, pull to sit, head movement in prone, passive movements, activity, cuddliness. This scale is designed so that very low or very high scores (1, 2, 8, and 9) fall outside of the range of tonus normal for a healthy, full-term newborn. Thus it is among the least differentiating scales, given a normal population.

1. The infant is flaccid, limp, like a rag-doll. There is extreme head lag with no adjustment. The baby offers no resistence when the Examiner moves his limbs.
3. Tonus is within normal limits, but the infant is rather flaccid and offers only weak resistence to movement of his limbs.
5. The limbs can be flexed and extended by the Examiner, but the infant offers definite resistence to these manipulations. The baby evidences ability to control postural adjustments, and this muscular action can be felt when the baby is handled. The infant may characteristically maintain a posture on the bed or examining table of flexion with the hands held closed, although this is not universal.
7. The baby's limbs are very resistent to extension, and there is a pronounced tensing of the muscles when held and handled; e.g., arching of the back, twisting, turning when held and placed in the prone position.
9. The baby's body is characteristically very tight, tense, rigid. It is difficult to move the limbs, and the limbs will spring back when extended. There may be extreme fistedness. An infant at this end of the scale must be distinguished from one with very strong muscles, but with more optimal tonus.

2. LABILITY OF SKIN COLOR   (9 point scale)

This scale measures the change in color and vascularity of the infant's skin during the course of the examination; e.g., the acrocyanosis or peripheral mild cyanosis when an extremity is left uncovered; the change from pink to pale or purple when the baby is undressed; mottling and a weblike appearance which may appear in an effort to maintain body heat. A normal newborn is likely to demonstrate mild color changes several times in an exam during which he has been undressed, disturbed, and upset. No change in color may be the result of a depressed or overstressed autonomic and vascular system, as seen in dopey, pale, or cyanotic infants. Marked changes which vary from minute to minute would be seen in prematures or in babies who were not yet adjusted to extra-uterine temperature changes, or in infants whose central and autonomic nervous systems were unable to master the change during an exam. Thus, scores of 1, 2, 8, and 9 on this scale fall outside of the normal Caucasian range. We have found that normal Navajo infants, however, are frequently scored 8. In darkly pigmented infants, of course, low scores are meaningless. Factors to be considered in arriving at a summary score for the infant are the *degree* of color change, the *rapidity* of that change, and the amount of time it takes to *return to normal color* when disturbing circumstances cease. Because crying produces maximal color change in most infants, it is important, for later interpretation of the rating of this scale, that an accurate rating of irritability be made.

1. There is no change in skin color during the exam. The baby is dopey, pale, or cyanotic and does not change from this condition.
3. The infant has healthy skin color, but does not change color when uncovered or handled. When the baby cries, there may be change of color, about the mouth or face, but it is not extreme and disappears as soon as crying stops.
5. The infant's skin changes color when the baby is uncovered or when he is crying. The face, lips, extremities may pale or redden, and mottling may appear on the face, chest, and limbs. However, original color returns quickly.
7. The baby's skin often changes color, perhaps to very red or very blue, when uncovered or crying. There is somewhat delayed recovery to original color.
9. The baby shows marked, rapid changes from original coloring to very blue or red, with little recovery to original color.

3. PEAK OF EXCITEMENT (9 point scale)

This scale is designed to give a measure of the infant's peak of excitement as observed during the course of the exam. Excitement may be a product of crying, and, often, an infant will reach his peak during an episode of distress. However, other indices of excitement can also be observed, such as sucking behavior and motor activity. As such, excitement must be distinguished from irritability and might generally be defined as overt responsiveness to stimulation. That stimulation might come from the environment, or it might be internal in nature. It is important to note that excitability is closely related to state. The kind of intense reactions which some infants demonstrate when they reach their peak of excitement shows an unavailability to the outside world, and must be scored high. Others are hardly to be jogged to respond at all, and should be scored low. An average optimal response falls in the moderate, reachable range, in which the infant can be brought to respond to stimuli in spite of a high degree of upset or excitement.

1. The infant doesn't go beyond a low level of excitement. There is no crying in response to disturbing stimuli. E unable to stimulate a response.
3. Some response to E's stimulation, but chronically low.
   Maximal degree of upset or activity is moderate.
7. Baby reaches point of greater involvement in own activity (e.g., crying, rooting, mouthing) than in responding to E, but infant can be reached.
9. The baby reaches a state of distress or activity in which the examiner cannot reach him to quiet him or to distract his attention. Ordinarily it will be very difficult to test an infant at this level of excitement.

4. LABILITY OF STATES   (9 point scale)

This scale measures the amount of movement from one state to another during the course of the exam; i.e., *how often* the baby changes from one state to another. A highly labile infant moves frequently and without too many in-between rests in responsive states. The lability may be triggered by appropriate stimuli, but as he over-reacts, the infant loses his capacity to respond for any period to a series of stimuli. At the low end of the scale, the infant cannot be moved from a steady state of crying, sucking, sleep, or, in a few cases, alertness. A moderately labile series of states is best suited to the maneuvers of the examination. Thus, lability is viewed in terms of the infant's own propensity for change in state, as well as his responsiveness to attempts by the examiner to effect change.

1. The infant cannot be moved or does not spontaneously move from a steady state of crying, sleeping, sucking, alterness.
3. The infant does not often move spontaneously from state to state. The examiner may effect change, but not readily. Not more than two state changes are observed.
5. There is some spontaneous movement from one state to another. The examiner usually effects a change. The infant remains in an attending state long enough to be receptive to stimulation by the examiner. Not more than three changes of state are seen.
7. The infant frequently moves from one state to another and four or five state changes may be observed.
9. The infant continuously oscillates from one state to another.

5. ALERTNESS (OPTIMAL)   (9 point scale)

This scale assesses the degree to which the infant is responsive to his environment during his period of greatest alertness (as defined by the gradated scale of states from S_3 to A_1). Alertness in this sense is defined in terms of the baby's auditory and visual attention to stimuli outside of himself. This stimulation may be presented by the examiner, but need not be. For example, some infants are most interested in looking about the Nursery. This scale excludes startles and reflexive, involuntary reactions to stimulation. It is important to note that the infant need not exhibit both visual and auditory alertness to be scored high on the scale.

1. The infant does not respond to any efforts on the examiner's part to attract his attention. Nothing in the environment seems to spontaneously attract or hold his interest.
3. In response to an auditory stimulus, there is brightening of the face, perhaps widening of the eyes, and quieting of activity. When responding to a visual stimulus, the baby will focus or stare fleetingly, catching the object visually and then losing it. He will lose sight of the object about 3/4 as much as he will stare at it.
5. The infant will brighten, still, and then attend to an auditory or visual stimulus for a short period of time. While it is possible to again catch his attention, interest span is repeatedly short. When presented with a visual stimulus, the infant will lose it or look away about $\frac{1}{2}$ of the time.
7. The infant will attend to a visual or auditory stimulus for a prolonged period of time. While he may occasionally lose it, his attention will be focused upon it for approximately 3/4 of the time that it is available to him.
9. The infant seems completely fascinated with any auditory and/or visual stimulus, and becomes engrossed, as if shutting out everything else around. The response seems almost mechanical, as if the infant is 'hooked onto' the stimulus and is unable to release it. If the infant is responding to the general environment, he will appear wide-eyed and his head and eyes turn freely as he 'drinks everything in'. He will exhibit repeated, pronounced attempts to locate sources of sounds.

6. FOLLOWING WITH HEAD AND EYES
(INANIMATE OBJECT)   (9 point scale)

This scale measures the infant's ability to focus upon a stimulus and follow its movement, with the eyes or with eyes and head, horizontally, vertically, and in a circular path. Assessment is also made of the continuity or 'smoothness' of that movement. Several objects may serve as stimuli: e.g., we generally use a red ball and a shiny chromed bell (silent). It is helpful to place the infant's head in midline when initially presenting a visual stimulus, to maximize the baby's ability to follow both sides. It is also *important that the lighting in the testing room be dim*, as young infants are very sensitive to bright light and may not be able to fully open the eyes in it. Most neonates will demonstrate some ability to fix on a visual object and follow it briefly in the horizontal plane. Vertical following seems to be of a higher order than horizontal following and usually is seen only when horizontal following is excellent. For maximal performance it is sometimes helpful to hold the infant or to prop him so that the head is higher than the feet. A suggestion: while we do not here distinguish between the amount of following and quality of following, it would be possible to develop two such scales in place of this one.

1. The baby does not focus upon or follow a stimulus object.
3. The infant will fixate upon an object, but will not follow with eyes or head.
5. The baby focuses and follows with the eyes for some distance horizontally for at least a 30° arc and/or vertically. The movement is jerky, and there may be some nystagmus of the eyes. The baby will lose the object intermittently, but will catch it again. He does not follow with the head at all.
7. The infant will follow with both eyes and head at least 60° horizontally, briefly vertically, or in a circle. However, movement is only partially continuous and he will lose the object from time to time.
9. The baby follows the stimulus continuously horizontally for at least 120° vertically and in a circle. Movement is smooth and well-coordinated.

7. REACTION TO SOUND
(USUALLY BELL AND RATTLE)   (9 point scale)

This scale measures the infant's reaction to auditory stimuli (excluding reaction to the examiner's voice). It is well to present more than one type of sound, as some infants seem to 'like' and, thus, to react better to some sounds than to others. However, it is also important not to present the stimuli one immediately after the other, as the infant is likely to habituate to the stimuli, thus effectively shutting them out. Rarely is there no reaction to sound, and normally, there is evidence of at least brief attention, such as respiratory change, blinking, slight change of attention. In more attentive babies, there will occur some shift of eyes and head, a decrease in other activity, and a more significant state-adjustment. In very attentive infants, there is a marked response, with head turning and even searching with the eyes, softening and alerting of the face, as the infant seems to search for the source of auditory stimulation.

Suggestion: Use standardized sound, e.g., hi C and lo C triangles, and score separately for high-pitched and low-pitched frequencies.

1. There is no observable response. The baby does not brighten, still, or look. This reaction is usually seen only in dopey, drugged or damaged babies.
3. The baby brightens and stills to the sound, but makes no effort to purposefully locate the source. Or, the infant may immediately shut out the stimulation.
5. The infant shows a definite, though involuntary, reaction to the sound. There may be quieting, brightening, an increase in respiration, and a decrease in other activity. There may be involuntary jerking of the eyes toward the stimulus whenever it is sounded, accompanied in some cases by involuntary head movements.
7. The infant shows what appears to be purposeful searching for the source of sound with the eyes. A general alerting of the face and searching expression in the eyes can be observed.
9. When the stimulus is presented, the infant alerts and turns eyes and head in the direction of the sound, searching for the source. This purposeful reaction is repeated over and over again whenever sound is presented.

8. DEFENSIVE MOVEMENT (CLOTH ON FACE)   (9 point scale)

This scale assesses the extent and effectiveness of the infant's attempts to remove a cloth which has been pressed *firmly* over the nose and mouth for a few seconds. If the cloth is merely placed on the face, a substantial number of infants will not react at all, and potential individual differences are lost. The important factors to be considered are the infant's degree of arousal and the degree of coordination in the withdrawal response. Most infants will respond with one or several of the following behaviors: (1) mouthing and rooting against the cloth (especially when hungry); (2) head twisting from side to side and, more vigorously, up and down; (3) twisting of the trunk of the body, and (4) swiping at the cloth with the arms and hands in a circular fashion. To be scored high on the scale, the infant must defend himself repeatedly and successfully with 'on target' movements. This is a mature response, as it contains a series of associated, complex behaviors.

1. There is no reaction to smothering. The baby makes no attempt to remove the cloth. This reaction is seen usually in very dopey or drugged babies.
3. The infant mouths, roots, sucks on the cloth, or simply tries to turn his head.
5. The infant will show mouthing, turning of the head, increased activity of the limbs, and ineffective swipes at the cloth with his hands and arms.
7. The infant reacts with mouthing, pronounced head turning, more vigorous movement in the trunk, and partially effective pushing movements of one or both arms.
9. The baby exhibits twisting of the whole body, perhaps arching of the back, vigorous head turning, accompanied by well-coordinated 'on target' pushing movements of both hands and arms. This response is consistently given.

9. IRRITABILITY   (9 point scale)

This scale gives a summary impression of the infant's fussiness and irritable crying as observed over the course of the examination. Some procedures in the exam would be expected to produce irritation (e.g., undressing, Moro, pinprick, smothering). Thus, it is the unusual infant who will exhibit no irritation at all. It is important to note crying behavior, even when the infant is not being handled.

1. The infant never cries, even in response to irritating stimulation.
3. The infant shows some distress, but only sporadically, and only in response to either extremely irritating or often repeated stimulation (e.g., Moro, pinprick, light on eyes).
5. The infant cries in response to some stimulation and not others; or the infant cries inconsistently in response to one type of stimulation. He may cry for short periods for no observable reason.

7. The infant often, or quickly, cries in response to stimulation, even those procedures which would not be expected to produce irritation. There may be frequent outbursts of crying and sucking on hands for no observable reason.
9. The infant spends much of the time crying, and characteristically responds to all stimulation with irritation.

10. SELF QUIETING ACTIVITY (9 point scale)

This scale yields a measure of the infant's ability to quiet himself after a period of upset. The repertoire of activities with which the infant actively modulates his state of irritation is considered, as well as the effectiveness and consistency of these actions. Techniques for self-quieting which are often seen in newborns are: placing the hand into the mouth (and sucking on it); sucking on other materials (as the bedding or examiner's gown); visually catching onto an object to quiet self; adjusting the head to a comfortable position and quieting; gradually attending to a repeated disturbing stimulus and quieting; shutting-off. If the infant does not cry at all, this item cannot be scored. However, since some computer programs cannot deal with absent data, it is perhaps permissable to score the few such infants as 9.

1. The infant cannot actively quiet himself. He always requires intervention. He exhibits no sign of attempting to quiet himself by any of above mentioned techniques.
3. Makes attempts, such as hand in mouth, but does not quieten.
5. The infant sometimes quiets himself and sometimes requires intervention. His ability is inconsistent. He clearly exhibits attempts to quiet himself but these attempts are frequently not successful. He shows at least one successful attempt at self quieting.
7. Successfully repeats self-quieting acts, but does not quieten for sustained periods.
9. The infant using one or several methods, consistently quiets himself quickly and for sustained periods of time. (Or, the infant does not cry at all.)

11. CONSOLABLE WITH SOCIAL INTERVENTION (9 point scale)

This scale measures the extent to which the baby, when irritated, quiets in response to the examiner's efforts at social soothing. Factors to be considered are: consistency of response, amount of soothing required to quiet the infant, rapidity of quieting, and whether or not the baby remains quiet (permanency of state change). In order of increased effort on the examiner's part soothing as we practise it consists of: (1) touching the baby, (2) talking to him, (3) picking the baby up, (4) cuddling, rocking and talking to him in the arms, and (5) bundling him. Soothing required in response to physiological needs (e.g., feeding when hungry, changing diaper when wet, or even giving the baby a pacifier) are not considered as part of social soothing. It is important to examine the baby, if possible, when he is dry and not hungry. Some infants require less 'intense' social soothing to quiet them effectively than do others, and may respond well, for example, to the sound of the examiner's voice or to the touch of the examiner's hand placed on the tummy. Most babies, however, require holding and cuddling. As in other studies cf. Lipton and Steinschneider (5)], we have found bundling to be quite effective.

In a very few instances, the infant cries when held, but quiets immediately when placed in the crib again. The examiner should note the method of soothing most effective for the infant in the summary paragraph, as it may well be one further clue to the baby's individual mode of responsiveness to stimulation. Rarely, an infant does not cry at all, so that this item cannot be properly scored.

1. The baby does not respond to any form of social soothing.
3. The examiner is able to sooth the infant only once or twice, or only after a very prolonged period of crying. Even then, the baby remains quieted for only a short time.
5. The baby quiets in response to soothing, at least half the time, but does so only after some delay. He usually does not remain quieted for long, and the examiner must repeat her attempts. E must usually pick-up, cuddle and talk to the baby to achieve soothing.
7. The baby almost always responds quickly to the examiner, but he may not always remain quieted. The examiner must therefore repeat attempts to sooth and usually must pick-up the baby. On the other hand, rocking and vocal soothing in the arms are not necessary.
9. The baby consistently and quickly quiets in response to the examiner and remains soothed. Simple touch or voice is usually sufficient, and the baby does not require picking-up.

1 2. PULL TO SIT   (9 point scale)

This scale measures the infant's ability to hold his head in midline and parallel to the body trunk when pulled from a supine position to sit. As such, it is an indirect measure of the musculature of the neck and shoulder girdle. Infants who make no attempt to bring up the head or adjust in the shoulder girdle with flexion as they are lifted rate a low score. The average infant cannot maintain his head as he comes up, but, when sitting, will right the head parallel with the body and maintain it in midline for brief, unsuccessful periods. A few strong infants can bring the head up parallel with the body as it is raised, and can maintain it upright for long periods in midline. They are rated at the upper end of the scale.

1. The baby's head falls back immediately when pulled from the prone. The infant does not correct this lag.
3. The baby's head lags back when pulled up, but the infant makes attempts, though unsuccessful, at righting it.
5. The baby's head lags back when pulled up, but it is righted to midline after some delay when the baby sits. The head then falls forward or back again, with the infant again attempting to correct the lag.
7. The baby's head does not lag back when he is pulled to sit. It does fall forward in the sitting position, but it is corrected by the infant and held in midline momentarily before it again falls forward; there is repeated attempt at correcting.
9. There is no head lag. The baby holds his head at midline as he is pulled up and maintains this position when held in the sitting position. The head does not fall forward.

1 3. HEAD MOVEMENT IN PRONE   (9 point scale)

This scale gives an assessment of the baby's ability to lift and turn his head when he is placed prone with head in midline and face pressed gently down into the bedding. Most infants will react by turning the head to one side, and often will put the fist into the mouth. Normal infants will often lift the chin from the bed; others will clearly lift the neck and head; and a few will push themselves up on the arms so that even the chest is freed from the bedding. It is important, in eliciting this response, to place the infant's arms to the sides and out from under the trunk, and to gently tuck the baby's head down into the bedding. It is also convenient to watch for crawling at this point, as that response is elicited by placing the infant on his stomach.

1. The infant's head remains in midline, tucked down into the bedding. There is no head movement or mouthing of the bedding.
3. The infant turns his head to one side by rolling around on the cheek and chin. He does not lift the chin.
5. The infant turns his head to one side by lifting the chin from the bedding.
7. The infant lifts his chin and neck from the bedding and turns his head to the side.
9. The infant pushes himself up with his arms, so that head and upper chest are free of the bed. He turns his head to the side.

14. ACTIVITY   (9 point scale)

This scale measures the amount of motor activity which the infant exhibits during the course of the exam. As a summary score, it includes all spontaneous activity, both when the infant is lying alone unclothed and clothed and when he is being held and handled. Examples of typical neonate motoric activity are: postural adjustments when being held and handled; spontaneous movement of hands, arms, legs, feet; pronounced extension and flexion of the limbs; head movement; twisting and turning of the trunk and arching of the back.

1. The baby exhibits little or no spontaneous motor activity, except postural changes for balancing during crying and when being handled.
3. The baby exhibits some low-order spontaneous movement of the limbs and head. Most activity, however, is stimulated by holding and handling.
5. The infant, when quiet and awake, exhibits frequent spontaneous movement of the limbs. There is some increased activity when the infant is handled.
7. In addition to limb movements, the infant exhibits active movement of the neck and trunk, especially in the prone position. Flexing of the back muscles may be noted. Spontaneous activity is frequent and prolonged.
9. The infant is hyperactive. Repeated and intense motor activity may or may not be accompanied by constant crying. There is movement of the limbs and trunk, including arching of the back and writhing with the entire body. While the infant may be reachable, it is often difficult to test him.

15. SOCIAL INTEREST IN THE EXAMINER
(ATTENDS FACE) (9 point scale)

This scale assesses the way in which the infant responds to the examiner's face, and includes focusing, staring, following, and exploring the face with the eyes (as, for example, during feeding). As a summary score over the length of the exam, the rating should reflect spontaneous interest which the infant exhibits, as well as responses actively elicited by the examiner. As with the other visual items, infants typically do considerably better in dim light.

While it is often necessary to speak to the infant to catch his visual attention initially, it is important to consider visual attention to the face only when unaccompanied by the voice. The face should be presented and moved across the infant's field of vision to encourage following. The examiner may smile or not as he wishes, unless he wishes to distinguish the baby's responses to the two facial configurations. Many babies do better when cradled in arms, and we, typically, sit with the infant propped in the lap.

1. The infant shows no interest in the examiner's face. He cannot be induced to focus upon the face or follow.

3. The infant will look at the face when presented, and may quiet. However, his glance continuously shifts away from the face. He shows little spontaneous interest in the face. He will not follow movement of the examiner's face with eyes or head.

5. The infant will focus on the presented face and follow with the eyes, but not with the head. Visual focus, however, is not continuous. There is some lag in following, so that it may be necessary to coax the baby to follow in a series of stop and start movements from one side to the other. The infant shows some spontaneous interest in the face and may focus on it for brief periods of time.

7. The infant alerts and brightens visibly when the face is presented. He focuses and follows with eyes and head from side to side, although following is somewhat discontinuous and the baby loses the face from time to time. He shows spontaneous interest in the face, focusing on and exploring it visually from time to time.

9. The infant repeatedly focuses intently on the presented face and follows smoothly with eyes and head as the examiner moves her face. The baby may spontaneously study the face intently at frequent intervals.

16. SOCIAL INTEREST IN THE EXAMINER
(ATTENDS FACE ACCOMPANIED BY VOICE)   (9 point scale)

The face should be moved slowly across the infant's field of vision, as in 15, with the examiner speaking to the baby all the while. Again, note should be taken throughout the examination period of any instances of spontaneous attention to the examiner's face when accompanied by the voice.

1. The infant exhibits no interest when the face and voice are presented simultaneously. The examiner is unable to engage the baby's visual or auditory attention.
3. When face and voice are presented together, the infant stills, brightens, and focuses on the face. However, his attention quickly shifts away. There is no attempt to follow the face with eyes or head. The infant seldom focuses on the face-voice configuration spontaneously.
5. The infant focuses on the face when the face and voice are presented together, and follows with the eyes. This may be accompanied by a few involuntary jerks of the head in the direction of the face. Following is only partially continuous, and the examiner may have to repeatedly catch the infant's attention. The baby shows occasional spontaneous interest in the face-voice configuration.
7. The infant stills, brightens, and focuses on the face when face and voice are presented. He follows with eyes and head from side to side, although movement may be somewhat jerky. The baby often attends to face and voice spontaneously.
9. The infant focuses intently on the face when face and voice are presented, and follows consistently with eyes and head in smooth coordinated movements. He is observed to spontaneously study the face intently at frequent intervals.

17. SOCIAL INTEREST IN THE EXAMINER
(ATTENDS VOICE)   (9 point scale)

This scale measures the extent and characteristic way in which the infant responds to the examiner's voice. The examiner speaks softly and close to the infant's ear, being careful to remain outside of the baby's visual field in order not to confound visual and auditory cues. This can be accomplished by raising the infant, face-up, above the head of E, so that all the baby can see to begin with is the ceiling. He must thus turn to the voice to see E. This is then repeated in the other ear.

1. The infant does not visibly react to the voice. There is no apparent change in behavior.
3. When the voice is presented, the baby stills and brightens, but does not purposefully search for the source.
5. The infant reacts to the voice by quieting and brightening. The eyes shift involuntarily toward the source, accompanied at times by involuntary head movements.
7. The infant stills to the voice and searches purposefully for the source of sound with his eyes. There is some head movement, in the correct direction, but no insistent turning-to.
9. The infant consistently turns the eyes and head toward the source of sound and focuses on the examiner's face.

18. SMILING

Smiles are seen in the neonate. They can be of a reflexive nature, as when the infant is dropping from an awake state into an S_2 state after a feed. They also occur 'appropriately' – in response to soft auditory and/or visual cues. Occasionally, when he is handled and restrained in a cuddling position, a smile comes across his face as the infant relaxes. Close replicas of 'social smiles' can be seen in the newborn period – when an examiner leans over his crib and talks softly to him. They are difficult to be sure of, may consist primarily of a softening and brightening of the infant's face with a reflex grimace thrown in, and they are always difficult to reproduce. Hence, one hesitates to call these social 'smiles', but they surely are the precursors of such behavior [see for example, Freedman (3)].

Number of smiles seen throughout the examination are counted.

19. PASSIVE MOVEMENT OF LEGS

20. PASSIVE MOVEMENT OF ARMS   (5 point scale)

These are measures of amount of resistance in the limbs when E extends them from the abducted position. E takes hold of both hands and slowly pulls the arms outward, then releases. Likewise with the feet and legs. Entering into a judgment of resistance are both the resistance experienced in the pull out and the amount of 'snapback' to the original position once the limb is released. Geber has reported differential resistance between arms and legs in a normal group of Ganda infants, and for this reason separate scales for each pair of limbs are used here.

1. Flaccid, completely malleable limb positions.
3. Definite resistance offered to limb manipulation, but snapback is moderate.
5. Great resistance and flexion, very high snapback.

21. RAPIDITY OF BUILD-UP
(FROM SLEEP TO AWAKE)   (5 point scale)

This scale assesses the characteristic speed and abruptness with which an infant moves from the sleep to the awake state, usually at the very start of the examination. Ideally the baby will be asleep when the exam starts; he should be carefully uncovered and undressed, and if still in an S state, the physical-ability items, such as 'pull to sit', may commence.

1. The baby may give signals which hint of an anticipated change, but these changes do not occur. Remains in S state.
3. The baby eases into the awake state, with the examiner observing some anticipatory signals followed by the expected transition.
5. Rapidly 'shoots' from S to A state. Because the changes are very sharp and quick, states can be clearly delineated one from another.

22. HABITUATION TO REPEATED STUMULATION
(SHUT-OFF MECHANISM) LIGHT ON EYES   (5 point scale)

One of the most impressive mechanisms in the neonate is the capacity to decrease responsiveness to repeated, disturbing stimuli, to a point, for example, where an S_1 state may replace an A_3. This scale is one measure of the infant's ability to shut out such irritating stimulation. Of three measures originally included in the examination to assess this capacity (repeated Moro, repeated pinprick, repeated presentation of bright light to the eye), only the latter has been retained. The first two procedures can be highly disturbing to particularly sensitive infants who startle easily and it was found that the process of habituation is often difficult to see clearly using the first two methods.

The light should be presented in short flashes directly into the infant's eye, and the scale is written in terms of the number of flashes required before the infant effectively shuts out the stimulus and no longer responds with eye blink, grimace, or turning of the head. When the infant continues to respond to the light in an obligatory, repetitive way, he is rated low on the scale. As he demonstrates quickly suppressed responses to the light, he is rated high.

This measure appears to be highly dependent on the infant's state, and in our experience an infant in the A_3 state habituates more quickly than others.

1. 12 or more flashes. The baby does not effectively habituate.
2. 9-11 flashes.
3. 6-8 flashes. The baby exhibits average habituation for a fullterm neonate.
4. 3-5 flashes.
5. 0-2 flashes. The baby rapidly habituates.

23. HAND-MOUTH FACILITY   (5 point scale)

This scale measures the infant's ability to bring his hand to his mouth and to successfully maintain hand-mouth contact. From birth, most infants mouth the hand in prone, and many do so in the supine position, especially when they are upset and are attempting to quiet themselves. If the examiner notes no attempts to bring the hand to the mouth, the scale should not be scored.

1. The infant makes unsuccessful attempts to bring his hand to his mouth.
3. The infant exhibits fairly good hand-mouth facility in prone and some successful attempts when lying on his back. He can maintain hand-mouth contact for short periods of time.
5. The infant repeatedly places his hand in his mouth, regardless of the position he is in. He is able to maintain the hand in the mouth for long periods of time.

24. AMOUNT OF MOUTHING   (5 point scale)

This scale gives a measure of the amount of time during the exam that the baby spends mouthing. The infant may suck on his fist, on the bedding, on the examiner's gown, or he may just make mouthing motions with the lips. Thus, *amount* of mouthing is not necessarily directly related to hand-mouth facility, although some infants mouth mostly on the hand. Mouthing behavior often increases as the baby becomes hungry, and, for that reason, it is important to note in the summary statement the extent to which the infant seemed to be hungry during the examination.

1. There is no mouthing. The infant did not mouth at all during the exam.
3. The infant mouths off and on during the exam, or mouths during one period of the exam.
5. The infant mouths the greater part of the time. Mouthing is a predominant feature of the infant's behavior during the exam.

25. TREMULOUSNESS   (5 point scale)

The newborn may exhibit a rapid trembling movement, tremulousness, in the chin and extremities during the first week of life. Some tremulousness is demonstrated at the end of a startle, or as a baby comes from sleeping to awake states. As the infant is dehydrated normally in the second, third, and fourth days, metabolic imbalances may cause tremulousness. Thus, tremulousness may be a measure of any of several things, e.g., CNS disturbance or depression, metabolic imbalance, or of immaturity.

1. Low.   The infant seldom or never exhibits tremulousness.
3. Medium. The infant may exhibit tremulousness momentarily as he wakes, or at the end of a startle. However, the reaction is quickly suppressed.
5. High.   The infant is very tremulous, and the reaction, once set off, is not quickly suppressed. The reaction may be so frequent or so intense as to disturb the infant and cause crying. At the extreme, the infant may have to be swaddled to control the tremulousness and assist him in maintaining equilibrium.

26. STARTLE   (5 point scale)

This scale assesses the extent to which the infant exhibits spontaneous startles during the course of the examination (and excludes the Moro elicited by the examiner which is scored instead under Elicited Movements). Startles may occur as the infant lies passively in the crib or on the examining table, or may occur as he is handled. Sometimes, such spontaneous startles may appear as full Moros, but at other times will consist of less intense 'abbreviated' extensions of the limbs away from the trunk of the body.

1. Low.   The infant never startles.
3. Medium. The infant startles only occasionally and usually in response to strong or sudden stimulation. Startles are usually discrete; one startle does not set off a chain reaction.

5. **High.**   The infant startles often and in response to many types of stimulation. Chain reactions may be observed, with the infant appearing to be at the mercy of the reaction.

27. VIGOR   (5 point scale)

This scale gives a measure of the kind of excitement or energy that the infant characteristically invests in his behavior throughout the test. Vigor is to be assessed, for example, in connection with motoric activity, sucking, crying, responses to reflex stimulation. An infant who appears lethargic or 'lazy' during the test will receive a low score, while the infant who appears to possess intense, driving energy will be scored high. In our experience most infants are rated three, and this has consequently been a minimally useful scale.

1. The infant reacts in a lethargic, perhaps 'dopey' fashion throughout the test. The cry is weak. There is little or no self-initiated, spontaneous motor activity. Elicited reflexes tend to be of low intensity.
3. The baby exhibits frequent self-initiated motor activity, and these movements are strong and show some force. The cry is lusty and strong. Reflexes are generally of moderate intensity.
5. The infant appears to be robust and energetic. Spontaneous motor activity is strong, forceful and frequent. The baby shows strong tensing and flexor adjustments in the neck, back, and shoulders. The cry tends to be persistently loud, and crying may be accompanied by arching of the back and writhing of the body. Elicited reflexes are of medium to high intensity.

28. CUDDLINESS   (5 point scale)

This scale yields a subjective measure of the infant's ability to relax with handling and 'fit' into the examiner's arms when held. Thus, the rating is an indirect measure of the infant's ability to make postural adjustments. Naturally some examiners will feel greater ease and less ambivalence in scoring this item than others.

1. The infant feels stiff when handled or held. The baby's body does not fit into the curve of the examiner's arm, the limbs do not relax or may stiffen and jab the examiner. The infant may actually arch the back and head when picked up.

3. The infant makes some postural adjustments when held and handled, but still feels somewhat stiff and resistent. Or, the baby feels stiff when first picked up, but eventually molds into the examiner's arms.
5. The infant molds quickly easily and completely into the examiner's arms when held. The back relaxes and limbs fold in close to the baby's body. When the baby's position is changed, he readily readjusts his trunk and limbs. When handled, his body is not stiff or awkward to manipulate.

SUMMARY DESCRIPTIVE PARAGRAPH

The summary paragraph should constitute the examiner's overall impression of the baby, and should incorporate, with attempts to explain, notations made on the test form during scoring. Any special characteristics of the infant should be discussed towards the end of establishing the infant's individual mode of responding and reacting. It is important, also, to make note of any factors which the examiner feels might have unduly influenced the baby's test performance, as: hunger, any signs of illness, undesirable conditions in the testing room (e.g., bright light, noise, interruptions), and hypothesize in what ways the infant's behavior might have been different. This will be the paragraph which will help the examiner to remember the baby later, and may be an important source for categorizing infants in a global fashion, for understanding the scores in the different categories, and for understanding meaningful constellations of these categories.

ELICITED MOVEMENTS

The elicited movements differ from the other observations, in that they generally require some specific manipulation or positioning of the infant on the part of the examiner. Unlike the other scales, the scoring refers specifically to the behavior of the infant once put into position. However, the scores should reflect the latency, intensity and reliability of elicitation of the response. An 'average' response is a 2; 3 implies hyperactivity i.e., clear cut short latency intense response; whereas, 1 indicates hypoactivity demonstrated by prolonged latency, unreliability of elicitation, lack of vigor and discreetness, or asymmetry in the behavior. The nature of the asymmetry should be noted. Absence of a response when an attempt has been made to elicit the response is scored a O, and X is used when no attempt has been made to elicit the response.

Placing: The examiner holds the infant with both hands under the arms and around the chest. The baby is then lifted off the surface and the top (dorsum) of one foot is gently rubbed against a protruding edge, such as a table top or the edge of a crib. When one foot is stimulated both feet are lifted by flexion in the knees and hips. Then the legs extend and the feet will be placed on a flat surface if it is provided. Each foot should be tested separately.

Straightening of Legs Reaction: The examiner holds the infant with both hands under the arms and around the chest. The infant is placed so that he is slightly angled forward and the soles of his feet are touching the mattress. When so placed the baby's legs may become rigidly extended and the trunk straighten as if to support his weight. The elicitation of this behavior may be facilitated if the baby is lightly 'bounced' up and down so that more of his weight is placed on his feet. The supporting reaction may occur without being followed by the automatic walk or stepping reaction.

Stepping Reaction (Automatic Walk): The position for eliciting the response is the same as for the supporting reaction. Tilting the body of the infant slightly forward is a precaution against the newborn assuming a backward position which inhibits the stepping response. The standing infant flexes one leg at the knee and hip. If the examiner follows this movement with the infant's body, the child places his foot down just beyond the extended one. In essence, reciprocal flexion and extension of the legs ensues. While the foot is being moved forward, it may leave the ground or drag over the surface. Infrequently, the legs are crossed. The toes are generally kept pointed out. These stepping movements of the newborn differ from real walking in that the legs alone are used.

Babinski Sign: The Babinski reflex is elicited by scratching the middle of the sole of the foot with a finger nail, moving from the toes toward the heel. Stimulation of the sole of the foot evokes overextension of the big toe and a spreading of the smaller toes.

Palmar Grasp Reflex: Stimulation of the palmar surface of the fingers and hand with the examiner's index finger or any other similarly sized object causes forceful grasping. The attempt to withdraw the finger makes the grip tighten. Illingworth (4) separates these two aspects, distinguishing between the grip reflex and the reflex due to traction. However, this distinction is not necessary for the purpose of the present scale. The grasp reflex should be elicited with the infant's head in the midline position as it may be elicited more easily on the side nearest the back of the head. Each hand should be tested separately.

Plantar Grasp Reflex: A similar grasping motion may be demonstrated with the feet by applying gentle pressure to the ball of the foot just behind the toes. Again, each foot should be tested separately.

Tonic Neck Response: When the infant is on his back (supine position) and not crying, he may be seen to lie with his head to one side with the arm and leg of this side extended. The opposite arm and leg are often flexed. Passive rotation of the head by the examiner elicites a shift in position so that the baby assumes the position which is the mirror image of the original one. This is due to an increase in tonicity on the side that the baby is facing. A similar shift will occur if the baby spontaneously changes his head direction. The position of the infant may not be maintained statically because of his voluntary movements, but there always exists a tendency to extend the limbs on the side the baby is facing and flex those on the opposite side.

Spontaneous Crawling: This score is concerned with spontaneous crawling movements that are observed in an infant placed in a prone position. Spontaneous crawling should be distinguished from crawling elicited as the result of pressure applied to the soles of the infant's feet.

Incurvation of the Trunk (Galant's Reflex): The examiner supports the infant on the palm of his hand and runs his finger nail along the infant's back parallel to the vertebral column. This results in the infant arching his body so that the concavity of the arch is on the stimulated side. The exact location along the back which will best elicit this incurvation varies with the infants. The examiner should try several times at different locations between the midline and extreme side of the back, stroking from the shoulder to the buttocks. The response may also be elicited when the infant is lying in a symmetrical prone position with his head centered in the midline. Both sides should be tested. There is very definite examiner-skill involved here, and some E's are able to elicit the response more frequently than others.

Withdrawal Reflex: Brisk flexion of the foot and leg of the infant occurs in response to a noxious stimulus such as a pin-prick applied to the sole of the foot. It should be applied when the baby is in a supine position with leg

NEWBORN BEHAVIORAL AND NEUROLOGICAL SCALES 129

extended. The response may be absent or weak in a baby born as a breech with legs extended. The response differs among babies in the degree to which the unstimulated leg and the rest of the body are involved. The examiner notes how much and how rapidly the whole body responds to the stimulus. In an immature or CNS damaged infant, the opposite foot (and the whole body) will withdraw as quickly as the stimulated foot (a demonstration of the all-or-none aspect of an immature organism). It is this aspect of the response to the pin-prick, called spread, which is scored high, medium, or low.

Doll's Eye Reflex: There are two means of releasing what is usually called the doll's eye. In one, the baby is supported by its back facing the examiner. It is then tipped backwards with the head supported and righted rapidly. The infant's eyes will close completely or partially when he is tipped back and open or widen briefly when he is again righted. The second method involves a delay in the movement of the baby's eyes after the head is turned from side to side by the examiner. In an adult the eyes normally move with the head.

Sucking Reflex: The stimulus consists of putting a nipple over the examiner's finger into the infant's mouth. This will usually be followed by vigorous sucking. This is extremely crude compared with electronic measures now possible [cf., Lipton and Steinschneider (5)].

Rooting Reflex: Touching or stroking the cheek or corner of the infant's mouth with a finger or smooth object induces opening of the mouth and turning in the direction of the stimulus. Infants may be seen to root on their blankets, clothing or almost anything which brushes across the cheek.

Rotation Test: The examiner holds the infant facing him with his hands around the infant's trunk and supporting his head. A comfortable position is with the infant's legs and buttock balanced against the examiner's body. While the examiner spins around, he should hold the infant in a nearly upright position or at an acute angle to his own body. From this position the head and eyes of the infant will turn in the direction of rotation during rotation, turning in the opposite direction when rotation ceases. Changes in the position of the infant may affect the direction of the head and eye movement. An infant who is held horizontally, will turn his head and eyes in the direction opposite to the direction of movement, reversing when rotation ceases. A quarter turn may be sufficient to elicit the reaction in some infants but others may need one or two full cycles. During rotation the infants may make short jerky eye movements back and forth known as nystagmus. The present scale is directed toward assessing nystagmus during rotation although nystagmus after rotation may also be observed.

Ankle Clonus: The infant is tested for clonus while supine. Pressure is applied to the sole of the foot so that the toes touch the leg and the position is held momentarily. Any tremor of the foot or leg is noted when the foot is released. The degree of tremulousness in the ankle is scored under ankle clonus and is used in conjunction with other observations of tremulousness to mark the scale for tremulousness.

Moro Reflex: This reflex can be elicited in several ways. One method is to place the baby supine with the back of the head supported in the examiner's hand. Rapid release of the head initiates the reflex; however, some babies are so strong in the neck that the head does not drop. The method we recommend as the most reliable is to lift the head of the baby's bassinet a few inches off its stand and drop it suddenly.

The Moro reflex consists of a rapid extension of the infant's lombs and their movement away from his body with a fanning of the digits. This is followed by a flexion of the extremities, a movement of the infant's arms across his chest and a closing of the hands. A score of 3 would indicate that the movements were all present and exaggerated. A tremor of the hands may occur. If the different parts of the reflex are all present but not exaggerated, it would be scored a 2. A score of 1 would be used if the movements of the arms are incomplete or the hands fail to open at the height of the reflex; or there is asymmetry on the response. The score of O is again used if the response cannot be elicited, whereas X refers to a test not given.

Kyphosis: To what extent does the back become convex during pull to sit?

Lordosis: The extent of arched concavity of back, between shoulders and rump, when baby is placed in prone or, when held in prone on palm of hand.

Scarf: Ease with which each arm can be drawn across the chest and over the opposite shoulder. A high score is obtained when elbow can be drawn past the baby's chin. A low score usually indicates high rigidity and/or strength of shoulder musculature.

SUGGESTIONS FOR GROUPING ITEMS

A. Infants in Supine (not necessarily in order)

1. Pull to sit
   a. Note degree of kyphosis
2. Hand grasp
3. Plantar grasp
4. Ankle tonus
5. Passive movement of arms
6. Passive movement of legs
7. T.N.R. Tonic neck reflex
8. Pin-prick
9. Defensive movements
10. Babinski
11. Scarf
12. Habituation
13. Sucking
14. Rooting

B. Erect position (support the infant with both hands under the arms around the chest)

1. Automatic walk
2. Straightening of legs
3. Placing

C. Prone position

1. Incurvation can be determined while infant is held prone on one palm
2. Amount of crawling should be observed
3. Head movement in prone can be assessed
4. Presence or absence of lordosis should be noted as well as degree if it is present

D. Infant in arms

1. Following with head and eyes
   a. Inanimate object
2. Sensitivity to sound
   a. Rattle
   b. Bell
3. Social interest in the examiner
   a. Face
   b. Face and voice
   c. Voice
4. Cuddliness

E. Standing with infant in arms

1. Doll's eye
2. Rotation test
3. Moro

F. The following items should be observed throughout the examination period

1. Predominate state
2. General tonus
3. Lability of skin color
4. Peak of excitement
5. Lability of states
6. Alertness
7. Irritability
8. Self quieting activity
9. Consolable with social intervention
10. Activity
11. Eyes closed smiling
12. Rapidity of build-up
13. Hand-mouth facility
14. Amount of mouthing
15. Tremulousness
16. Startle
17. Vigor

REFERENCES

1. Prechtl, H. & Beintema, D., *The neurological examination of the full term infant.* London 1964.
2. Beintema, D. J., *A neurological study of newborn infants.* New York 1969.
3. Freedman, D. G., Smiling in blind infants and the issue of innate vs. acquired. *J. Child Psychd. Psychiat.* 5, 171 (1964).
4. Illingworth, R. S., *The development of the infant and young child; normal and abnormal,* Baltimore 1966.
5. Lipton, E. L. & Steinschneider, A., Studies on the psycho-physiology of infancy. *Merrill-Palmer Quarterly* 10, 102 (1964).

MOTOR BEHAVIOUR IN RELATION TO BRAIN STRUCTURE

H. F. R. PRECHTL

INTRODUCTION

By development of motor behaviour is meant the sequence of systematic changes of the repertoire of motor patterns in infancy and childhood. These changes are directly or indirectly related to the growth and maturational process of the nervous system. They are an expression of the structural and functional development of the brain. The development of the nervous system lasts longer than that of many other organ systems of the organism.

The term 'development' is not unequivocally defined. It is indeed difficult to find a definition of the term development that would be common to all the fields in which it is used. However, we are dealing with particular biological processes, and in this much narrower context the term can reasonably be defined as meaning the sequential changes which continuously transform any biological system of relatively simple organization into one of increasing complexity and differentiation until a final stable stage is reached. This definition would also fit the term 'ontogeny'.

I shall deal with two problems in this paper: first with the descriptive aspect of motor development, as it is employed in developmental diagnostic procedures, and secondly with the development of the neural functional organization of motor behaviour.

THE PHENOMENOLOGY OF DEVELOPING MOTOR PATTERNS

Attempts to describe and list the specific motor patterns in infancy and childhood have been made for the past 100 years. Preyer (1), Peiper (2), McGraw (3), Gesell (4) and others have carried out careful studies of the normal development of motor behaviour. Thanks to them the phenomenology of motor development is relatively well-known. However, much less is known about the developmental course of motor behaviour. Only single reflexes and responses have been followed but normative data from longitudinal representative population studies are practically non-existent. Data from the usual developmental tests such as from Arnold Gesell and their modifications by Bühler-Hetzer (5), Griffith (6), Knobloch (7), Illingworth (8) or the Denver test (9) are too eclectic to provide a comprehensive picture of the development of motor functions. In addition we know from the developmental tests only which of the arbitrarily selected items are attained by 50% of children at a particular age. As soon as one wishes to know the interrelationship in the complex changes of motor functions these results will not provide an answer. Most of the published data are based on transectional studies of groups of children and most of them are based on Gesell's material. Data on the ages in which particular responses mature can therefore only be used as crude approximations in clinical work. Still missing are normative data of motor development of many behaviour patterns which are presented in medians and percentiles such as those used in growth and weight curves. The first example, and to my knowledge the only one, is provided by Neligan and Purdham (10) and is shown in figure 1, which illustrates the maturation of sitting and walking. The application of these data to other populations, however, must be made with caution. Genetic and cultural differences may cause different developmental courses.

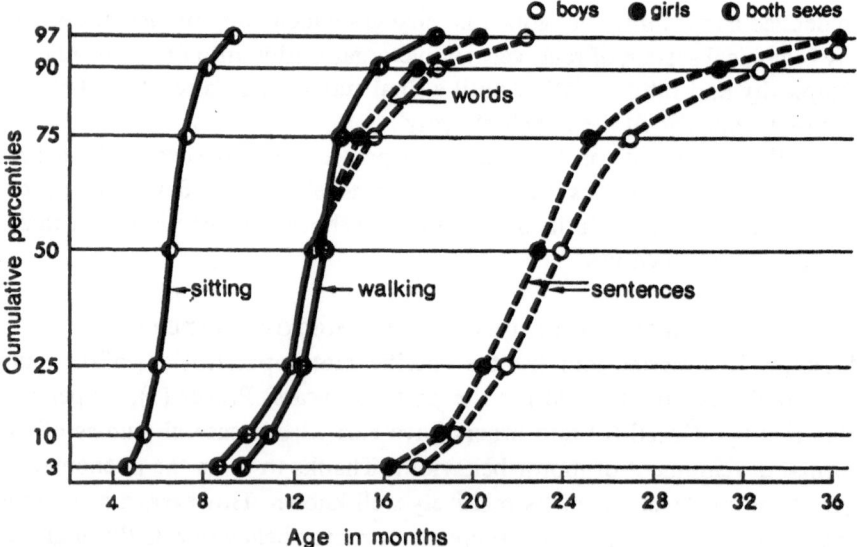

Fig. 1. Distributions of cumulative percentiles for sitting, walking and speaking sentences from a representative sample of children from Newcastle upon Tyne. Data from Neligan and Purdham (10).

During the last few years motor behaviour has also been employed to separate the small-for-date infants from true preterm infants. This topic will be dealt with extensively by Dr Casaer.

MECHANISMS OF EARLY MOTOR BEHAVIOUR

Let us turn now to the details of motor development. I will not emphasize the phenomenology of the developing motor patterns but I shall rather deal with the functional processes of the different motor patterns.

Motility begins in the human long before birth. Hooker (11) and Humphrey (12) have observed in the human foetus of $8\frac{1}{2}$ weeks postmenstrual age the first consistently elicited movements. Mechanical stimulation of the perioral skin in the maxillary and mandibular branch of the N. trigeminus leads to a generalized extension of trunk and extremities as well as to a sideward flexion of the head (Fig. 2). This is the first and only successful input to the nervous system because stimulations of other areas and with other modalities do not yet produce responses. Two or three weeks later localized and circumscribed responses can be elicited first from the proximal areas such as the skin of the back and later from the hand and the foot. In the case of the trigeminal reflex the relationship between the maturation of structure and function is explored in detail (Fig. 3). The nervous apparatus and the central connections are differentiated at $8\frac{1}{2}$ weeks to such a degree that they are functional. The comparison of the somatotopic representation in the brain stem of the embryo (Fig. 4) and the adult (13) (Fig. 5) demonstrates the fundamental differences in the morphology. This study and a few others are the only ones in which correlative studies of structural and functional maturation have been carried out in human embryos. On the other hand we are much better informed about the embryos of other vertebrates. Coghill (14) has devoted his life work to the study of the larva of Amblystoma. He formulated the theory for motor development, namely that the specific reflex movements differentiate later from a primary total pattern due to 'individuation'. This was widely accepted as a general rule in the literature and can now be found in most textbooks on developmental psychology. This presents, however, a striking example of fallacious generalization from one species to another, since studies of other species of Amblystoma indicated a completely different developmental course (15). Also Hooker's interpretation must be seen now in a different light. In the baby the total pattern remains in the form of startles and does not disappear when local responses occur.

An important question is now: what is the significance of prenatal motor

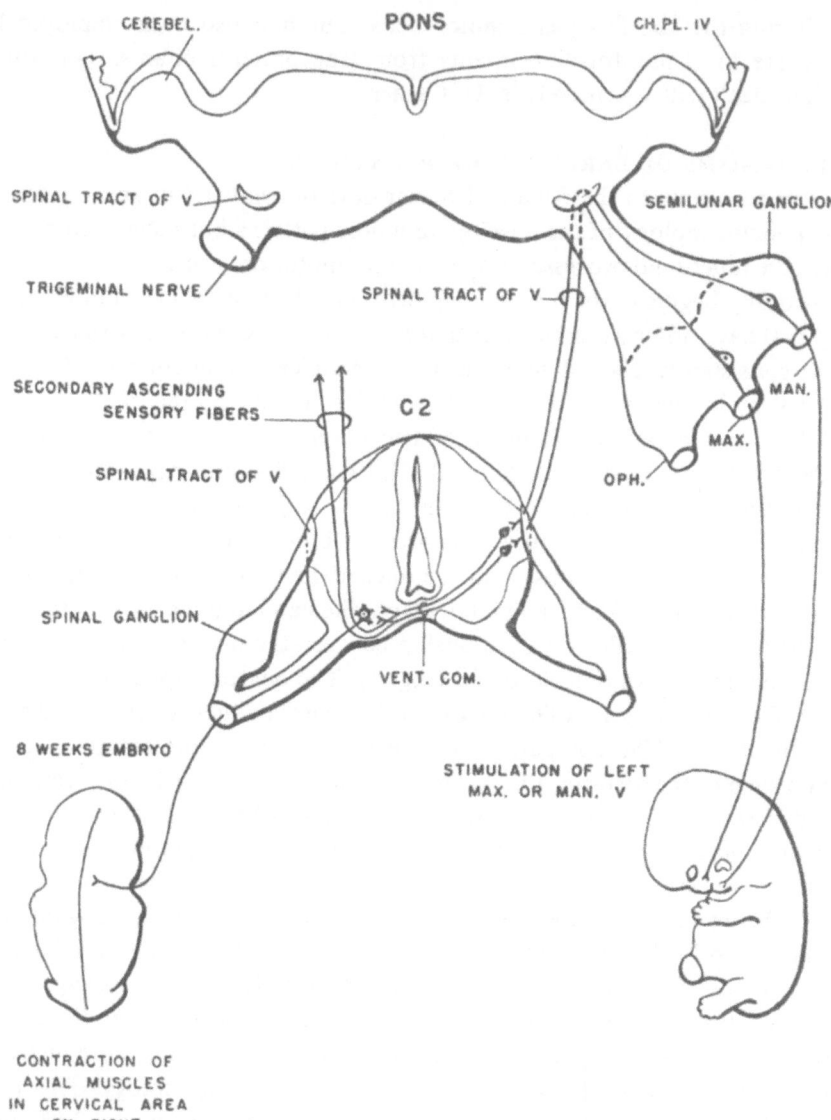

Fig. 3. A diagram to illustrate the probable pathway for the nervous impulses resulting in the early contralateral flexion in the cervical region following perioral stimulation. From Humphrey (12).

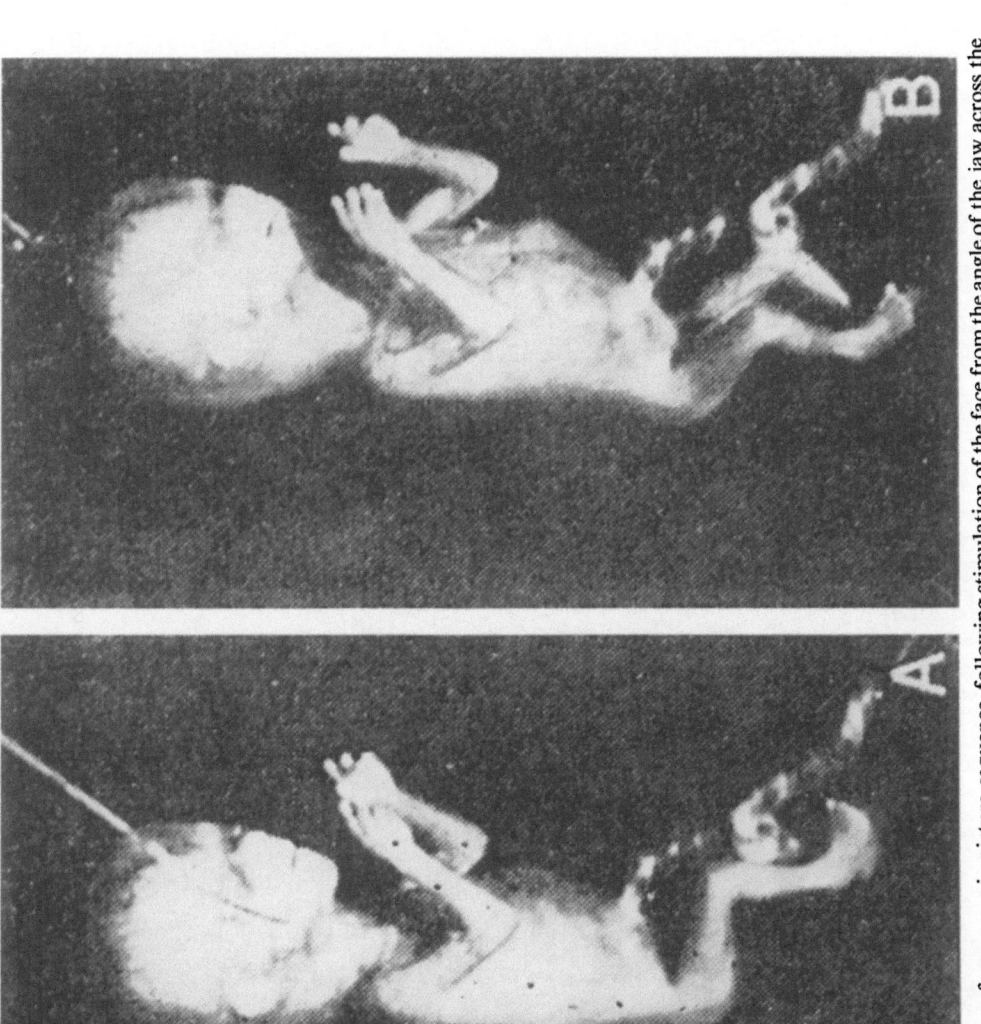

Fig. 2. Two frames from a movie picture sequence following stimulation of the face from the angle of the jaw across the right cheek and eyelids to the forehead of a human foetus of 13 weeks of menstrual age (88.5mm CR).From Humphrey(12).

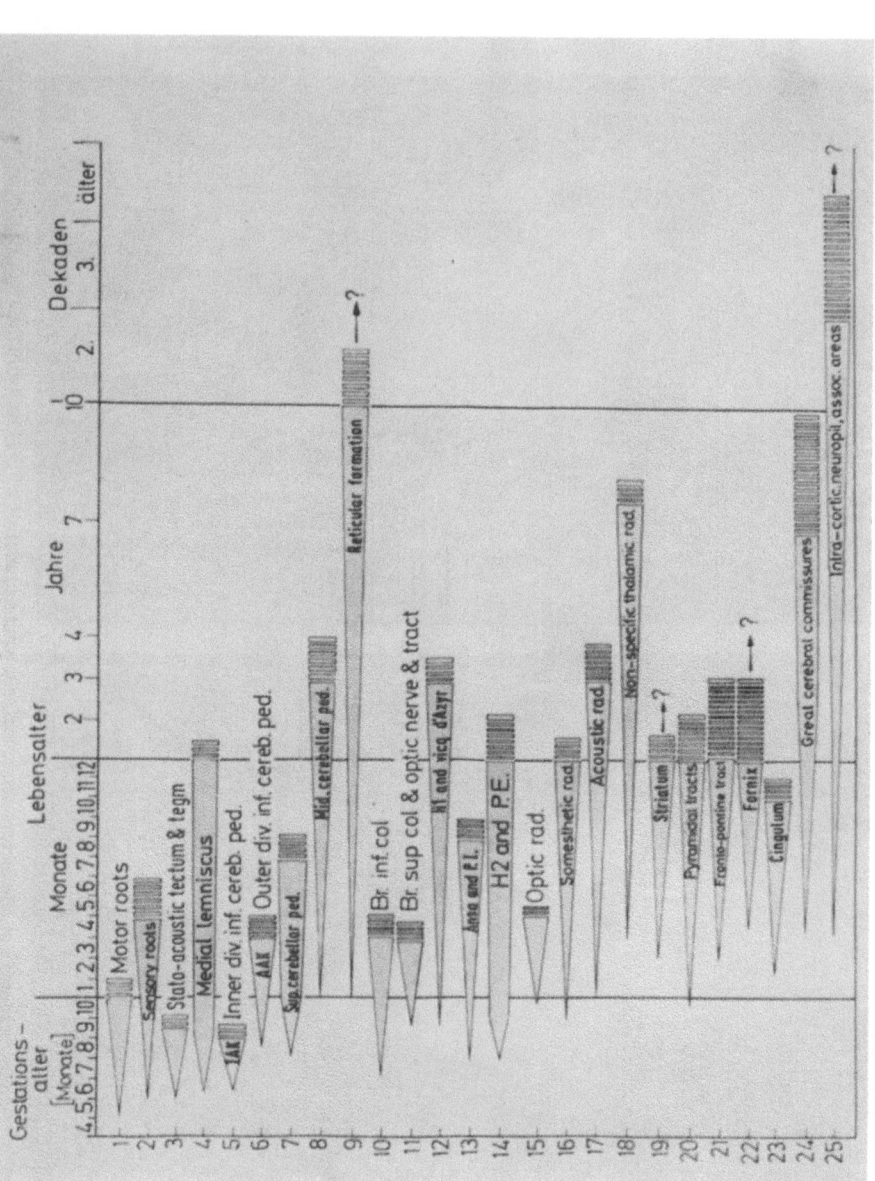

Fig. 7. Course of myelination of various brain structures according to the study by Yakovlev and Lecours (25). From Joppich and Schulte (28).

activity? First of all nervous activity itself could have an effect on the maturation of the nervous system. For the early stages this seems unlikely since Crain and his coworkers (16) have demonstrated that embryonic nervous tissue differentiates normally even if it is anaesthetized with xylocaine in tissue culture. While the early developmental phases may be strongly determined by genetical programming, this may not exclusively be the case for later development. Additionally, motor activity may have an effect on the development of musculature and of the joints, though this is only proven for chick embryos (17). Another aspect is that motor activity very likely has a significant influence on the stabilization of the intra-uterine position of the foetus, especially throughout the last month of pregnancy as Langreder (18) has pointed out.

The newborn baby needs a rather extensive repertoire of motor patterns. These mechanisms must mature at an earlier age to be ready to act right at the change to the extra-uterine environment at delivery (19, 20). Therefore it may not be surprising that the neural maturation starts early in foetal life. In order to explain these infantile behaviour patterns in the newborn one needs to see them in the context of child-mother interaction. Indeed, seen in this context the newborn infant is not at all a helpless creature (21): he breathes, he roots for the nipple, he sucks, he grasps, he has spatial orientation, he

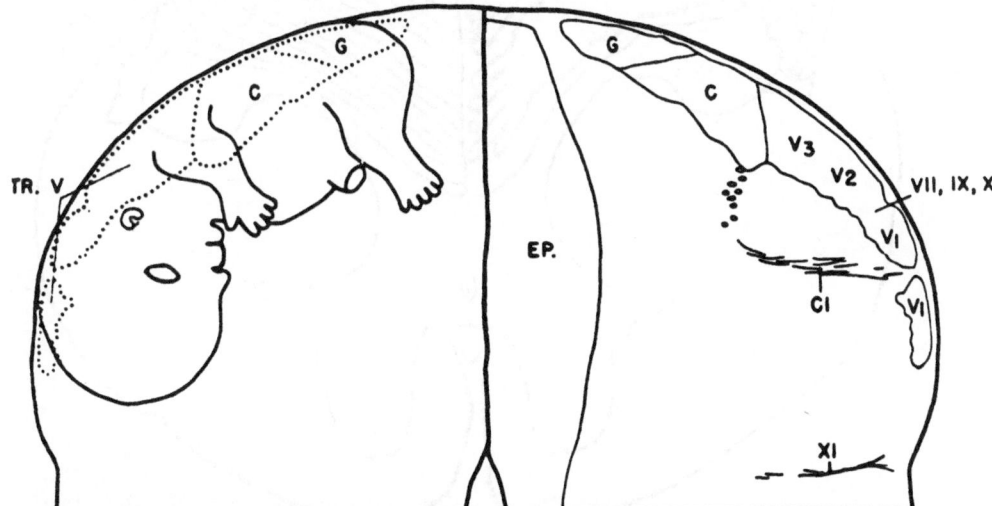

Fig. 4. Transverse section of the spinal cord of an 8½-week old human foetus at the level of segment cervical 1. Somatotopic representation of the spinal tract of trigeminal nerve and dorsal funiculus. From Humphrey (13).

shows distinct sleep and wakefulness cycles and he communicates with his caretaker by crying. In summary, all observations demonstrate the gradual unfolding of prenatal motor behaviour which enables the newborn infant to fulfil all his vital functions under the normal care of his mother.

DETERMINANTS OF EARLY MOTOR BEHAVIOUR

Now, which factors influence the prenatal motor development? First of all the *milieu interne* must be optimal in order to insure normal, genetically programmed maturation of the nervous system. A long list of factors is known which endanger the structural development of the brain. In addition to that there are other factors which may influence nervous functions. Several years ago we found one of the possibilities in infants who are born in breech presentation (22). They showed a change of the withdrawal reflex of the

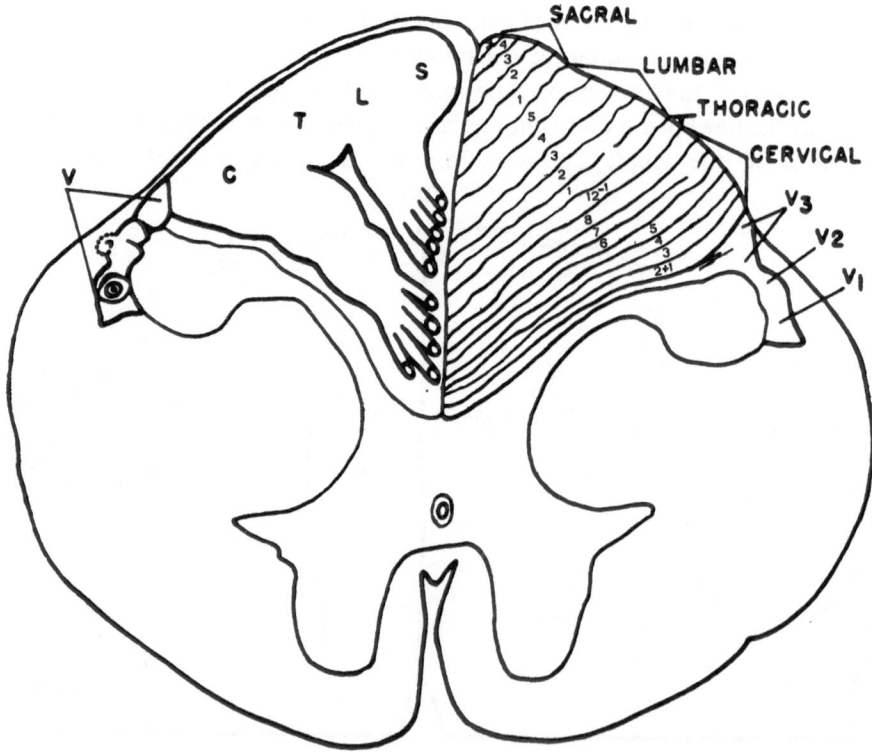

Fig. 5. Transverse section of the first cervical segment of the spinal cord of adult man. From Humphrey (13).

legs as well as of the magnet response (Fig. 6). Babies who are born with extended legs showed a decrease of the flexion reflex and an increase of the magnet response, while infants born with footling position showed an increase of the withdrawal and a decrease of the magnet reflex. These changes

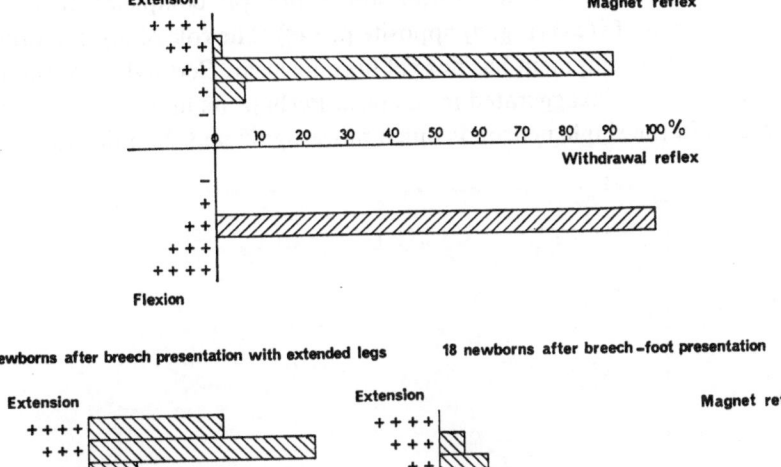

Fig. 6. Quantitative results of the magnet reflex and the withdrawal reflex in human infants, born in vertex presentation and born in breech presentation with extended legs and breech foot presentation respectively. Data from Prechtl and Knol (22).

may remain for months after delivery. The intra-uterine position of the legs plays a significant role in the formation of seemingly inborn and simple reflexes.

An interesting opportunity to study effects of environmental influences on the development of motor behaviour is offered by preterm infants when they reach the postmenstrual age of 40 weeks. Very few studies have been carried out so far, yet the similarity of the preterm at 40 weeks with the full-term infant at 40 weeks is striking (23). But Michaelis (24) demonstrated recently differences in all those motor patterns which involve muscle power such as raising the head in prone, standing and stepping etc.

As is generally known, the morphological maturation of the nervous system is not complete at birth but continues over years. Myelination of different brain structures such as the large cerebral commissures, the intra-cortical connections and the reticular formation is not yet completed before the 7th-10th year of life (25) (Fig. 7, opposite p. 135). The role of myelination for the functional development has not yet become clear. Certainly its significance has been greatly exaggerated in the past. Perhaps its importance for spike generation in the single neuron is much more significant than the increase in

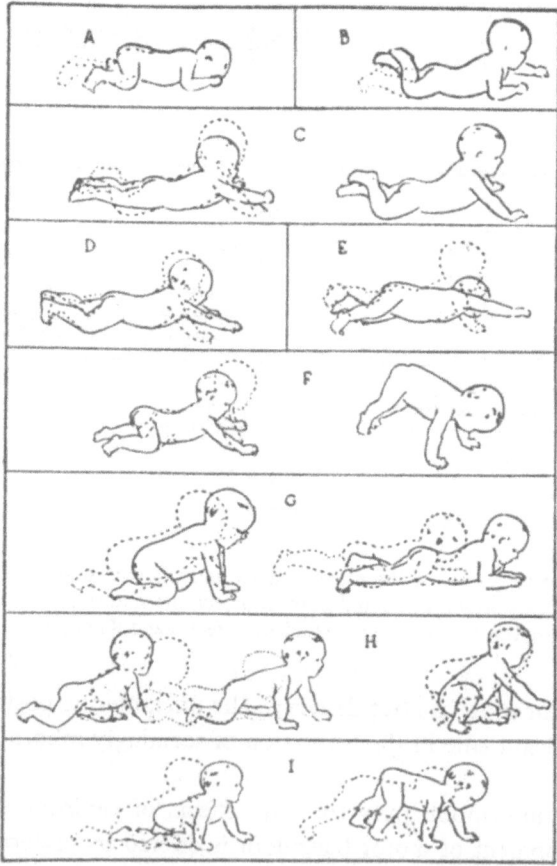

Fig. 8. Nine phases in the development of prone locomotion as described by McGraw (26).

nerve conduction velocity. How can the tremendous changes of neural functions found during development of say, the first years of life be explained simply by an increase in nerve conduction velocity? The development of dendritic structures and especially of the synapses and enzyme systems must play crucial and decisive roles, though, unfortunately, systematic data is still scarce. To me it also seems very unlikely that the development of sitting, standing, walking etc. is due to learning alone without profound changes in

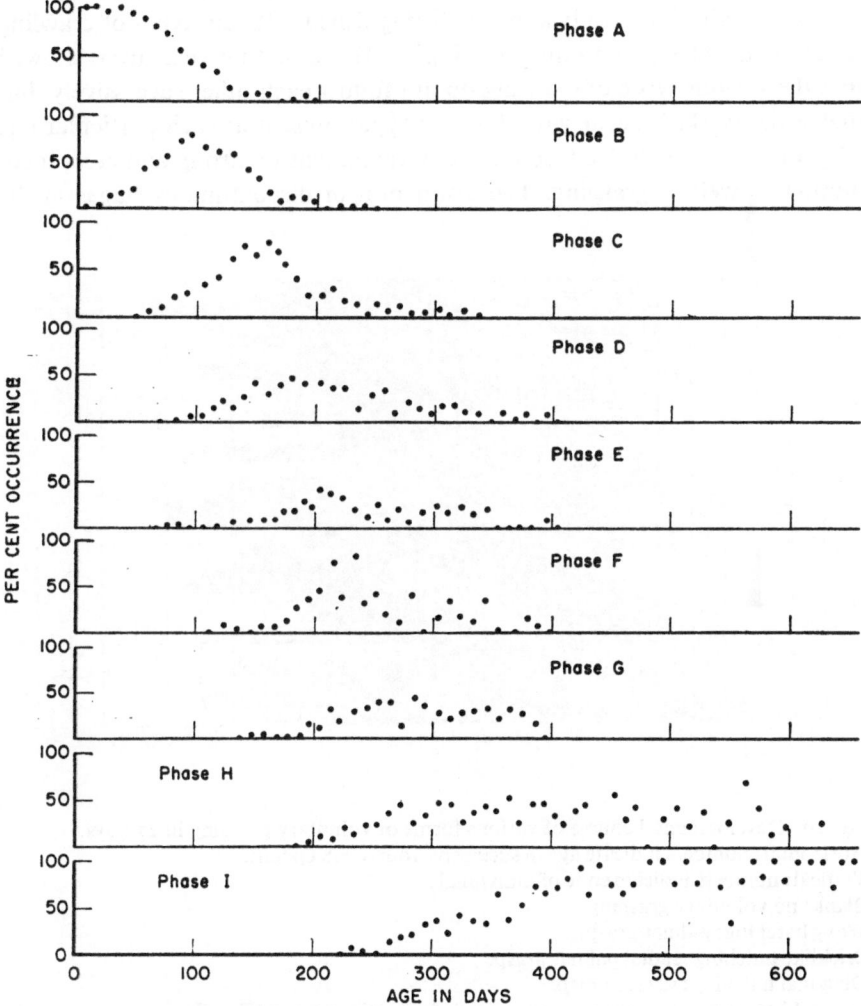

Fig. 9. Percentage distribution of each of the nine phases of prone locomotion analysed in a group of 82 infants by McGraw (26).

the neural structure involved. Obviously the time table of the developmental course is too rigid to be explained by environmental factors only.

CONTINUOUS OR STEPWISE DEVELOPMENT?

While from the morphological point of view the nervous system develops in a continuous, gradual process, psychologists have emphasized, on the other hand, jumps and stages in the development of motor patterns. Mc-Graw (26), for instance, has examined the development of crawling in a detailed longitudinal study and she distinguished different types of crawling which occur throughout ontogeny (Fig. 8). Her quantitative analysis showed that the various types of crawling do not follow each other successively, but that wide overlaps occur with different types present at each particular age (Fig. 9). The same holds true for the development of sitting and erect loco-motion as well as grasping. The distinction of discontinuous stages in the

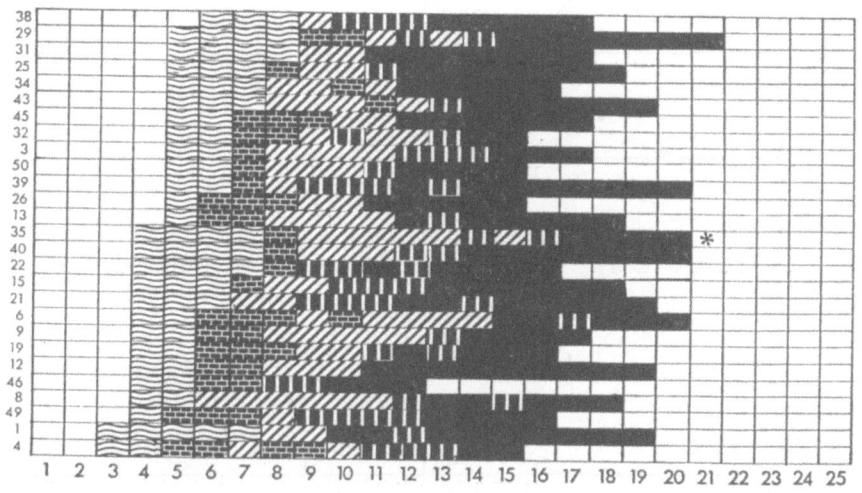

Fig. 10. Developmental course of various forms of voluntary grasping in 27 boys.
Horizontal: numbers indicate age in successive four-week epochs.
Vertical: numbers indicate code of individuals.
Blank: no voluntary grasping.
Wavy hatching: palmar grasp.
Bricklike hatching: radial palmar grasp.
Diagonal hatching: scissor grasp.
Vertical hatching: scissor-pincer grasp (= inferior pincergrasp (Gesell).
Black bar: pincer grasp. (right end: end of the examination)
Data from Touwen (27).

developmental process are methodological artefacts. Touwen (27) found in a recent longitudinal study of the neurological development throughout the first year of life that the changes from one type of grasping to the other or the dissolution of particular reflexes such as the Moro response are not clear-cut but may fluctuate over months (Figs. 10 and 11).

RULES OF MOTOR DEVELOPMENT

Are there general rules of motor development? Between foetal life and adolescence there is a continuously changing age-specific motor repertoire. This includes dissolution of existing motor patterns as well as formation of new ones. Simultaneously there is an increase in complexity of existing motor patterns and of their goal directedness. There is also a decrease in the irradiation of motor activity, this means a decrease in associated movements which are irrelevant for the motor act, which facilitates isolated movements. There is finally a decline in motor instability in the form of overflow activity and other types of motor restlessness. All these changes are genetically programmed and occur at particular ages. The role and importance of environmental influences in these developmental processes are different from motor

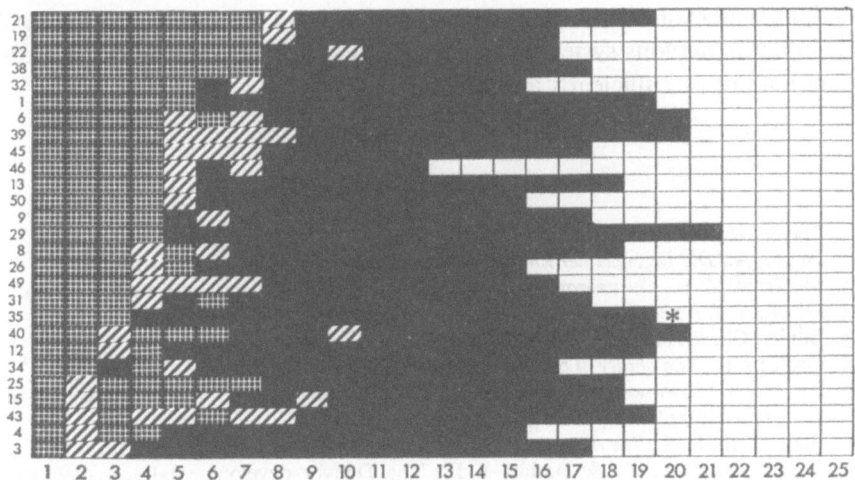

Fig. 11. Developmental course of the Moro response elicited by a hit on the surface the baby is lying on. Only the extension and abduction component of the arms is considered. Cross-hatching: full response.
Diagonal hatching: weak and inconsistent response.
Black bar: absent response. (right end: end of the examination)
Data from Touwen (27).

pattern to motor pattern. One extreme is the dissolution of the baby's stepping movements which is completely uninfluenced by training and excercise, and the other extreme is the acquisition of motor skill which is purely dependent on learning.

This list is not at all complete, I only wanted to point out a few aspects. Many detailed studies in developmental neurology will be necessary to clarify the causal mechanisms of these phenomena. Methodologically we must start from the fact that the nervous system of the young infant is qualitatively different from that of the adult. We still know very little about the interrelationship of the brain's structural changes and overt behaviour. It is an urgent task for us to reevaluate critically our theories about human motor development. Only too often have they been extrapolated from the final stage of development, namely from the adult. Furthermore many motor patterns are seen as analogues from the results of animal experiments such as decerebrated and decerebellated dogs. As in the course of the postural reflexes, one obviously searched only for patterns which had been found previously in animal experiments, but not for the normal repertoire of infants in their daily behaviour.

Motor behaviour is only one aspect of neural functions but motor behaviour is an exquisite example which demonstrates the special properties of the infantile nervous system. The consequences for neuropediatrics are obvious but not yet sufficiently appreciated.

REFERENCES

1. Preyer, W., *Die Seele des Kindes*, Leipzig 1882.
2. Peiper, A., *Die Eigenart der kindlichen Hirntätigkeit*, (3. Aufl.) Leipzig 1961.
3. McGraw, M. B., *The neuromuscular maturation of the human infant*, New York 1969.
4. Gesell, A. & Amatruda, C. S., *Developmental diagnosis*, New York 1969.
5. Bühler, Ch. & Hetzer, H., *Kleinkindertests*, Leipzig 1932.
6. Griffiths, R., *The ability of babies*, London 1954.
7. Knobloch, H., Pasamanick, P. H. B. & Sherard, E. S., A developmental screening inventory for infants. *Pediatrics* 38, 1095 (1966).
8. Illingworth, R. S., *The development of the infant and young child*, Edinburgh 1966.
9. Frankenburg, W. K. & Dodds, J. B., The Denver developmental screening test. *J. Pediat.* 71, 181 (1967).
10. Neligan, G. & Purdham, D., Norms for four standard developmental milestones by sex, social class and place in family. *Develop. Med. Child Neurol.* 11, 413 (1969).
11. Hooker, D., *The prenatal origin of behaviour*, Lawrence 1952.
12. Humphrey, T., Some correlations between the appearance of human fetal reflexes and the development of the nervous system. *Progr. Brain Res.* 4, 93 (1964).
13. Humphrey, T., Pattern formed at upper cervical spinal cord levels by sensory fibers of spinal and cranial nerves. *Arch. Neurol. Psychiat.* 73, 36 (1955).

14. Coghill, G. E., *Anatomy and the problem of behavior*, Cambridge 1929.
15. Faber, J., The development and coordination of larval limb movements in triturus taeniatus and amblystoma mexicanum. *Arch. Neerl. Zool.* 11, 498 (1956).
16. Crain, S. M., Bornstein, M. B. & Peterson, E. R., Maturation of cultured embryonic CNS tissues during chronic exposure to agents which prevent bioelectric activity. *Brain Res.* 8, 363 (1968).
17. Drachman, D. B. & Sokoloff, L., The role of movement in embryonic joint development. *Devl Biol.* 14, 401 (1966).
18. Langreder, W., Über Fötalreflexe und deren intra-uterine Bedeutung. *Ztschr. Geburtsh. Gynäkol.* 131, 237 (1949).
19. Prechtl, H. F. R., Die Entwicklung und Eigenart frühkindlicher Bewegungsweisen. *Klin. Wschr.* 34, 281 (1956).
20. Prechtl, H. F. R. & Beintema, D. J., The neurological examination of the full-term newborn infant. *Clin. Develop. Med.* no. 12, London 1964.
21. Prechtl, H. F. R., *Die Entwicklung der frühkindlichen Motorik I.* Nahrungsaufnahme. Film C. 651. Inst. Wiss. Film, Göttingen.
    Idem, *Motorik II.* Körperhaltung und Fortbewegung. Film C. 652.
    Idem, *Motorik III.* Greifen und andere Bewegungsweisen. Film C. 653.
    Prechtl, H. F. R., Die Kletterbewegungen beim Säugling. *Mschr. Kinderheilk.* 101, 519 (1953).
    Prechtl, H. F. R., The directed head turning response and allied movements of the human baby. *Behaviour* 13, 212 (1958).
    Prechtl, H. F. R., Problems of behavioural studies in the newborn infant. *Adv. Study Behav.*, 1, 75 (1965).
    Prechtl, H. F. R. & Lenard, H. G., Verhaltensphysiologie des Neugeborenen. In: *Fortschritte der Pädologie*, Band II, p. 88 Linneweh, F. (ed.), Berlin 1968.
22. Prechtl, H. F. R. & Knol, A. R., Der Einfluss der Beckenendlage auf die Fusssohlenreflexe beim neugeborenen Kind. *Arch. Psychiat. Zsch. Neurol.* 196, 542 (1958).
23. St.-Anne Dargassies, Neurological maturation of the premature infant of 28–41 weeks gestational age. In: *Human Development*, Falkner, F. (ed.), Philadelphia 1966.
24. Michaelis, R., Schulte, F. J. & Nolte, R., R., Motor behavior of small for gestational age newborn infants. *J. Pediat.* 76, 208 (1970).
25. Yakovlev, P. I. & Lecours, A. R., The myelogenetic cycles of regional maturation of the brain. In: *Regional development of the brain in early life*, p. 3, Minkowski, A. (ed.), Oxford 1967.
26. McGraw, M. B., Development of neuromuscular mechanisms as reflected in the crawling and creeping behavior of the human infant. *J. Genet. Psychol.* 58, 83 (1941).
27. Touwen, B. C. L., A study of the development of some motor phenomena in infancy. *Dev. Med. Child, Neurol.* 13, 435 (1971).
28. Joppich, G. & Schulte, F. J., *Neurologie des Neugeborenen*, Berlin 1968.

DISCUSSION

Stoelinga: You showed the variation in the appearance or disappearance of the Moro-test. Cases that show reflexes at older ages were asleep or did they show variations in activity while you tested them? In other words, does the result of the test depend on the activity state of the child at a particular moment?

Prechtl: I think this is one of the crucial aspects of the neurological examination: that one controls for state. For a long time students of the neurology of the young baby have not been aware of the tremendous effect of the state. Now all these babies have of course been examined with a standardized technique, which includes state control. So they are all in the same comparable state.

Sander: Could you summarize what you feel at present about activity types in babies. There has been a considerable use of this idea of highly active and less active babies.

Prechtl: You mean normal babies or abnormal?

Sander: Normal.

Prechtl: Some are more active than others. Very little is known, however, about normative data and the best data I know are from Sander. So I can only refer you to your own publications. You, as a psycho-analyst, would like to attribute these differences to differences in temperament. There is a wide range in the amount of motor activity displayed by babies. There is one concept in the literature which always bothers me and this is 'mass-activity', introduced I think, by Irwin. A baby is swaying his arms and legs in supine position, but what else should he do? Why is this an unorganized 'mass-motor-activity'? If you put a beetle on its back it will make these 'uncoordinated' movements with all its limbs too. And if you put the baby in prone you see that all his limb movements are well organized, well coordinated. And I think, keeping the baby in supine and watching it for his motor-activity is an unfair position for the baby.

Widdowson: I noticed in one of the early slides that you showed, that girls speak words and put sentences together sooner than boys. This was so, was it not? Can you relate this to any other aspect of brain development?

Prechtl: The girls' brains are genetically different from the brains of the boys. It is a very trivial answer and unfortunately I am unable to give a more meaningful answer. This is a thing which puzzles us tremendously, this enormous sex-difference in behavioural development.

Freedman: I just want to refer to Conel's work on brain post-mortems in which he finds, at least in a few cases, there is earlier differentiation of the hemispheres (in terms of myelinization) in girls' brains than boys' brains (Conel, J. L., *The postnatal development of the human cerebral cortex.* Volumes I through VI. Cambridge (Mass.) 1939-1963). In addition there is the study of Kimura which also shows that there is an earlier right-left dominance in girls in terms of perceiving sounds. (Kimura, D., Functional symmetry of the brain in dichotic listening. *Cortex* 3, 163, 1957). Thus there is a certain amount of evidence that there is more rapid cerebral differentiation occurring in girls than in boys, which may, in fact, underlie the precocious sentence-construction and verbalization of girls.

Van der Werff ten Bosch: I should like to point out that a sex difference at birth is not necessarily due to a difference in chromosomes. I am thinking of work in which the hormonal status of females has been altered before birth and where you can find differences between the sexes caused by such manipulations. And I would hesitate off-hand to attribute any of the sex differences at birth to chromosomes without considering hormones first.

NEUROLOGICAL CRITERIA FOR THE ESTIMATION OF THE POST-MENSTRUAL AGE OF NEWBORN INFANTS

P. CASAER AND Y. AKIYAMA

INTRODUCTION

The title of this paper could be rephrased as a question: can the developing brain tell us something about the age of the newborn? Since the true age of the newborn, i.e. the interval from conception to birth, cannot be determined, the first day of the last menstrual period (LMP) is commonly used as the reference day (see fig. I). The interval between the first day of the LMP and ovulation varies. In women with regular menstrual cycles (28-30 days)

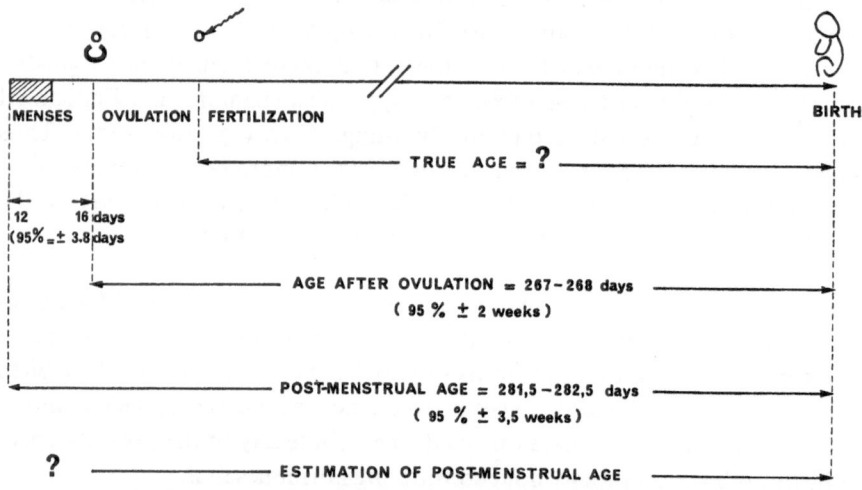

Fig. I. A schematic representation of menses, ovulation, fertilization, and birth. The true age, i.e. the time since conception, is unknown. The interval between the first day of the last menstrual period and the ovulation varies (mean 13th day, 95 per cent limit ± 3.8 days, 75 percent between 12th and 16th day). The time between ovulation and birth varies (mean 267-268, 95 per cent limit ± 2 weeks). The time between the first day of the LMP and birth varies (mean 287 days, 95 per cent limit ± 2.5-3.5 weeks). In cases with doubt concerning the first day of the LMP, other time references for the estimation of the PM age must be determined.

the peak of ovulations falls on the 13th day, 75 per cent of the ovulations fall between the 12th and 16th day, and the 95 percentile range is $\pm$ 3.8 days (1). The time between ovulation and birth also varies. In studies based on basal temperature curves the mean was 267 days and the 95 percentile range $\pm$ 2 weeks (1, 2). These two factors account for the variation between the first day of the LMP and birth. In selected cases with regular cycles the mean has been reported as 287 days, the 95 percentile range as $\pm$ 2.5-3.5 weeks (1). Cases in which there is doubt as to the first day of the LMP and/or irregular cycles require other criteria, based on phenomena related to the developmental changes in various organ systems. We must keep in mind that in all studies on criteria for age estimation this biological variation can never be overcome. This means that the level of accuracy in such studies can never lie higher than within a total range of 5 to 7 weeks.

Despite this variation of $\pm$ 2 to 3 weeks, the age remains an essential factor in perinatal clinical work, research studies, and follow-up projects.

On the basis of age, newborns can be classified as pre-terms (PT), full-terms (FT), and post-terms (PST), and each of these categories can be subdivided by weight into small (SPD), normal, and large for date (LFD) infants.

Neonatal mortality is more dependent on age than on birth weight. Clinical problems differ in infants with comparable weight but different ages. Pre-term infants with a normal weight for their age show, for instance, immaturity of enzyme systems, immature lungs, capillary fragility, and susceptibility to infection. Infants with comparable weights but born at term, that is SFD-FT, have quite different clinical problems, including deficiency of energy reserves, polycythemia, and massive pulmonary haemorrhage (for detailed references see Casaer and Akiyama (3).

Since physiological functions may be strongly dependent on age, research studies on neonatal physiology must be done in infants with an accurately determined postmenstrual age. A good example of this is provided by the study on temperature control and evaporative water loss done by Hey and Katz (4), who demonstrated that newborns older than 37 weeks postmenstrual age have greater sweating capacities than younger infants, a finding they would not have made if the comparison had been based solely on weight or surface area.

In follow-up studies of developmental processes the selection of the subjects should be based on the PM age; and a further subdivision into weight per age categories can then be made (5, 6, 7). For developmental tests, Gesell and Amatruda (8) pointed out that for the developmental score in the young infant not the age since birth but rather the post-menstrual age is relevant;

this fact has recently been stressed again by Parmelee and Schulte (9), although it is still ignored in other studies.

Of the various parameters available (see table 1), the developmental neurological parameters and the parameters related to the skin are the most helpful at present (3). In this paper the discussion is limited to the developmental neurological criteria (see table 2).

Table 1. Estimation of the post-menstrual age I. Developmental non-neurological parameters

	Prenatal	Postnatal
Body growth	fundus height	body weight/length
Bone growth	ossification centres (radiological technique)	ossification centres (radiological technique)
Developmental changes in the skin	vernix amniotic fluid cell cytology changes in resistance media expressed as changes in R wave amplitude (EKG) radiological outlining of the skin covered with vernix	external characteristics of skin and appendages
Developmental changes in the heart	foetal heart tones changes in heart rate changes in EKG pattern changes in phonocardiogram	changes in EKG pattern
Physico-chemical changes	amniotic fluid ($\pm$ extracellular)	tissue and plasma (intra- and extracellular)

Table 2. Estimation of the post-menstrual age II. Developmental neurological parameters

	Prenatal	Postnatal
Brain/skull growth	estimation of biparietal diameter of the skull (ultrasound technique)	head circumference
Neuro-motor function	quickening	neurological tests polygraphic data
Electro-physiological		nerve conduction velocity (reflex arc latency) EEG evoked response
Visual system		eye fundus electro-retinography and photically evoked responses

During the last half of pregnancy, the developing brain rapidly increases in weight, surface area, volume, number of gyri and sulci, complexity of the cyto-architecture, myelinization, and the activity of enzymes involved in neural transmission (10, 11, 12, 13, 14, 15). The brain weight is less affected than the weight of the heart, liver, and thymus in intra-uterine growth retardation (14), and shows better correlation with PM age than with birth weight (16, 12). Radiological studies of the skull (17) demonstrated the same trend for the brain volume. Once formed, myelin is relatively stable and independent of changes in the environment (11). On the basis of these findings it was to be expected that the functional aspects of the nervous system would best reflect the developmental age of the infant.

PRENATAL CRITERIA

The earlier the pregnant mother comes under the obstetrician's care, the more likely he will be to get a reliable history of the first day of her last menstrual period, and he can also begin to follow the changes in the fundus height before the 14th week. When there is doubt as to the precise age of the foetus, the obstetrician must resort to other means to obtain this information, since the age has great importance for treatment of the foetus and pregnancy. Although a combination of neurological parameters and the parameters related to the skin-vernix is the most promising in this respect, we will discuss here only the neurological parameters: the onset of quickening and the determination of the biparietal diameter with ultrasound.

THE ONSET OF QUICKENING

The onset of the foetal movements is an indicator for a certain degree of neuromotor development (see paper by Prof. H. F. R. Prechtl in this monograph), and is invariably felt by the mother between the 16th and 20th week after the first day of the LMP.

In a recent study, Rawlings and Moore (18) evaluated the onset of quickening for prediction of the expected day of delivery, and compared this predictability to that based on the first day of the last menstrual period. Both dates were recorded in 291 primiparae and in 165 multiparae. The first day of the last menstrual period was recorded in a group of 383 consecutive pregnancies. Pregnancies resulting in babies younger than 36 weeks foetal age or smaller than 5.5 pounds were excluded as well as pregnancies artificially terminated for reasons other than postmaturity.

The mean time from the first day of the last menstrual period to quickening was 19 weeks 5 days for the primiparae (1 standard deviation = 16.4

days) and 18 weeks 3 days for the multiparae (1 standard deviation = 15.2 days). The mean time from the onset of quickening to delivery was 20 weeks 3 days for the primiparae (1 standard deviation = 14.9 days) and 21 weeks 3 days for the multiparae (1 standard deviation = 16.5 days). The mean duration of pregnancy (1st day of LMP to delivery) in the 383 consecutive mature pregnancies was 40 weeks 3 days (1 standard deviation = 13.9 days).

On the basis of the onset of quickening, the expected day of delivery was accurately predicted ($\pm$ 1 week) in 38 per cent of the pregnancies, whereas on the basis of the first day of the last menstrual period the percentage was 48. When the two predictions were combined the percentage rose to 58. The recording of the onset of quickening is 'a simple, painless, non time consuming operation' (18) and is very helpful in combination with the first day of the last menstrual period.

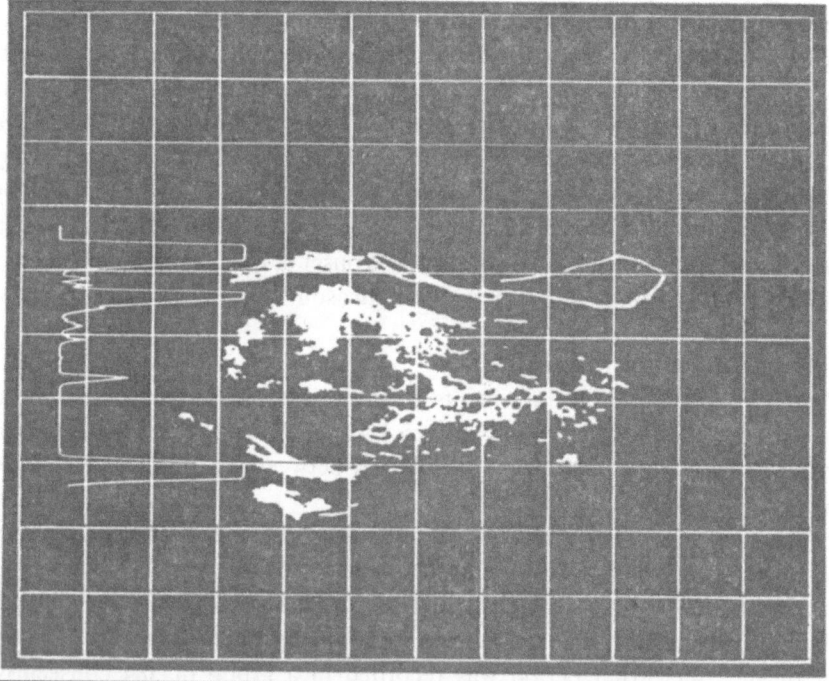

Fig. 2. A montage of a one-dimensional (left side) and a two-dimensional (right side) ultrasound display of the transverse section of foetal head in vertex position with the ultrasonic beam passing through the biparietal eminences at right angles to the phalx. The biparietal diameter is measured on the one-dimensional display. (Photograph courtesy of H. J. Huisjes, Department of Obstetrics, University Hospital, Groningen, The Netherlands).

THE DETERMINATION OF THE BIPARIETAL DIAMETER OF THE FOETAL
HEAD BY AN ULTRASONIC TECHNIQUE

The growth of the brain, expressed in weight and volume, is less affected by
adverse intra-uterine conditions than are body weight and length. The
measurement of the biparietal diameter, a parameter for skull growth, is
therefore one of the more reliable indices of the PM age. In a recent review,
Donald (19) summarized the basic principles of the technique.

Intermittent or pulsed sound waves of very high frequency, above the
range of human hearing, are emitted by a crystal, under directional control,

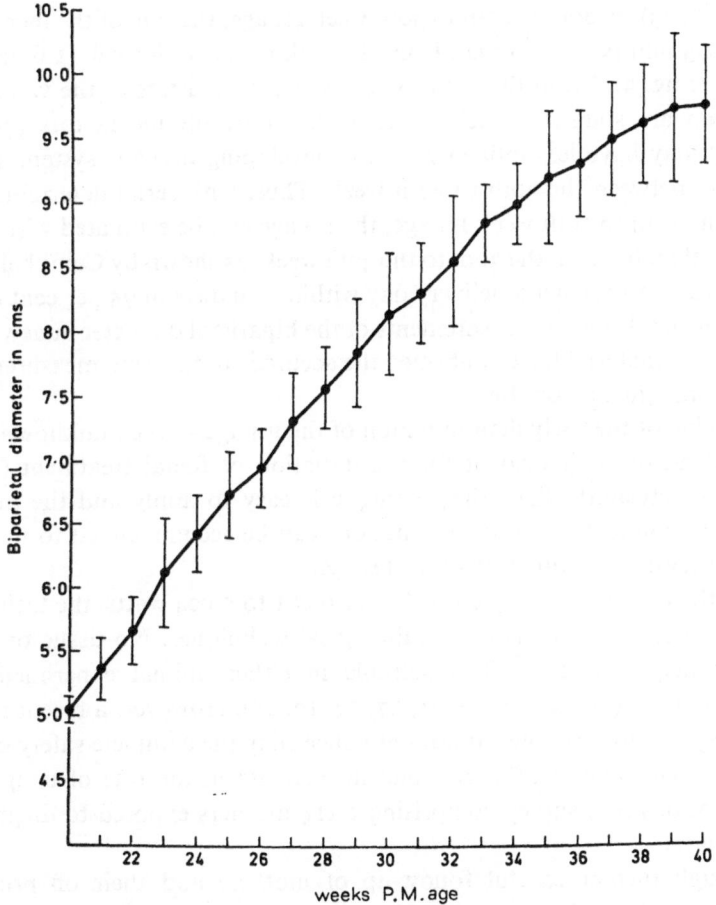

Fig. 3. Means and ± two standard deviations of the foetal biparietal diameter for each
week of PM age measured by the ultrasonic technique in 186 normal pregnancies (471 individual measurements). (Courtesy of S. Campbell, 24).

as beams of small packets of energy. Echos of the sound waves are picked up from the junctions or interfaces between tissues having different physical properties, and detected by the same crystal. The echo signals are made visible as tracings up the face of a cathode-ray tube or screen, a two-dimensional picture of the intra-uterine content being built up progressively as the ultrasonic scanning beam transverses the abdomen. Time-exposure polaroid photography or a memory scope converts a transient image to a more permanent record. After the two parietal bones have been identified, the biparietal diameter can be measured (see fig. 2).

The biparietal diameter increases from the 20th to the 40th week PM age (20, 21, 22, 23). From the 20th to 30th week PM age, the rate of the increase is higher (2.5 mm per week) than from the 30th to the 40th week (1.6 mm per week) (see fig. 3). From the 20th to 30th week the scatters of the values per age group are smaller, which suggests that intra-uterine factors (growth support) may have less influence on the developing nervous system at this time than between the 30th to 40th week. Thus, with serial determinations during the 20th to 30th week PM age, the PM age can be estimated with more accuracy than between the 30th to the 40th week, as shown by Campbell (24), who was able to predict a delivery day within ± 9 days in 95 per cent of the cases. Postnatal caliper measurements of the biparietal diameter in newborns and autopsy material have confirmed the accuracy of the echo measurements made *in utero* just before birth.

The value of the early determination of the PM age – when unknown from maternal history – is evident for the initiation of foetal treatment (intrauterine transfusion). Since the technique is easy to apply and the mother feels no discomfort, serial determinations can be recommended to increase the accuracy of the estimation of the PM age.

With the use of energy levels as low as 0.001 to 0.004 watts, the technique is reported to be safer than the radiological techniques. No tissue or functional damage has been demonstrable in either animal experiments or clinical practice (25, 22, 23, 26, 21, 27, 24, 19, 28). However, a recent report by Serr *et al.* (29) raises new questions concerning the complete safety of this technique. Hellman *et al.* (30) found no increase in the rate of congenital malformations in a survey comprising 1,114 mothers exposed to diagnostic ultrasound.

Although further careful follow-up of mothers and their offspring as well as research on the influence of low energy exposure at the microcellular level are needed, at present the ultrasonic technique may be considered as reasonably safe (31).

POSTNATAL CRITERIA

When a newborn infant's PM age is unknown, a number of techniques are available to the physician to estimate its age (Tables I and 2). And even when the PM age is thought to be accurate, assessment of this age should still be made in the neonatal period, since any discrepancies in the results of the estimations would alert the physician to an unreliable history or a pathological situation.

NEUROLOGICAL TESTS

Gesell and Amatruda (8), Söderling (32), and Bergström *et al.* (33) noted the difference in behaviour between PT and FT infants, and later investigators have suggested that neurological tests might be helpful in differentiating PT from SFD-FT. Saint-Anne Dargassies (34, 35, 36, 37), using the neurological examination technique developed by Thomas and associates (38, 39), clearly demonstrated that surprisingly similar neurological findings are made in infants regardless of whether they have reached 40 weeks PM age *in utero* or were born earlier and developed *ex utero* (40, 41, 42, 15). The neurological technique of Saint-Anne Dargassies and coworkers assesses muscle tone as a fundamental criterion by describing the resting posture, 'passive tone' (resistence to movements as felt by the examiner and the range of movements of extremities), and 'active tone' (postural movements in response to stimuli) as follows.

Resting posture: Under 32 weeks PM age, the extremities of the infants are usually in extension; between 32-36 weeks there is usually extension of arms and flexion of legs in the supine position and flexion of arms and extension of legs in the prone position; after 36 weeks, flexion of arms and legs in prone and supine position.

Resistance to movements and range of movements: The range of movements of the hips (heel to ear), knees (popliteal angle), and shoulder (scarf sign) decreases with increasing PM age, and the resistance to movements increases.

Postural responses: Placing the infant on his feet in an upright position results in the straighthening of the legs only at 32 weeks PM age; the legs and trunk after 36 weeks; and legs, trunk, and head at 40 weeks (37). The 'roll reflex' is seen after 35 weeks, and head-righting in the prone position and crawling after 40 weeks PM age (43).

The developmental course of the resting posture, resistance to passive movements, range of movements, and postural responses have been similarly described by different investigators (37, 40), although exceptions were noted (43). It would be interesting to have quantitative data on premature behaviour to see whether some of these phenomena could be helpful in distinguishing infants of various PM ages.

Robinson (44) investigated twenty reflexes and responses according to the method proposed by Prechtl and Beintema (45), standardized for sequence of elicitation of the responses, semi-quantitative scoring, in a group of infants strictly selected for known first day of the mother's last menstrual period. The five responses he found to be the most helpful in the estimation of PM age were as follows.

Pupil reaction to light: The contraction of the pupil to a standard light source was positive in 2/16 infants under 31 weeks PM age and in 43/43 infants older than 31 weeks PM age.

Glabella tap reflex: A blink response of the eye-lids to a finger tap on the glabella was positive in 4/21 infants under 32 weeks PM age and in 28/36 infants older than 32 weeks PM age.

Traction response: When a full-term infant is pulled up by the wrists from the supine position, a flexing of the elbows and bracing of the shoulders, anterior flexing of the neck, and raising of the head can be observed. This response was present in 2/20 infants under 33 weeks PM age and in 10/11 infants older than 33 weeks PM age.

Neck-righting reflex: In the supine baby, when the head is rotated, the trunk follows in the same direction. This reflex was present in 4/32 infants younger than 37 weeks PM age and in 6/9 infants older than 37 weeks PM age.

Head-turning to light: When diffuse light falls on one side of the face of a quiet alert full-term infant, the eyes and the head turn slowly toward the light. This response was absent in 6/6 infants under 32 weeks PM age and present in 18/24 infants older than 32 weeks PM age.

In infants older than 26 weeks PM age, the optical blink, Galant reflex, Moro response (abduction and extension components), withdrawal of the feet, and palmar and plantar grasp were always present (13). The crossed-extension response was present after 36 weeks PM age and the adduction phase of the Moro was present between 32 and 36 weeks, but the ranges of the time of appearance of these two responses were wide and the correlation with PM age was weak (13). The characteristics of the Moro reflex were studied electromyographically by Schulte *et al.* (46), who concluded that this method is not suitable for estimation of the PM age because the overlapping of the values for different ages is too great.

The majority of the exteroceptive reflexes (total number: 82) investigated in a group of 30 infants (age range: 30-40 weeks PM age) were present in all infants independent of age (47).

The interscorer and intertest reliability of the evaluation of reflexes and responses (13) is based on earlier studies in full-term infants (45). The reliability is better with semi-quantitative scores than with descriptions (48).

The five reflexes (see tabel 3) not only show a relationship with PM age but in addition their appearance at a particular age in the developmental course

Table 3. Reflexes of value for the assessment of the post-menstrual age (Robinson, 44).

Reflex	Stimulus	Positive Response	PMA (in weeks) if reflex is Absent	Present
Pupil reaction	Light	Pupil contraction	< 31	29 or more
Traction	Pull up by wrists from supine	Flexion of neck or arm	< 36	33 or more
Glabellar tap	Tap on glabella	Blink	< 34	32 or more
Neck-righting	Rotation of head	Trunk follows	< 37	34 or more
Head-turning	Diffuse light from one side	Head-turning to light	Doubtful	32 or more

is very abrupt, thus permitting distinction between infants under 31 weeks PM age, over 34 weeks PM age, and over 37 weeks PM age. The absence of the responses to light under the 31th week PM age is probably due to the presence of the pupillary membrane; the onset of positive responses may be indicative of the onset of the disappearance of this membrane.

Instead of a combination of neurological items, Dubowitz et al. (49) proposed that a simple sum of individual neurological scores be used. A scoring system for 'gestational age', based on 10 neurological and 11 'external' (skin and appendages) criteria was applied to a group of 167 unselected newborns; only newborns too sick to be examined or lacking the Moro reflex were excluded. The 'external' score (identical to the 'physical external characteristics' proposed by Farr et al. (50) showed a slightly better correlation with the PM age than did the neurological score. The neurological score consisted of 10 items selected on the basis of the results of a pilot study (n = 133) for their independence of state and pathology: posture (0-4), square window (0-4), dorsiflexion of the foot (0-4), arm recoil (0-2), leg recoil (0-2), popliteal angle (0-5), heal to ear (0-4), scarf sign (0-3), head lag (0-3), and ventral suspension (0-4); total neurologic score (0-35).

As logically to be expected, a combination of the two scores to form a total score gave the best correlation. The method gave more consistent results in the first five days of life than the score obtained in the first 24 hours. The test-retest reliability and interobserver reliability were reported to be high. The accuracy of the estimation of the PM age was reported as ± 2 weeks (95 per cent confidence limit), however further work needs to be done to verify this accuracy (see addendum).

Up to this point we have been concerned with the estimation of the PM age in normal newborns. In a group of healthy small-for-dates (n = 25) the pupil reaction, glabellar tap, traction, neck-righting, head-turning to light, were found to appear at the same time as in a control group of infants with normal weight for age (44). This statement does not mean that the neurological behaviour of SFD infants is identical to that of normal weight for age infants. Schulte et al. (46) and Michaelis et al. (51) reported that SFD (38-42 weeks; n = 22) have a weaker adduction and flexion of the Moro, a more marked asymmetric tonic neck reflex of the legs, frequent windmill movements of the arms, poor or absent head-lifting and poor rhythmic turning of the head in prone, and poor or absent standing and stepping movements, as compared to normal full-terms (39-41 weeks; n = 25). These differences between SFD and normal weight for age babies could perhaps be explained in some cases of chronic foetal distress by adverse influences on the synaptic and conduction properties of the nervous system (51), but the difference in weight and in muscle mass and their mechanical implications should also be taken into account.

In pathological conditions in which the nervous system is directly involved (hyperbilirubinaemia, hypoxia, hypoglycaemia, dehydratation, and electrolyte disturbances) it would appear that the PM age tends to be falsely underestimated (52, 53).

POLYGRAPHIC STUDIES

Behaviour as an indicator of central nervous system maturation was first studied by observation. The percentages of sleep and wakefulness during a 24-hour period was reported to change with age (8, 54, 55, 56). Prematures were found to be more active than FT infants during sleep (8).

A polygraphic technique was developed to study various parameters of infant behaviour and their interrelationships. Multi-channel recordings of the respiration (with a thermister or pneumograph), electrocardiogram, electro-oculogram, electro-encephalogram, and electromyogram (with surface electrodes) are made on paper and stored on magnetic tape for further analysis. Recording is usually continued for several hours to obtain a series of behaviour cycles. During such recording periods, temperature, light, sound, and time of feeding should be standardized (57).

Sleep was noted to have two phases in the FT infant (see also review: Lenard, 58). The following terms are applied to two comparable periods of sleep in the literature: no eye movement sleep, eye movement sleep (59), regular sleep, irregular sleep (60, 57), stage I, stages 2 and 3 (61); deep sleep, light sleep (62); Phase II, Phase I (63); State I, State 2 (45); quiet sleep, active sleep (64, 65); stages b and c, stages a and d (paradoxical sleep (66).

In this paper the terms regular sleep and irregular sleep will be used. Regular sleep is characterized by regular respiration, regular heart rate, closed eyes, absence of eye movements, high-amplitude discontinuous EEG, and no body movements except for occasional startles; irregular sleep is characterized by irregular respiration, irregular heart rate, closed eyes, eye movements, low-amplitude continuous EEG, and body movements (see table 4).

Table 4. Sleep-cycle characteristics in full-terms.

Regular sleep		Irregular sleep	
Observation	Polygraphic phenomena	Observation	Polygraphic phenomena
Regular respiration	Regular respiration Regular heart rate	Irregular respiration	Irregular respiration Irregular heart rate
Eyes closed	No EOG activity	Eyes closed	EOG activity
No eye movements		Eye movements	REM superimposed on slow EM
	High amplitude discontinuous EEG Traçé Alternant* Predominant codes: 405-407-403-402**		EEG: low amplitude Predominant codes: 402-403**
No movements	Slight EMG activity	Movements	EMG activity
Rhythmic oral movements	Startles	Startles	Startles
Startles		Twitches	
		Mass movements	

According to Prechtl and co-workers.
*Samson-Dolfuss (82), Dreyfus-Brisac *et al*. (81).
**EEG codes according to Parmelee *et al*. (85).

Periods of sleep not satisfying the above criteria are classified by some authors as transitional sleep (64, 65).

The changes in the duration of the sleep periods and in the physiological variables of the two sleep phases with increasing age will be discussed in relation to their usefulness for the distinction between different PM ages.

Duration of sleep phases: Between the 24th and 28th week PM age, it is difficult to apply the criteria of regular and irregular sleep as used in full-terms to the observed behaviour of the infant (67). The division of sleep into

Table 5. Sleep-cycle characteristics in relation to post-menstrual age.

Dreyfus–Brisac (67, 69)
Dreyfus–Brisac & Monod (64)
Dreyfus–Brisac et al. (68)
Monod & Pajot (106)
Monod et al. (72)
Eliet-Flescher & Dreyfus-Brisac (70)

24 – 28 weeks: sleep cycle absent
30 – 36 weeks: some correlations between different parameters appear periodically
37 weeks: dual sleep cycle

Petre-Quadens (73, 66, 74, 75)
6½ months 13.5% Paradoxal Sleep
> 8 months 37-40% Paradoxal Sleep

Parmelee et al. (65)

Weeks PM age	Irregular Sleep (%)	Transitional Sleep (%)	Regular Sleep (%)	N
29	84	0	16	1
31-32	–	–	–	0
33-34	68 (63-72)*	14 (13-16)	18 (16-21)	2
35-36	60 (55-68)	18 (12-28)	22 (12-32)	4
37-38	60 (53-69)	20 (7-42)	20 (4-41)	4
39-40	58 (44-79)	16 (7-30)	25 (5-41)	7
53-(3 months)	36 (28-42)	13 (7-21)	52 (40-59)	6

Regular Respiration
32 weeks   10% in Regular Sleep**   4% in Irregular Sleep
36 weeks   25% in Regular Sleep   5% in Irregular Sleep
40 weeks   58% in Regular Sleep   10% in Irregular Sleep

Weinmann et al. (78)
35 weeks – 40% in Regular Sleep**
> 38 weeks – 60% in Regular Sleep

*Total ranges
**Percentage of sleeping time with regular respiration of the total time in regular or irregular sleep

regular and irregular sleep becomes more distinct between the 30th and 36th week PM age. The maturational course has been reported as showing an increase in regular sleep, a decrease in irregular sleep, and a decrease in transitional sleep (68, 69, 70, 71, 72, 73, 66, 74, 75, 76, 77). In a longitudinal study of 24 infants (29-53 weeks PM age) the percentages of regular sleep showed an increase from 16 at 29 weeks PM age to 52 at 53 weeks PM age, for irregular sleep a decrease from 84 at 29 weeks PM age to 36 at 53 weeks PM age, and for transitional sleep a decrease from 20 at 37 weeks PM age to 13 at 53 weeks PM age (65) (see table 5).

Respiration: Parmelee *et al.* (65) found that the amount of regular respiration increases and regular respiration becomes more prevalent in regular sleep between the 32nd and 40th week PM age. Similar trends were reported by Weinmann *et al.* (78) in prematures (35 weeks PM age and older).

For the estimation of the PM age of the newborn, the length of the sleep periods and the descriptions and percentages of the respiratory patterns seem to be of minor help, because there is too much overlapping of the values for the different age groups. Transitions from awake to sleep and from irregular to regular sleep and the interrelationships between the physiological parameters were disturbed in sick newborns (71, 72). Schulte *et al.* (53) reported that children of diabetic mothers have less stable sleep cycles, resembling a younger sleep pattern, than would be expected for their PM age.

The introduction of automatic data analysis, has made it possible to distinguish objectively and quantatively between certain aspects of neurologically normal and abnormal infants (79), but objective and quantified data on the maturational changes of sleep obtained by automatic data analysis are lacking.

Electro-encephalogram (EEG): EEG patterns for regular and irregular sleep are described in terms of amplitudes, frequencies, rhythmicity, continuity or discontinuity, and spatial organization over the different areas of the skull.

In general, the maturational changes in the EEG for irregular sleep take the form of a decrease in the amplitude and a trend toward higher frequencies, resulting in a low voltage, rapid continuous activity at the 40th week PM age (see codes 322, 323, 361, 401, 402 and 403 in fig. 4), and for regular sleep, bursts of high-amplitude slow waves alternating with periods of very attenuated EEG activity gradually change to bursts of high-amplitude slow wave activity with faster and sharper waves superimposed, alternating with a less attenuated EEG activity with mixed frequencies at the 40th week PM age

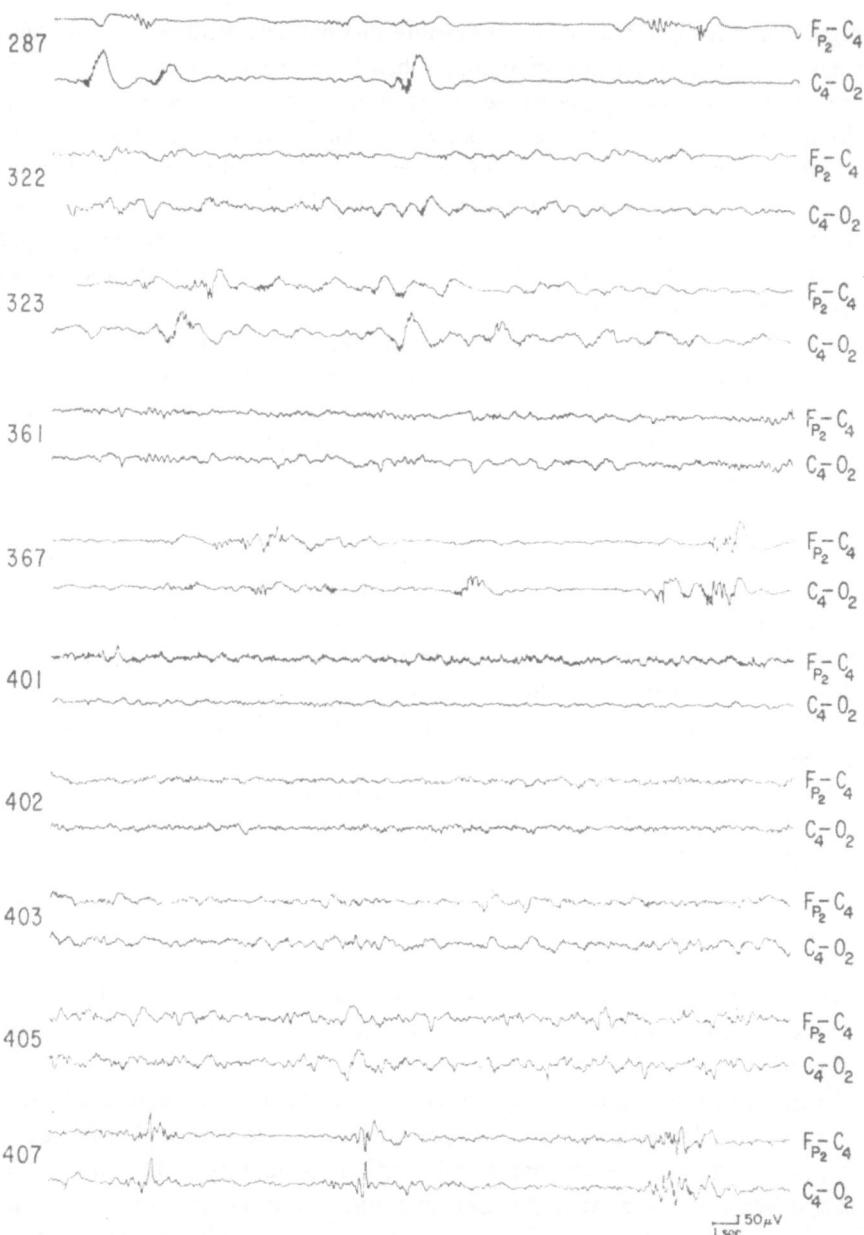

Fig. 4. Illustrations of EEG codes. The first two digits indicate the PM age at which a variation in the EEG patterns (indicated by the third digit) is seen. (EEG electrodes: F_{P_2}-C_4 = right frontocentral, C_4-O_2 = right centro-occipital.). (Courtesy of A. H. Parmelee Jr *et al.* (85).

(see codes 287, 367, 407 in fig. 4), described as Schlafgruppen (80), tracé alternant (81, 82), and episodic patterns (83). The descriptions of the EEG were reported to be surprisingly similar for infants at a particular PM age whether their development had taken place intra-uterinely or extra-uterinely (69, 84, 82). To study the developmental aspects of the EEG by quantitative analysis, Parmelee *et al.* (85) proposed a 3-digit coding system: the first 2 digits indicate the PM age at which a variation of the EEG pattern indicated by the third digit is observed (see fig. 4). The distribution of the EEG codes for regular and irregular sleep were determined in 32 infants between 30th and 40th week PM age (see fig. 5). On the basis of the distribution of the EEG codes and without knowledge of the infants, the examiners estimated the PM age correctly within ± 2 weeks in 85 per cent of the cases.

To avoid the observer bias usually present in visual interpretation, the

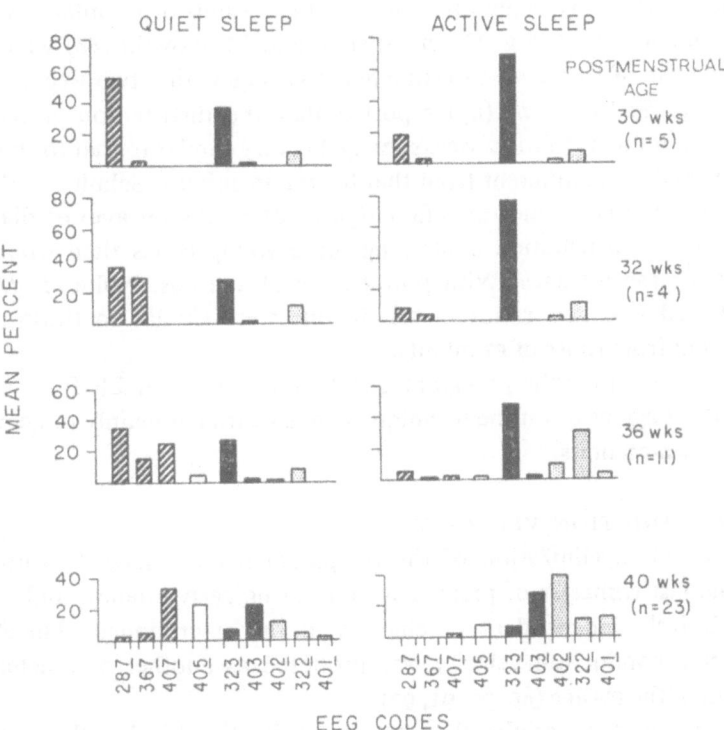

Fig. 5. Distribution of EEG codes in regular and irregular sleep at different PM ages. Basic EEG patterns are shaded similarly at each age level. (Courtesy of A. H. Parmelee Jr. *et al.* (85)).

EEG was further investigated by frequency analysis by Nolte *et al.* (86, 87) who computed the power spectra, i.e. the numerical value for the squared amplitude of the EEG in different frequency bands. A total power spectral score (sum of the power spectral values for each frequency interval) was calculated for regular and irregular sleep and the interrelationship expressed as an irregular to regular sleep ratio. In 36 infants (30 to 42 weeks PM age) the ratio was reported to decrease from about 1.5 at 34 weeks PM age to 0.7 at 40 weeks PM age, reflecting the inverse maturational changes in the amplitude in these two sleep phases. In 8 pairs of twins ˙(34 to 42 weeks PM age; weight range 850 to 2700 g), despite inter-pair differences in the birth weight ranging from 0-50 per cent, irregular to regular sleep ratios were almost identical for each pair of twins (mean inter-pair differences = 9.7 per cent).

The use of the EEG for the estimation of the PM age is the best criterion yet available for the polygraphic parameters. In a group of 96 infants with a birth weight under 2500 g, Dreyfus-Brisac and Minkowski (88) were able in 76 per cent of the cases to estimate the PM age within two weeks of the true age. Parmelee *et al.* (85) reported that the distribution of the EEG codes of SFD infants (38 to 42 weeks PM age) is very similar to that for normal full-terms and quite different from that for the PT infants. Schulte *et al.* (53) showed that the EEG codes of infants (36 to 41 weeks PM age) of diabetic mothers had a distribution containing more young codes than would be expected for the PM ages. With power spectral analysis, Nolte *et al.* (87) demonstrated that EEG ratios of SFD infants were similar to those of FT and different from those of PT infants.

At the present time the polygraphic technique is not suitable for the estimation of PM age as a routine technique and is restricted mainly to neonatal care and research units.

NERVE CONDUCTION VELOCITY

The degree of myelinization of the peripheral nerves increases with age during the last trimester of pregnancy and during early infancy, and seems to be relatively independent of changes in the environment. Therefore, motor nerve conduction velocity was proposed as another parameter for estimation of the PM age (89, 90, 91, 92).

In this method a peripheral motor nerve is stimulated with a supramaximal square pulse from a skin electrode at a proximal and distal point along the nerve. The evoked muscle action potential is recorded by skin or needle electrodes. The distance between the two stimulation points is measured and the conduction times between the two stimulus artefacts and the muscle action potential are determined. The conduction velocity of the nerve is calculated by dividing the distance between two stimulus points by the difference between the two conduction times. For the material of the

Table 6. Nerve conduction velocities (in m/sec).

	Schulte et al. (92)	Ruppert & Johnson (91)	Blom & Finnström (89)	Dubowitz et al. (90)
N. ulnaris				
Full-terms	30.4 ± 3.40	—	29.5 ± 4.52	29.6 ± 1.3
Pre-terms	25.9 ± 4.00	20.8 ± 3.9	20.7 ± 2.53	24.8
Small-for-dates (38-42 weeks PM age)	32.4 ± 7.25	29.5 ± 1.4	—	—
N. tibialis				
Full-terms	25.8 ± 2.00	—	25.2 ± 3.57	24.8 ± 1.3
Pre-terms	18.6 ± 3.71	18.9 ± 4.3	17.8 ± 1.76	20.1
Small-for-dates (38-42 weeks PM age)	23.6 ± 4.02	30.0 ± 3.1	—	—

various investigators, which was carefully selected for known PM age, the mean conduction velocities (see table 6) range for the ulnar nerve in FT from 29.5 to 30.4 m/sec (S.D. 1.3-4.5 m/sec), for the PT from 20.7 to 25.9 m/sec (S.D. 2.5-4.0 m/sec), and for SFD (38-42 weeks PM age) from 29.5 to 32.4 m/sec (S.D. 1.4-7.2 m/sec).

The mean conduction velocities of the tibial nerve in the FT range from 24.8 to 25.8 m/sec (S.D. 1.3-3.5 m/sec), for the PT from 17.8 to 20.1 m/sec (S.D. 1.7-4.3 m/sec), and for SFD (38-42 weeks PM age) from 23.6 to 30.0 m/sec (S.D. 3.1-4.0 m/sec).

The values of the conduction velocities reported by the different authors for FT and SFD (38-42 weeks PM age) are significantly higher than the values reported for PT.

Nerve conduction velocities have a higher positive correlation with PM age than with birth weight, as clearly shown in twins with the same PM age but different birth weights (92). Although the correlations are high, the scatter of the conduction velocities per age group are wide, and the scatter of ages for a particular nerve conduction value, is even wider. For example, a value of 22 m/sec is found in infants with an age range of 32 to 40 weeks.

The determination of nerve conduction velocities seems to be a benign technique, although slightly uncomfortable for the infant. Special equipment, strict temperature control, and care in measuring are necessary. The great advantage of this technique is that results were reported to be reliable in abnormal conditions such as SFD, LFD, toxemia, Rh-incompatibility, maternal diabetes, hydrocephalus and spina bifida (93, 53) and in jaundice and hypoxia (89, 93, 53).

With use of the mechanical stimulator to tap on the biceps tendon, the time between the stimulus and the first biceps muscle depolarization was measured to evaluate the time required for an impulse to transverse a spindle afferent, intraspinal synapse, motor afferent, and myoneural junction. This reflex-arc latency was then related to a standard skeletel measurement to compute a 'reflex velocity'. In a group of 59 newborns these reflex velocities were positively correlated with the postmenstrual age, as were the nerve conduction velocities. The overlap of the values of different ages groups was, however, wider for the reflex velocities than for the nerve conduction velocities (Eisengart, 94).

EVOKED RESPONSES

Photic, acoustic, proprioceptive, somasthetic, and pain stimuli have been shown to induce potential changes in the EEG; maturational phenomena were reported for photically and acoustically evoked responses. The suitability of these factors for determining PM age will be discussed in this section.

The EEG changes can sometimes be visually observed on the write-out, especially after photic stimuli. However, they can be observed more easily if a series of the responses (50-150) to photic, acoustic, or external stimuli are superimposed on an osciloscope or are analysed by a special-purpose computer (computer of average transients). The averaged evoked responses can be quantitatively studied by measuring the amplitudes and latencies from the stimulus to the onset of the first or subsequent peaks of the evoked response wave.

The latencies of the photically evoked responses become shorter with increasing PM age (95, 96, 97, 98). In a group of PST infants (n = 15) a significantly shorter latent period after photic stimuli was found as compared with the latencies found in FT infants (n = 341) (97).

The latencies of the acoustically evoked responses do not show consistent maturational changes with increasing PM age (99, 100, 101). The shape of the response wave to acoustic stimuli was proposed by Graziani et al. (100) as a qualitative assessment of the PM age. In FT infants (n = 10) the amplitudes of

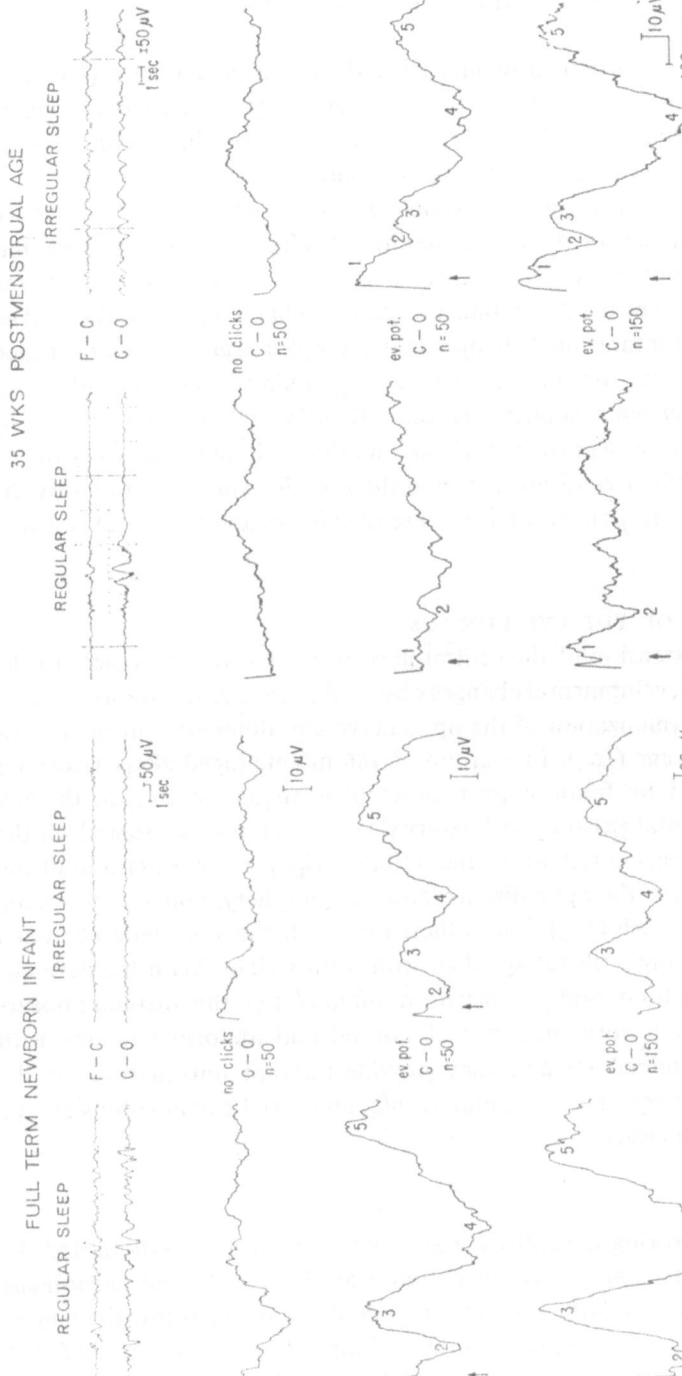

Fig. 6. Acoustically evoked responses in a normal full-term infant and a premature (35 weeks PM age) infant in regular and irregular sleep obtained from 50 and 150 clicks (n = number) as compared with 50 samples of background EEG without clicks (no clicks). Arrows mark the point of stimulus presentation (EEG electrodes: F-C = fronto-central, C-O = centro-occipital). The acoustically evoked response in the full-term infant has higher peak amplitudes in regular than in irregular sleep; the premature infant has higher peak amplitudes in irregular sleep than in regular sleep. (Courtesy of Y. Akiyama *et al.* (101).

the responses were higher in regular sleep than in irregular sleep (101) (see fig. 6). The acoustically evoked response of an SFD (birth weight 1800 g, 39 weeks PM age) resembled the evoked response observed in FT infants more closely than that of PT infants with comparable birth weight.

Several factors are probably responsible for the changes in the evoked responses with increasing PM age. In addition to changes in the synaptic time of the central nervous system, changes with age in the background EEG are reported to influence the developmental changes characteristic of the evoked response (101). Maturational changes in the receptor organ, as demonstrated for the retina by electroretinography (102, 103) could also be relevant.

The use of evoked responses for the estimation of PM age seems to be promising, but at present the experience and the equipment necessary to obtain reliable results free of artifacts and the need for studies to quantify the variability of the responses, limit the use of this method to special research units.

EXAMINATION OF THE EYE FUNDUS

The eye is an extension of the central nervous system readily visible to the examiner. The developmental changes observed in the eye fundus may reflect the degree of myelinization of the optic nerve and differences in the micro-circulation with age (104). In a group of 186 infants (aged 28-41 weeks PM age) investigated by fundoscopy because of a history of oxygen therapy during the neonatal period, the 'maturity' of the fundus was scored on the basis of the increasing redness of the retinal periphery, the extension of the retinal vessels from the optic disc towards the periphery, and the increasing diameter of the vessels (105). The authors found a higher correlation between their maturity score with PM age than with birth weight. With the development of retinal photography in newborn infants (104), this method appears promising. Future work on series of normal and abnormal infants with accurately determined PM age, may provide relevant information for the estimation of PM age. The technique is safe, and serial examinations can be performed rather easily.

DISCUSSION

Phenomena appearing abruptly at particular ages are ideal criteria for the estimation of the PM age, since the presence or absence of these phenomena makes it possible to distinguish between infants above or below these ages. The five neurological tests proposed by Robinson (13) are examples of such criteria. With respect to the other neurological criteria, there is good evidence in the literature that they permit assessment of post-menstrual age with an accuracy of ± 2.5-3.5 weeks for the 95 percentile range. To approach a solution to the problem of the accuracy more closely, future studies will have to be based on samples with a more equal distribution over the various age groups, especially the younger groups. In practice, an evaluation of the infant is made and then the PM age is estimated from the results; therefore, for the practical application of these techniques the results should be displayed with the age as the dependent variable and the measurement as the independent variable.

Although the value of a combination of criteria in normal and abnormal samples requires further investigation, it is clear that they can be helpful, since pathology does not affect the different organs to the same degree. Furthermore, the consistencies or discrepancies in the ages estimated by various criteria may identify particular groups of newborn infants, such as normal pre-term, neurologically sick pre-term, small-for-date, large-fordate, and normal full-term infants (see illustration of hypothetical cases in fig. 7).

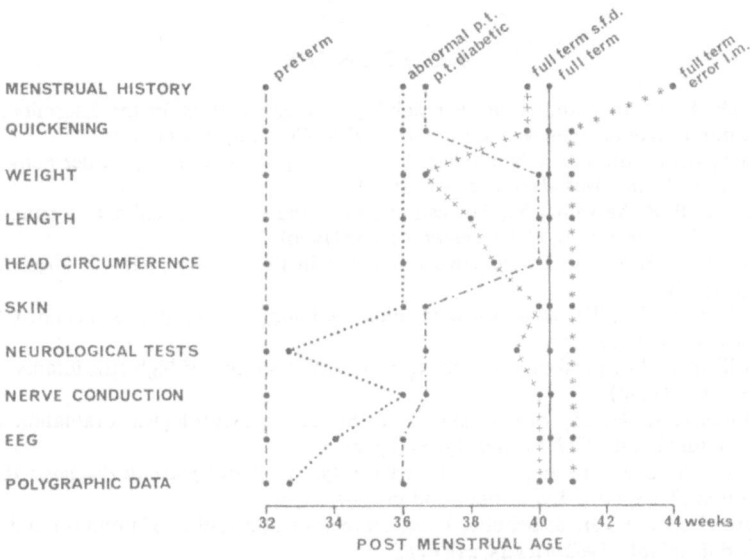

Fig. 7. Consistencies and discrepancies in the results of a combination of parameters for the estimation of the PM age illustrated by hypothetical cases: a normal pre-term (32 weeks PM age), a neurologically abnormal pre-term (36 weeks PM age), a large-for-date pre-term of a diabetic mother (36 weeks PM age), a small-for-date full-term, a normal full-term, and a normal full-term with an error in the pregnancy history as to the first day of the last menstruation (full-term, error l.m.).

In summarizing of the foregoing, it may be said that the developing brain can tell us something about the age of the newborn. A combination of assessments of developmental changes in the brain and other organ systems, especially the skin, can be a perinatal diagnostic tool.

ACKNOWLEDGEMENTS

We wish to express our sincere gratitude to Professor H. Prechtl for his advice, criticism, and comments on this paper. Our thanks are also extended to O. Finnström, A. Gramsbergen, H. Huisjes, A. Kalverboer, A. Parmelee Jr, R. Robinson, F. Schulte, B. Touwen, J. Vos-Niël and J. Vos for their comments and stimulating discussions, and to Miss F. van der Velde, Mrs H. Versteeg, and Miss W. van Dijk for their assistance.

This study was partly supported by a grant from the Organization for Health Research T.N.O. (The Netherlands).

REFERENCES

1. Brody, S., Further studies on the reliability of a new method for the determination of the duration of pregnancy. *J. Obst. Gynec. Brit. Cwlth.* 67, 819 (1960).
2. Bolte, A., Kessler, J. & Winkhaus, I. Zur Reifegradbestimmung in der Schwangerschaft. *Geburth. Frauenheilk.* 30, 616 (1970).
3. Casaer, P. & Akiyama, Y., The estimation of the postmenstrual age: a comprehensive review. *Devl. Med. Child Neurol.* 12, 697 (1970).
4. Hey, E. & Katz, G., Evaporative water loss in the newborn baby. *J. Physiol.* 200, 605 (1969).
5. Drillien, C. M., The small-for-date infant: etiology and prognosis. *Pediat. Clin. N. Amer.* 17, 9 (1970).
6. Drillien, C. M., Fresh approaches to prospective studies of high risk infants. *Pediatrics* 45, 7 (1970).
7. Parmelee, A. H. Jr., Minkowski, A. & Stern, E., Neurological evaluation of the premature infant. *Biol. Neonat.* 15, 65 (1970).
8. Gesell, A. & Amatruda, C. S., Praematurity. In: *Developmental diagnosis* (Second Edition), New York, Evanston, London 1947.
9. Parmelee, A. H. Jr. & Schulte, F. J., Developmental testing of pre-term and small-for-date infants. *Pediatrics* 45, 21 (1970).
10. Himwich, W. A., Bernardon, H. B. W. & Tucker, B. E., Metabolic studies on perinatal brain. In: *Mental Retardation*, 173. Bowman P. W. & Mautner H. V. (eds.), New York 1960.
11. Davison A. N. & Dobbing, J., Myelinisation as a vulnerable period in brain development. *Brit. Med. Bull.* 22, 40 (1966).
12. Larroche, J. C., The development of the central nervous system during intrauterine life. In: *Human Development*. Falkner, F. (ed.), London 1966.

13. Robinson, R. J. & Tizard, J. P., The central nervous system in the newborn. *Brit. Med. Bull.* 22, 49 (1966).
14. Gruenwald, P., Growth pattern of the normal and the deprived fetus. In: *Aspects of praematurity and dysmaturity*, 38. Jonxis, J. H. P., Visser, H. K. A. & Troelstra, J. A. (eds.), Leiden 1968.
15. Joppich, G. & Schulte, F. J., *Neurologie des Neugeborenen*, Berlin 1968.
16. Larroche, J. C., Quelques aspects anatomiques du développement cérébral. *Biol. Neonat.* 4, 126 (1962).
17. Vignaud, J., Radiological study of the normal skull in premature and newborn infants. In: *Human Development* Falkner F. (ed.), London 1966.
18. Rawlings, E. E. & Moore, B. A., The accuracy of methods of calculating the expected date of delivery for use in the diagnosis of postmaturity. *Amer. J. Obstet. Gynec.* 106, 676 (1970).
19. Donald, I., Sonar as method of studying prenatal development. *J. Pediat.* 75, 326 (1969).
20. Donald, I. & Brown, T. G., Demonstration of tissue interfaces within the body by ultrasonic echo sounding. *Brit. J. Radiol.* 34, 539 (1961).
21. Hibbard, L. T. & Anderson, G. V., Clinical applications of ultrasonic fetal cephalometry. *Obstet. Gynecol.* 29, 842 (1967).
22. Willocks, J., Donald, I., Duggan, T. C. & Day, N., Foetal cephalometry by ultrasound. *J. Obstet. Gynaec. Brit. Cwlth.* 71, 11 (1964).
23. Thompson, H. E., Holmes, J. H., Gottesfeld, K. R. & Taylor, E. S., Fetal development as determined by ultrasonic pulse echo techniques. *Amer. J. Obstet. Gynec.* 92, 44 (1965).
24. Campbell, S., The prediction of fetal maturity by ultrasonic measurement of the biparietal diameter. *J. Obstet. Gynaec. Brit. Cwlth.* 76, 603 (1969).
25. Andrew, D. S., Ultrasonography in pregnancy, an enquiry into its safety. *Brit. J. Radiol.* 37, 185 (1964).
26. Durkan, J. P. & Russo, G. L., Ultrasonic fetal cephalometry: accuracy, limitations and implications. *Obstet. Gynecol.* 27, 399 (1966).
27. Bernstine, R. L. Safety studies with Ultrasonic Doppler Technic: A clinical follow-up of patients and tissue culture. *Obstet. Gynecol.* 34, 707 (1969).
28. Kratochwil, A., Die Bedeutung der Ultraschalldiagnostik für Geburtshilfe und Gynäkologie. *Schweiz. Med. Wschr.* 99, 992 (1969).
29. Serr, D. M., Paden, B., Zakut, H., Shaki, R., Mannor, S. M. & Kalner, B., *Studies on the effects of ultrasonic waves on the foetus.* Second European Congress for Perinatal Medicine. London 8-10 April 1970. (Abstract.)
30. Hellman, L. M., Duffus, M., Donald, I. & Sundén, B., Safety of diagnostic ultrasound in obstetrics. *Lancet* 7657, 1133 (1970).
31. Editorial. Safety of sonar in obstetrics. *Lancet*, 7657, 1158 (1970).
32. Söderling, B., Pseudoprematurity. *Acta Paediat.* 42, 520 (1953).
33. Bergström, A. L., Gunther, M. B., Olow, L. & Söderling, B., Prematurity and pseudoprematurity studies of the developmental age in underweight newborns. *Acta Paediat.* (Uppsala) 44, 519 (1955).
34. Saint-Anne Dargassies, S., Methode d'examen neurologique du nouveau-né. *Etude Neonat.* 3, 101 (1954).
35. Saint-Anne Dargassies, S., A propos d'un enfant né au 6e mois de la gestation, *Etude Neonat.* 6, 11 (1957).
36. Saint-Anne Dargassies, S., Le nouveau né à terme aspect neurologique. *Biol. Neonat.* 4, 174 (1962).
37. Saint-Anne Dargassies, S., Neurological maturation of the premature infant of 28 to 41 weeks' gestational age. In: *Human Development*, Falkner, F. (ed.), London 1966.

38. Thomas, A. & Saint-Anne Dargassies, S., *Etudes neurologiques sur le nouveau-né et le jeune nourrisson*. Paris 1952.
39. Thomas, A., Chesni, Y. & Saint-Anne Dargassies, S., Neurological examination of the infant. *Little Club Clinics Dev. Medicine* 1, London 1960.
40. Brett, E. M., Estimation of fetal maturity by the neurological examination of the neonate. In: *Gestational age, size and maturity*. Dawkins M. & Mac Gregor B. (eds.), Clinics in Dev. Medicine, no. 19. London 1965.
41. Koenigsberger, M. R., Judgment of fetal age: Neurologic evaluation. *Pediat. Clin. N. Amer.* 13, 823 (1966).
42. Amiel-Tison, Cl., Neurological evaluation of the maturity of newborn infants. *Arch. Dis. Childh.* 43, 89 (1968).
43. Meitinger, Ch., Vlach, V. & Weinmann, H. M., Neurologische Untersuchungen bei Frühgeborenen. *Münchener Med. Wschr.* 20, 1158 (1969).
44. Robinson, R. J., Assessment of gestational age by neurological examination. *Arch. Dis. Childh.* 41, 437 (1966).
45. Prechtl, H. F. R. & Beintema, D., The neurological examination of the full-term newborn infant. Clinics in Dev. Medicine, no. 12, London 1964.
46. Schulte, F. J., Linke, I., Michaelis, R. & Nolte, R. E. M. G., Evaluation of the Moro-reflex in preterm, term and small-for-dates newborn infant. *Dev. Psychobiol.* 1, 41 (1968).
47. Vlach, V., Weinmann, H. M. & Meitinger, Ch., Exterozeptive Reflexe bei Frühgeborenen. *Z. Kinderheilk.* 107, 53 (1969).
48. Prechtl, H. F. R., Neurological findings in newborn infants after pre- and paranatal complications. In: *Aspects of Praematurity and Dysmaturity*. Jonxis, J. H. P., Visser, H. K. A., Troelstra, J. A. (eds.), Leiden 1968.
49. Dubowitz, L. M. S., Dubowitz, V. & Goldberg, C. Clinical assessment of gestational age in the newborn infant. *J. Pediat.* 77, 1 (1970).
50. Farr, V., Kerridge, D. F. & Mitchell, R. G., The value of some external characteristics in the assessment of gestational age at birth. *Develop. Med. Child Neurol.* 8, 657 (1966).
51. Michaelis, R., Schulte, F. J. & Nolte, R., Motor behavior of small for gestational age newborn infants. *J. Pediat.* 76, 208 (1970).
52. Schulte, F. J., Michaelis, R., Nolte, R. & Linke, I., Der Einfluss pränataler Störungen auf die Reifung zentralnervöser Funktionen. *Mschr. Kinderheilk.* 116, 243 (1968).
53. Schulte, F. J., Michaelis, R., Nolte, R., Albert, G., Parl, U., Larsson, U. & Jürgens, U., Brain and behavioural maturation in newborn infants of diabetic mothers. *Neuropädiatrie* 1, 24 (1969).
54. Parmelee, A. H. Jr., Sleep patterns in infancy. *Acta Paediat.* 50, 160 (1961).
55. Parmelee, A. H. Jr., Schultz, H. R. & Disbrow, M. A., Sleep patterns of the newborn. *J. Paediat.* 58, 241 (1961).
56. Roffwarg, H. P., Muzio, J. N., Dement, W. C., Ontogenetic development of the human sleep-dream cycle. *Science* 152, 604 (1966).
57. Prechtl, H. F. R., Akiyama, Y., Zinkin, P. & Kerr Grant, D., Polygraphic studies of the full-term newborn infant. I. Technical aspects and qualitative analysis. In: *Studies in infancy*. Bax, M. C. O. & Mac Keith, R. C. (eds.), Clinics in Dev. Medicine, no. 27, London 1968.
58. Lenard, H. G., Sleep studies in infancy. *Acta Paediat. Scand.* 59, 572 (1970).
59. Aserinsky, Y. E. & Kleitman, N. A., A motility cycle in sleeping infants as manifested by ocular and gross bodily activity. *J. Appl. Physiol.* 8, 11 (1955).
60. Wolff, P. H., Observations on newborn infants. *Psychosom. Med.* 21, 110 (1959).
61. Dittrichová, J., Nature of sleep in young infants. *J. Appl. Physiol.* 17, 543 (1962).
62. Dreyfus-Brisac, C., The electroencephalogram of the premature infant and the full

term newborn normal and abnormal development of waking and sleeping patterns. In: *Neurological and electroencephalographic correlative studies in infancy*, Kellaway, P. & Petersen, I. (eds.), New York 1964.

63. Goldie, L. & Van Velzer, C., Innate sleep rhythms. *Brain* 88, 1043 (1965).
64. Dreyfus-Brisac, C. & Monod, N., Sleep of premature and full-term neonates: a polygraphic study. *Proc. Roy. Soc. Med.* 58, 6 (1965).
65. Parmelee, A. H. Jr., Wenner, H., Akiyama, Y., Schultz, M. & Stern, E. Sleep states in premature infants. *Dev. Med. Child. Neurol.* 9, 70 (1967).
66. Petre-Quadens, O., On the different phases of the sleep of the newborn. With special reference to the activated phase, or phase d. *J. Neurol. Sci.* 3, 51 (1966).
67. Dreyfus-Brisac, C., Sleep ontogenesis in early human prematurity from 24 to 27 weeks of conceptional age. *Develop. Psychobiol.* 1, 162 (1968).
68. Freyfus-Brisac, C., Samson, D., Saint Anne Dargassies, S. & Ziegler, T., Veille, sommeil et réactivité chez le prématuré, *Electroenceph. clin. Neurophysiol.* 16, 418 (1965).
69. Dreyfus-Brisac, C., The bioelectrical development of the central nervous system during early life. In: *Human Development*, Falkner, F. (ed.), London 1966.
70. Eliet-Flescher, J. & Dreyfus-Brisac, C., Le sommeil du nouveau-né et du prematuré. *Biol. Neonat.* 10, 316 (1966).
71. Monod, N., Dreyfus-Brisac, C., Eliet-Flescher, J., Pajot, N. & Plassart, E., Les troubles de l'organisation du sommeil chez le nouveau-né pathologique. *Rev. Neurol.* 115, 469 (1966).
72. Monod, N., Eliet-Flescher, J. & Dreyfus-Brisac, C. Le sommeil du nouveau-né et du prématuré – Ill. *Biol. Neonat.* 11, 216 (1967).
73. Petre-Quadens, O., Etude du sommeil chez le nouveau-né normal. In: Le sommeil de nuit normal et pathologique, *Electroencephalographie et Neurophys. Clin.*; Nouvelle Serie nr. 2, 149 (1965).
74. Petre-Quadens, O., Ontogenesis of paradoxical sleep in the human newborn. *J. Neurol. Sci.* 4, 153 (1967).
75. Petre-Quadens, O., *Contribution à l'étude de la phase dite paradoxale du sommeil.* Thesis, Brussels-Antwerp 1969.
76. Polikanina, R. I., *Development of the higher nervous activity, in prematurely born babies during the early postnatal period of life.* Thesis, Leningrad 1966.
77. Dubois-Dalq, M., Contribution à l'étude du fonctionnement du système nerveux du nouveau-né à terme. *Acta Paediat. Belg.* 21, 257 (1967).
78. Weinmann, H. M., Meitinger, C. & Eiggler, G., Sleep states in the premature. *Electroenceph. clin. Neurophysiol.* 26, 466 (1969).
79. Prechtl, H. F. R., Weinmann, H. & Akiyama, Y., Organization of physiological parameters in normal and neurologically abnormal infants: comprehensive computer analysis of polygraphic data. *Neuropädiatrie* 1, 101 (1969).
80. Schroeder, C. & Heckel, H., Zur Frage Hirnstätigkeit beim Neugeborenen. *Geburtsh. Frauenheilk.* 12, 992 (1952).
81. Dreyfus-Brisac, C., Samson-Dolfus, D. & Fischgold, H., L'activité électrique cérébrale du prématuré et du nouveau-né. *La semaine des hôpitaux de Paris*, 31 1783 (1955).
82. Samson-Dollfus, D., *l'Electro-encéphalogramme du prématuré jusqu'à l'âge de 3 mois et du nouveau-né à terme.* Thesis, Paris 1955.
83. Harris, R. & Tizard, J. P. M., The electroencephalogram in neonatal convulsions. *J. Pediat.* 57, 501 (1960).
84. Dreyfus-Brisac, C., Flescher, J. & Plassart, E., L'EEG critère d'âge conceptionnel du nouveau-né à terme et du prématuré. *Biol. Neonat.* 4, 154 (1962).
85. Parmelee, A. H. Jr., Schulte, F. J., Akiyama, Y., Wenner, W. H. Schultz, M. & Stern, E., Maturation of electroencephalographic activity during sleep in premature infants. *Electroenceph. clin. Neurophysiol.* 24, 319 (1968).

86. Nolte, R., Schulte, F. J., Michaelis, R. & Juergens, U., Power spectral analysis of the electroencephalogram of newborn twins in active and quiet sleep. In: *Clinical EEG of children*, Kellaway, P., & Petersen, I. (eds.), London 1968.

87. Nolte, R., Schulte, F. J., Michaelis, R., Weisse, U. & Gruson, R., Bioelectric brain maturation in small-for-dates infants. *Dev. Med. Child. Neurol.* 11, 83 (1969).

88. Dreyfus-Brisac, C. & Minkowski, A., Maturation électroencéphalographique et trop faible poids de naissance. *Rev. Neurol.* 119, 299 (1968).

89. Blom, S. & Finnström, O., Motor conduction velocities in newborn infants of various gestational ages. *Acta Paediat. Scand.* 57, 377 (1968).

90. Dubowitz, V., Whittaker, G. F., Brown, B. H. & Robinson, A., Nerve conduction velocity. An index of neurological maturity of the newborn infant. *Dev. Med. Child. Neurol.* 10, 741 (1968).

91. Ruppert, E. S. & Johnson, E. W., Motor nerve conduction velocities in low birthweight infants. *Pediatrics* 42, 255 (1968).

92. Schulte, F. J., Michaelis, R., Linke, I. & Nolte, R., Motor nerve condition velocity in term, preterm and small-for-dates newborn infants. *Pediatrics* 42, 17 (1968).

93. Schulte, F. J., Albert, G. & Michaelis, R., Gestationsalter und Nervenheitsgeschwindigkeit bei normalen und abnormen Neugeborenen. *Dt. Med. Wschr.* 94, 599 (1969).

94. Eisengart, M. A., Reflex arc latency measurements in newborn infants and children. *Paediatrics* 46, 28 (1970).

95. Ellingson, R. J., EEG of normal full-term newborns immediately after birth with observations on arousal and visual evoked responses. *Electroenceph. clin. Neurophysiol.* 10, 31 (1958).

96. Hrbek, A. & Mareš, P., Cortical evoked responses to visual stimulation in full-term and premature newborns. *Electroencephalograph.* 16, 575 (1964).

97. Engel, R. & Benson, R. C., Estimate of conceptional age by evoked response activity. *Biol. Neonat.* 12, 201 (1968).

98. Umezaki, H. & Morell, F., Developmental study of photic responses evoked in premature infants. *Electroenceph. clin. Neurophysiol.* 28, 48 (1970).

99. Engel, R., Electroencephalographic responses to sound and light in prematures and full-term neonates. *Lancet* 87, 181 (1967).

100. Graziani, L. J., Weitzman, E. D. & Velasco, S. A., Neurologic maturation and acoustic evoked responses in low birthweight infants. *Pediatrics* 41, 483 (1968).

101. Akiyama, Y., Schulte, F. J., Schultz, M. A. & Parmelee, Jr, A. H., Acoustically evoked response in premature and full-term, newborn infants. *Electroenceph. clin. Neurophysiol.* 26, 371 (1969).

102. Horsten, G. P. M. & Winkelman, J. E., Electrical activity of the retina in relation to histological differentiation in infants born prematurely and at full term. *Vision Res.* 2, 269 (1962).

103. Samson-Dollfus, D., Développement normal de l'électrorétinogramme depuis l'âge foetal de sept mois et demi jusqu'à l'âge de quatre mois après la naissance à terme. *Bull. des Soc. d'Ophtalmologie de France*, no. 4, 1 (1968).

104. Bulpitt, C. J. & Baum, J. D., Retinal photography in the newborn. *Arch. Dis. Childh.* 44, 499 (1969).

105. Lomicková, H. & Melichar, V., Eye background findings in premature and hypotrophic newborns. *Biol. Neonat.* 12, 170 (1968).

106. Monod, N. & Pajot, M., Le sommeil du nouveau-né et du prématuré – I. *Biol. Neonat.* 8, 281 (1965).

ADDENDUM

A series of six articles under the title *Studies on maturity in newborn infants* by Dr Orvar Finnström, Umea, Sweden are in press; they concern the anthropometric findings external characteristics, neurological examination, postnatal radiological examination of epiphyseal centres, and motor conduction velocity in a series of 174 newborn infants. *Prediction models* for the estimation of 'gestational age' constructed from the results of this material were tested in a second series of 28 infants.

1. Finnström, O., Studies on maturity. I. Birth weight, crown-heel length, head circumference and skull diameters in relation to gestational age. *Acta Paediat. Scand.*, in press.
2. Finnström, O., Studies on maturity in newborn infants. II. External characteristics. *Acta Paediat. Scand., in* press.
3. Finnström, O., Studies on maturity in newborn infants. III. Neurological examination. *Neuropädiatrie* 3, 72 (1971).
4. Finnström, O., Studies on maturity in newborn infants. IV. Postnatal radiological examination of epiphyseal centers. *Neuropädiatrie*, in press.
5. Blom, S. & Finnström, O., Studies on maturity in newborn infants. V. Motor conduction velocity. *Neuropädiatrie*, in press.
6. Finnström, O., Studies on maturity in newborn infants. VI. Comparison between different methods for maturity estimation. *Acta Paediat. Scand.*, in press.

DISCUSSION

Marshall: May I just come back to my hobby-horse of age and maturity here. This question of estimating gestational age, postmenstrual age or whatever you choose to call it, is an excellent example of this problem. The more criteria we have the more likely we are to get close to the age. But until we have more evidence of the amount of variation there is between children in each criterion at each age, it will not be clear if they provide a satisfactory means of estimating the age of an individual child. But this does not matter, I think, because we are really barking up the wrong tree in most cases in trying to estimate age at all. This comes from the historical idea that age in fact represents maturity, which it does not. What we really want to measure in relation to pathology, growth, or anything else is the maturity of the infant and not its age. This in fact is what we are doing by these criteria.

Casaer: Thank you Dr. Marshall for these comments. But I think that at present the only thing we can do is to put the findings on a time scale. I agree that ultimately we would like to estimate maturity – or age appropriate functioning. But then we must answer first some questions like: maturity in what respect? For the lungs it is easy, adequate gas exchange; for the liver we get some idea, but for many other systems we don't know at this moment what in new-borns should be mature to what purpose. And so I think now we have simply to line all these things up and perhaps something will emerge.

Barth: Dr. Casaer, I would like to ask you if you are really confident as to the estimation of the nerve conduction rate as a good index of, let's say, foetal age. Protein– calorie malnutrition early in development may influence myelinization of the central nervous system. Now the nerve conduction rate seems to be related to the thickness of peripheral nerves. Is there any indication that this factor really does not have any influence?

Casaer: There are people much better qualified to answer your question than

I in the audience. I just tell you a story. When I started doing this review I thought it was the thickness. Somewhat later I became aware of the fact that the distances between the nodes of Ranvier are very important and now it appears, and I do ask Dr Dobbing to take this argument further, that perhaps it is the enzyme maturation in the nodes that is the really important thing.

Dobbing: It is nice to speculate about the functional consequences of 10% deficits in overall concentration of myeline substances but really this may have very little to do in the end with nerve impulse conduction rates compared with the factors that you mentioned like inter-nodal distances and so forth. I am a little less happy about Dr Marshall's remarks that we are only interest in maturational, in developmental age in these things. After all there is a big clinical difference between the fate of the small-for-date baby which has the same age as the full-term normally growing baby. And here I think we have to distinguish developmental age from chronological in the clinical sense; there is a clinical difference, we have to make judgements about this.

Marshall: In my opinion, the exact period of time it spent in utero, i.e. the baby's age, is not the primarily important factor. The important thing is, is this baby at birth a mature baby or an immature one? This is what in my view would decide its fate. Whether it is mature enough to survive; the right size to its maturity; or small for its maturity and so on.

Dobbing: This would be true if they were all born after the same length of gestation. But they are not.

Marshall: That is correct. They are not. I agree. But it is unusual to have a full-term baby which is grossly immature. It may be small, small-for-date, but it is in many respects mature, in spite of its smallness. I think it may be quite mature in many aspects of its neurological development. The typical small-for-date full-term baby is different from the premature baby in the sense that it has spent more time in utero, but also in the sense that it is genuinely more mature at birth. Maybe we are coming round to a problem of semantics rather than physiology.

Polman: I would like to raise a question about the EEG in premature infants. Do you have experience with such EEG's? In many of these children we find metabolic disturbances like hypocalcaemia, hypoglycaemia and others. In the EEG this can give errors and more or less specific disturbances. Is anything known about that?

Casaer: No answer to your question, just a comment. There are two authors of this paper and there is a dramatic increase in competency between the first and the second, so I would like to ask Dr Akiyama to comment on the EEG.

Akiyama: As far as the EEG's are concerned we should first qualify the examples that have been shown as those which were taken from what we considered normal prematures except for their premature birth. The problem with disturbed infants is again another question that has not yet been fully answered. I think we are beginning to see more of this type of data from Dr Schulte's group in Göttingen as he begins describing more infants of hypoglycaemia, infants of diabetic mothers, infants of toxaemic mothers, infants of phenylketonuria, but these again are not all prematures.

NEUROLOGICAL FOLLOW-UP OF INFANTS BORN AFTER OBSTETRICAL COMPLICATIONS

B. C. L. TOUWEN

Children with learning and/or behavioural difficulties are often described as suffering from 'minimal brain damage' or better, from 'minor brain dysfunction'. Moreover, they are often said to be born after complications in pregnancy and/or delivery, which may have damaged their nervous system.

What evidence do we have that children who are labeled as patients with minor brain dysfunction do actually show distinct neurological signs? The literature is very vague about this point with one recent exception: The Isle of Wight study by Rutter and coworkers (1).

When these neurological signs are reported in the literature, they are often called 'soft' or 'minor'. They are called soft or minor, because they are said to be very difficult to demonstrate reliably on different occasions. Moreover, their significance is often unknown.

The presence of such minor signs can only be demonstrated reliably with a standardized, refined and descriptive method of examination. Their validity in respect to behavioural disorders can only be evaluated in a study in which the neurological examination and the analysis of behavioural phenomena are kept strictly separated and therefore not contaminated.

In the present report I shall present to you data of a blind follow-up study of five year old children, who have been neurologically examined in the newborn period and who had a large variety of pre- and perinatal complications.

The follow-up examinations were carried out with a specially designed examination technique, which is age-specific, descriptive, quantitative and highly standardized (2). Since the ordinary gross clinical criteria failed for a meaningful data-processing, the concept of neurological optimality was adopted.

It is extremely difficult to establish a meaningful relationship between any one complication during pregnancy or delivery and the neurological condition of the newborn infant, due to the multifactorial structure of obstetrical complications. Therefore Prechtl proposed in 1967 in his analysis of a group

of 1378 infants the concept of optimality of the pre- and paranatal conditions (3). If one tries to define exactly complications and their weight, one
runs inevitably into major problems. On the other hand it is relatively easy
to define what the optimum is. By summing the number of optimal obstetrical
conditions each child obtained an optimal obstetrical score.

All these children have been examined extensively with the method described by Prechtl and Beintema in 1964 (4). This examination method is
specially designed for full-term newborn infants, it is highly standardized,
quantitative and descriptive. Similarly to the difficulties with the obstetric
data, a meaningful distinction between neurologically 'normals' and 'ab-
normals' created great problems. Here again it is easier to define 'optimality'. By counting the number of optimal responses each baby obtained an
optimal neurological score.

Prechtl demonstrated that the obstetrical optimal score shows a clear
relationship with the neurological optimal score in the neonatal period.

I have examined 167 five year old children, their ages ranging from 4

Table 1. Frequency of the main non-optimal obstetrical findings.

Bleedings during pregnancy:	21	cases
Infections during pregnancy:	22	–
Rhesus-antagonism:	31	–
AB-O incompatibility:	4	–
Toxaemia, moderate or serious:	15	–
Bloodpressure above 140/90:	57	–
Prolonged unwanted sterility:	9	–
Maternal chronic diseases:	16	–
Instrumental delivery:	33	–
Duration first stage > 24 hours:	24	–
Duration second stage > 2 hours:	8	–
< 4 minutes:	17	–
Weak contractions:	4	–
Drugs used by mother:	25	–
Intrauterine position non vertex:	24	–
Foetal presentation non vertex:	14	–
Amniotic fluid non clear:	25	–
Cardiac irregularity:	10	–
Foetal heart rate during 2nd stage < 100:	24	–
> 160:	2	–
Tight cord strangulation:	14	–
Onset of respiration after first minute:	29	–

years 9 months to 5 years 2 months. Of these 167 children, 88 were boys and 79 were girls. All of them were born at full term in the obstetrical department of our hospital and there were no cases with vital neonatal conditions.

Employing the concept of obstetrical optimality in this group of children, about a quarter of them (26%) have had a pregnancy and delivery without or with at most one non-optimal condition. In two-thirds of them (66%) two to six obstetrical conditions deviated from optimal, and only in 8% seven or more non-optimal conditions had been present (Table I). These latter 8% constitute the obstetrical high risk group. This does of course not mean that the children are brain damaged.

As far as the neonatal neurological findings are concerned half of the cases (52%) showed five or less deviations from optimal, in the other half of the cases (48%) six or more neurological items deviated from the criterium. By means of this arbitrarily chosen dividing line we call the first group neonatally optimal, and the second non-optimal.

I want to stress the point that this definition of 'optimal' is not identical with a clinical diagnosis of 'normality', but it helps to identify within the normal range a clearly defined group.

Among the non-optimal babies a large variety of neurological symptoms was present. None of the newborns, however, suffered from major neurological conditions such as hemiplegia, neonatal convulsions, etc. Therefore the chance to find in the follow-up examination of this group children with severe neurological handicaps is small. In fact only two of the 167 children showed major neural dysfunction, one being a hemiplegic patient, the other a slightly spastic oligophrenic. Both children acquired their handicap after a severe interval complication, both of them belonging to the optimal group in the neonatal period.

In the neurological follow-up examination the children were examined using a specially designed method (2).

None of the children or parents had complaints which requested medical help, except the two cases already mentioned. Hence these children represented so to say a clinically 'normal' group. Despite this fact wide variations within each neurological item were found.

It seemed meaningful to apply again the concept of optimality. Optimal ranges have been defined for 37 items of the neurological examination such as for the muscular system, posture, kinesia and motor coördination.

Table 2 contains the neurological findings and the optimal range, and figure 1 shows the percentage distribution of the optimal scores. Below each score is given the corresponding number of non-optimal conditions. The

Table 2. Optimal ranges for the neurological findings at five years.

Resistance to passive movements	moderate
Muscle power	moderate, strong
Muscle consistency	moderate
Contractures	absent
Knee jerk	moderate, symmetrical
Ankle jerk	– –
Radius periost reflex	– –
Biceps reflex	– –
Triceps reflex	– –
Footsole reflex	indifferent, plantar flexion
Other superficial reflexes lower leg	absent
Abdominal skin reflex	present, symmetrical
Position of feet, in sitting posture	neutral, symmetrical
Posture of extended arms	no vertical deviation <30° horizontal deviation
Posture of trunk, standing	straight, symmetrical
Posture of legs, standing	neutral, symmetrical
Walking	symmetrical, constant gait, width of gait 11-20 cm, short abrupt pelvis movements, alternating knee flexion extension
Posture during walking	straight, symmetrical
Finger-tip nose test, eyes closed	smooth; correct placing
Rebound phenomenon	0-5 cm
Response to push, sitting	balance without help of arms
Choreiform movements	absent
Facial musculature	symmetrical in rest and during movement
Eye movements	smooth, symmetrical; no nystagmus
Convergence	strong, symmetrical

main non-optimal findings consisted of choreiform movements, deviations from straight symmetrical posture and sensori-motor asymmetries.

For practical purposes the optimal scores were subdivided into three classes, class I zero to two, class II three to seven, class III seven or more non-optimal findings.

Figure 2 shows the relation between the three categories of optimality and sex. It is evident that in this group of children more girls belong to category I and more boys to category III. The difference is statistically significant at a 1% level of confidence.

For the relation of the follow-up findings with the neonatal neurological scores the risk of brain damage due to interval complications has to be taken into account. As interval complications were considered head injury, measles encephalitis, meningo-encephalitis etc. One third of the children had one or more interval complications in their history, as reported by their mother. Slightly more interval complications occurred in the neonatally non-optimal group.

In a group of children with minor neurological signs it may be expected

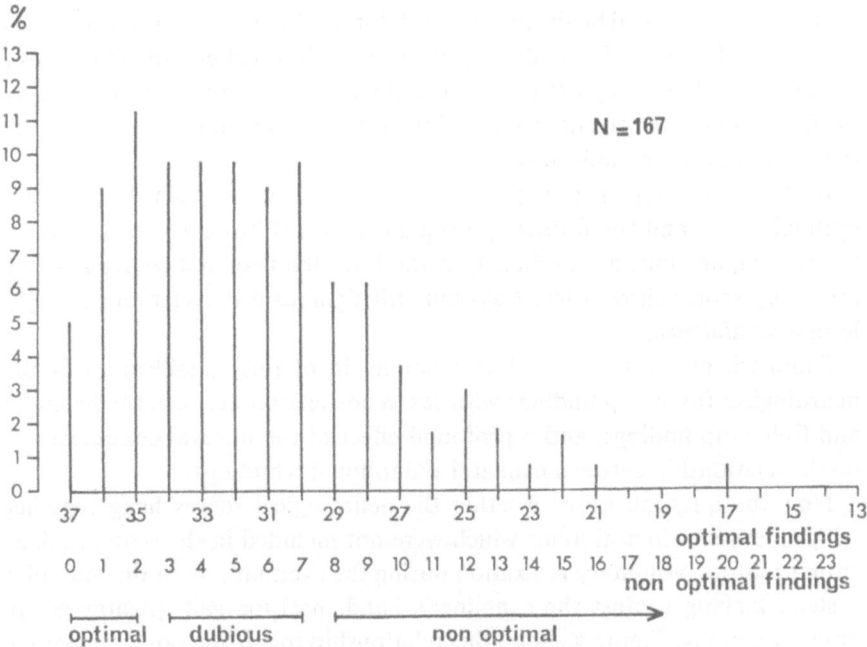

Fig. 1. The percentage distribution of the neurological optimal scores at 5 years. Below the scores the corresponding numbers of non-optimal findings are given.

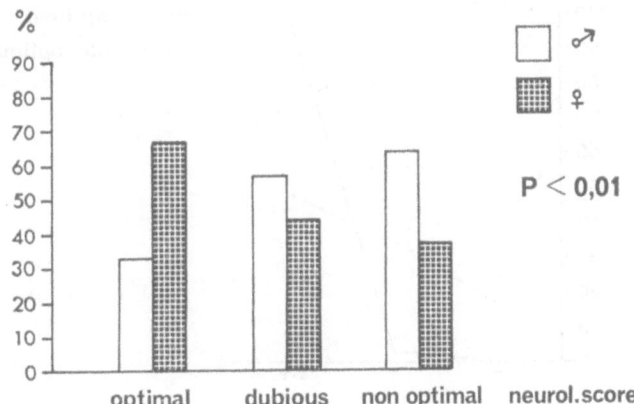

Fig. 2. The relationship between the neurological optimal scores and sex.

that the relationship after 5 years between neonatal and follow-up results is weak.

Two main reasons may be given. Firstly, many children who did not function optimally at birth may improve during their development. The chance of complete recovery will be the highest in children with the least severe neonatal nervous dysfunction. Secondly, the sequelae of interval complications may obscure the relationship between neonatal and follow-up results. The longer the interval between the neonatal and the follow-up examinations the higher the risk of interval complications.

In the total group there is no clear-cut correlation between the neonatal optimal scores and the follow-up optimal scores. If however cases with interval complications are excluded, in the boys the neonatal scores and the follow-up scores show a low (.28) but still significant correlation at a $2\frac{1}{2}\%$ level of confidence.

Summarizing we found a clear relationship of this classification of the neurological follow-up findings with sex, a correlation between the neonatal and follow-up findings, and a profound effect of the interval complications on the relationship between neonatal and follow-up findings.

Now the question arises whether the neurological scores hang together with other neurological items which were not included in the score, such as sitting posture, voluntary relaxation during the examination of the muscular system, kicking against the examiner's hand, heel-toe gait, plantar grasp, ankle clonus etc. Figure 3 shows this relationship for sitting posture, figure 4 illustrates kicking and figure 5 shows the relationship for the heel-toe gait.

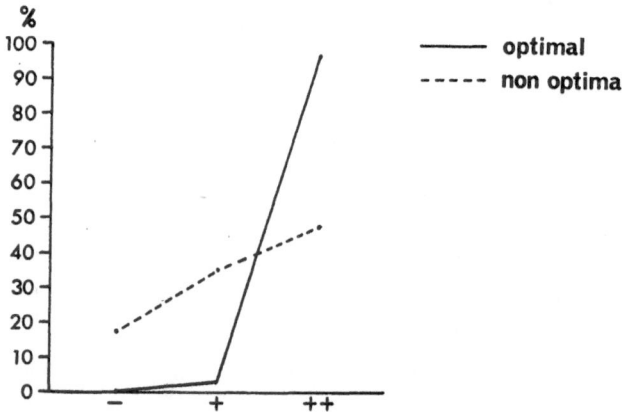

Fig. 3. The distribution of the qualitative scores for sitting in the neurologically optimal and non-optimal group.

If a maturation score is designed consisting of six motor functions (dia-dochokinesis, heel-toe gait, walking on tiptoe and heels, hopping and standing on one leg), a striking relationship with the neurological scores is found (Fig. 6).

Concluding one can say that an optimal score obtained in this way shows a clear-cut differentiation within a group of so-called clinically 'normal' children.

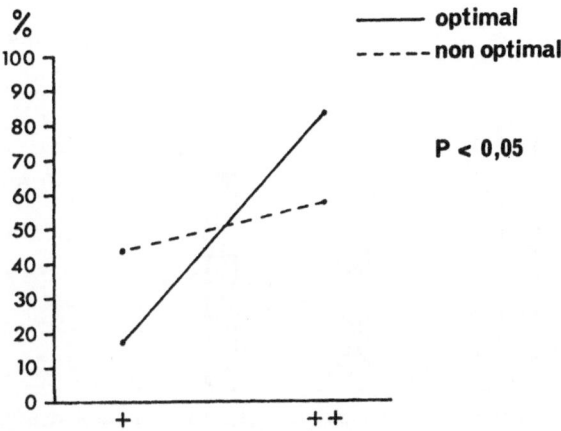

Fig. 4. The distribution of the scores for kicking in the neurologically optimal and non-optimal group.

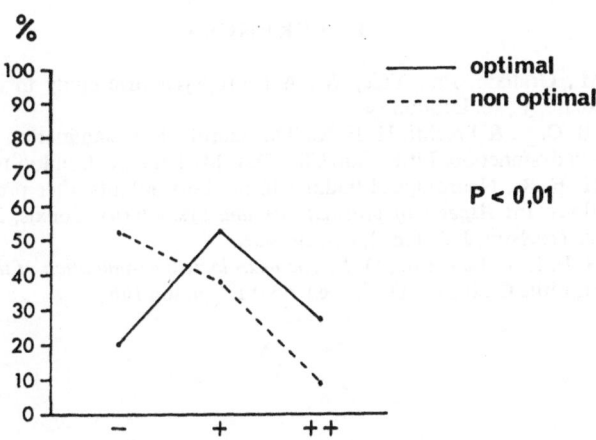

Fig. 5. The distribution of the scores for heel-toe gait in the neurologically optimal and non-optimal group.

Does this mean only a kind of typology of individual characteristics of normal children, or is this rather a gradation of neurological functioning with clinical significance? If so, our non-optimal children would represent cases suffering from minor brain dysfunction, but now within a strict neurological connotation, and not based on vague and ill-defined criteria. This question can be answered by means of other external criteria, such as behaviour (see p. 187).

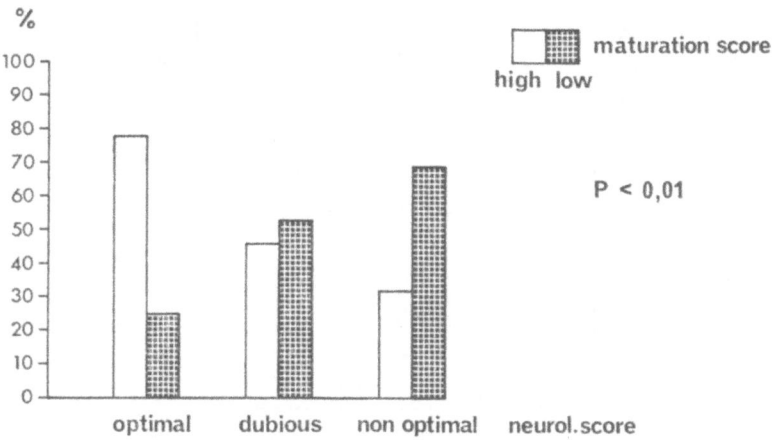

Fig. 6. The relationship between the neurological optimal scores and the maturity scores.

REFERENCES

1. Rutter, M., Graham, Ph., Yule, W., A neuropsychiatric study in childhood. Clin. Devl. Med. no. 35/36. London 1970.
2. Touwen, B. C. L. & Prechtl, H. F. R., The neurological examination of children with minor brain dysfunction. Little Club Clin. Dev. Med. no. 38, London 1970.
3. Prechtl, H. F. R., Neurological findings in newborn infants after pre- and paranatal complications. In: *Aspects of praematurity and dysmaturity.* Jonxis, J. H. P., Visser, H. K. A. & Troelstra, J. A. (eds.), Leiden 1968.
4. Prechtl, H. F. R. & Beintema, D. J., *The neurological examination of the full term newborn infant.* Little Club Clin. Devl. Med. no. 12. London 1964.

OBSERVATIONS OF FREE-FIELD BEHAVIOUR* IN PRE-SCHOOL BOYS AND GIRLS IN RELATION TO NEURO-LOGICAL FINDINGS**

A. F. KALVERBOER

INTRODUCTION

In his article 'Psychiatric implications of brain damage in children', published in 1957, Eisenberg put forward the view that the sequelae of brain damage are determined by 1. the alterations in the brain produced by the damage, 2. the reorganization of the personality in face of the deficit and 3. the influence of the social environment (1). Since then very little has been added to our knowledge of the association between brain damage and behavioural disturbances in children.

In general it is extremely difficult to determine how these three factors have been interacting, whenever a certain behavioural disorder becomes manifest. This is particularly true if the alterations in the brain are unknown, acquired in a life period in which the personality is not yet organized and in which the social environment has the profoundest influence on the behavioural organization.

This is the case in syndromes such as 'minimal brain dysfunction', 'minimal brain damage' etc., in which complex behavioural disorders are described as related to minor neurological dysfunctions. In this area there is an abundance of clinical descriptions, but a lack of experimental investigations. Behavioural, neurological and environmental variables have been badly defined or insufficiently controlled. Often children without any neurological signs are considered as suffering from 'minimal brain dysfunction', solely on the basis of behavioural phenomena, even though the relationship of the phenomena to the integrity of the nervous system is unclear (2).

* In a strict sense the term 'free-field behaviour' should be applied only for the behaviour in a natural environment. In human as well as in animal research this term is also used for the behaviour shown by a freely moving subject in a laboratory-setting (where the subject is only limited by the specific structure of the environment). In this paper we use the term in this last connotation.
** This project was supported by a grant from the Organization for Health Research T.N.O. (The Netherlands).

187

It is a fair estimate that approximately 10% of the children in a normal pre-school population are 'at risk' to develop learning and behavioural disturbances, which in one way or the other may be related to 'minor' neurological disorders. For the early detection and help of this group-studies in which objective and quantitative methods are applied for the assessment of nervous system and behaviour are necessary. In the follow-up project in pre-school children of which we present some first results here, an attempt has been made to meet these requirements.

As a technique for the evaluation of the nervous system we applied the method as described by Touwen and Prechtl (3).

To obtain information on 'clinically relevant' behaviours in our group of pre-school children, we analysed their 'free-field' behaviour in differently structured laboratory situations, applying descriptive categories.

This last method has been applied by ethologists in studies of exploratory behaviour in animals and recently by Hutt, Hutt and Ounsted in studies in brain damaged children (4). In such observations of spontaneous behaviour the investigator can focus on aspects of behaviour relevant in the study of brain – behaviour relationships in children, which are just interfering during psychometric testing, as there are motor-inconsistency, distractability, fluctuations in activity level, etc. Moreover, aspects of behaviour can be observed in the context of a larger behavioural repertoire, so that the complexity of the behavioural phenomena can be taken into account. The use of video- and audio-magnetic tape recordings enhances the refinement and reliability of the behavioural analysis.

In the course of the follow-up project on which we report here, carried out at the Department of Developmental Neurology, the 'free-field' behaviour of 150 pre-school children (between 4;10 and 5;3 years of age), all born in the University Hospital in Groningen, was systematically observed in a laboratory setting. Of each child detailed obstetrical data and results of neonatal neurological examination were available. Subjects for this follow-up study were selected on the basis of the neonatal neurological symptomatology: half of the group had shown minor neurological symptoms in the neonatal period, such as hyperexcitability, hypo- and hypertonia etc., the other half had not. At pre-school age all children lived in their homes. According to clinical citeria only two of them would have been considered as 'neurologically abnormal' (one hemiplegic and one imbecile boy). These cases were excluded from the analyses reported here.

Of the total group of children visited by a social case worker to participate in this study the drop-out percentage was as low as 10%.

The main objective of this project was to study the consequences of pre- and perinatal complications for the development of nervous system and behaviour. As a part of this study relationships between neurological and behavioural variables were thoroughly studied. In this presentation we focus on these relationships. As the statistical analysis of the data is still in progress only a few preliminary results can be reported here.

In this presentation we firstly mention some of the main differences observed in free-field behaviour between the total groups of boys and girls we observed and inspect if children with a different number of neurological signs contribute differently to these results. Secondly we focus on differences in free-field behaviour within the boys and the girls as related to the presence of minor neurological signs. Data are presented on relationships between a neurological optimality score, as given to each child and measures of motor, visual and verbal aspects of free-field behaviour.

Finally we briefly deal with the implications for complex behaviour of a single neurological symptom, specifically choreiform dyskinesia, a symptom which has led to some controversies in the literature (6, 7).

EXPERIMENTAL DESIGN

1. *General procedure*

Apart from the neurological examination and the behavioural observations mentioned already, each child had a psychometric examination focussing on intellectual and visuo-motor functions. Furthermore data on the social situation of the family and on the behaviour of the child at home and in school were collected. Behavioural, neurological, psychometric and social data were gathered by different examiners independent of each other and without knowledge of the obstetrical and neonatal neurological findings.

2. *The observation of free-field behaviour*

Each child was observed in a playing room on the floor of which there was a checkerboard pattern (Fig. 1). This room was in many respects similar to that employed by Hutt, Hutt and Ounsted (4). Video-recordings were made from behind a one-way mirror and with a fixed camera in the room, sound was recorded with a (hidden) microphone.

Each child was observed in 6 experimental conditions, always in the following sequence:

1. Together with mother in the empty room (3 min.). The mother was sitting on a stool on square a_4 (Fig. 1) and was asked not to interfere with the child's behaviour.
2. Alone in the empty room (3 min.).
3. With a box of blocks on square b_2 and a passive observer sitting on square d_6 (10 min.).
4. Alone in the empty room (3 min.).
5. Alone with a variety of toys (15 min.).
6. Alone with only one 'non-motivating' toy (5 min.): only the least manipulated toy of the previous condition was left in the room.

In all experimental conditions the child was allowed to move around freely.

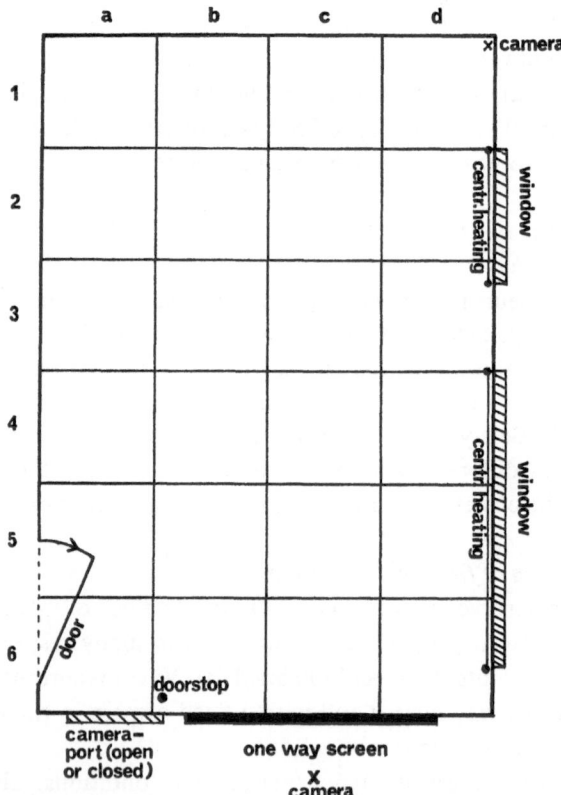

Fig. 1. Plan of the observation room. The squares represent the block pattern on the floor. Each square is 80 × 80 cm.

3. *Behavioural variables*

Aspects of motor, visual and verbal behaviour, as listed in table I, were scored from video-audio tapes. In situations in which toys were present additional scores were given for level of play activity and number of play objects, handled by the child. To score contact with mother the categories, as listed at the bottom of table I, were applied. Most of the behavioural variables were continuously scored throughout the entire observation period, so that for each of these variables a total score for each observation period was obtained. For more refined analyses the observation time was split up into 10 second epochs. In this paper only differences between the *total scores* will be reported.

For all these scores the interobserver-agreement was above 70% (the highest for locomotion: approx. 95%; the lowest for visual fixations: approx. 75%)*.

4. *The neurological optimality score*

In each child the condition of the nervous system was expressed in a so-called 'optimality score' (see Touwen, p. 179 of this volume). For each child such a score was obtained by summing-up those items out of a pre-determined list of 37 items of the neurological examination on which the child's score was within a previously defined optimal range. Items are included on motor coordination, kinesia, muscle tone, etc.

According to the optimality score the total group was divided into three sub-groups: an 'optimal group' with 35 or more optimal conditions, a 'medium group' with 30-34 optimal conditions and a 'non-optimal group' with less than 30 optimal conditions. Cutting points between classes were set by the neurologist independent of the results of the behavioural analysis. In this report we mainly focus on differences in 'free-field' behaviour between the *optimal* and the *non-optimal* group. Between these groups no significant differences in IQ, social class and rank-number at birth were found.

[Knowledge of the functional significance of these minor neurological signs for behaviour and of their interrelationships is scarce, normative data for children of different ages are not yet available. Therefore we feel it as a good strategy to start our analysis with the application of this optimality-score as a *quantitative overall measure* for the intactness of the nervous functions. As will be pointed out at the end of this presentation it allows for a more refined inspection of relationships between neurological and behavioural phenomena in later phases of the analysis.]

* In a later publication on the methodology of these observations more detailed data on the statistical properties of these measures will be presented.

Table 1. Categories applied in the observation of 'free-field' – behaviour in children.[a]

Behavioural category	Operationalization	Example
Locomotion	Number of 'blocks' covered.	
Postures	Number of times a posture is observed from a list of postural categories.	Standing upright, lying.
Types of movement	Number of times a type of movement is observed from a predetermined list.	Walking, hopping.
Object-manipulations	Number of times the child manipulates fixtures in the room (stool included).	Tapping the radiator, twisting the doorstop.
Self-manipulations	Number of times the child manipulates his own body or clothes.	Scratching his face, fumbling in his pocket.
Gestures	Number of times non-verbal, communicative movements are observed.	Pointing at an object, arm movements in relation to verbalization.
Additional movements	Number of times, movements are observed, which are not part of movement-patterns of locomotion, manipulation or communication.[b]	Waving his arms, rocking.
Visual fixations	Number of times the child looks at an object for 1" or longer.	
Visual scanning	Number of times the child looks around, without focussing a specific object for 1" or longer.	
Spatial contact with mother	Number of 10" epochs in which the child covers a block, adjacent to block a-4 (see fig. 1).	
Visual contact with mother	Number of 10" epochs in which the child looks at the mother for 1" or longer.	
Tactile contact with mother	Number of 10" epochs in which the child touches the mother.	
Verbal contact with mother	Number of 10" epochs in which the child talks to the mother.	

[a] This categorization is partly based on the work of Berkson (8) and Hutt et al. (4).
[b] Movements towards the one-way mirror are scored in a separate category.

RESULTS AND COMMENTS

1. *Boys' vs girls' behaviour: differences between total groups and between comparable optimality classes*

In a previous paper we reported differences in behaviour between boys and girls in an unfamiliar room in presence of the mother, the 1st condition in our series of observations (5). In subsequent analyses differences between the sexes were also found in the other five experimental conditions.

Here we only report some of the main findings (a detailed publication on these results is in preparation).

a. In all conditions *without toys* the boys showed more manipulations of 'fixtures' in the room, whereas in girls more manipulations of their own clothes and body were observed.

b. In all conditions *with toys* boys showed far more locomotion and variability in movement patterns and body postures than girls (a difference independent of the particular toys chosen by boys and girls).

c. In the condition '*alone with one non-motivating toy*', (labelled for convenience as: non-motivating condition) in boys more low-level activities were observed (such as: throwing toys away, simply piling up blocks etc.) than in girls, whereas in the other play-condition no such differences between boys' and girls' playing-level could be found. It appeared that the boys reacted stronger to the lack of motivating stimuli than the girls.

In the light of our topic 'free-field behaviour in relation to neurological findings' it is especially interesting to inspect in how much each of the neurological classes contributed to the differences between the total groups of boys and girls. A comparison of the same neurological classes in boys and girls (opt. boys vs opt. girls, medium boys vs medium girls, non-optimal boys vs non-optimal girls) gave the following interesting results.

– Differences in manipulations of fixtures (more in boys) and self-manipulations (more in girls) were found between the optimal, the medium, as well as the non-optimal groups.

– Differences between the *optimal* groups in *amount* and *variability of gross motor activity* were only found *in two of the play-conditions* (with blocks, with a variety of toys), whereas between the *non-optimal* groups such differences were present *in each of the 6 experimental conditions*: non-optimal boys showed invariably more changes in body postures and movement patterns than non-optimal girls, irrespective of the presence of play objects. It seems *plausible that the differences between the optimals merely reflect the normal differences in playing behaviour between the sexes, whereas differences in handling the toys can only partly explain the differences in motor-activity between the non-optimal groups.*

– Play activities at a low level in the 'non-motivating' condition were found more in the medium and non-optimal classes in the boys than in the same classes in the girls. This aspect did not discriminate between the optimal classes in boys and girls.

Other differences were found between the total groups to which the optimality classes contributed differently, but these will not be reported here. The main point we wish to make from the examples given here is that *in our study the non-optimal groups contributed more to the overall differences between boys and girls than the optimal groups.* In a random sample of boys the number of children with minor neurological dysfunctions is higher than in such a sample in girls. This factor can partly account for behavioural differences between such groups.

2. *Differences between 'optimals' and 'non-optimals' within each sex-group*
In the tables 2, 3 and 4 data are presented on the differences in behaviour between optimal and non-optimal groups in boys and girls.
     A global inspection of the data shows clear-cut differences between the results in boys and girls: the number of significant differences between optimals and non-optimals is much higher in boys than in girls. Out of 60 differences on motor and visual activity measures tested for significance (see table 2), in the boys 26, in the girls only 10 are significant below 10% level. Out of 21 differences on measures of play-activity (see table 3) 8 were significant below 10% for boys, only 3 for girls.
     Since there are a number of intercorrelations between the behavioural variables we must be careful in drawing conclusions (here we can not go into the details of these interrelationships). Nevertheless *these results may indicate that the neurological condition, as operationalized in an optimality score has a stronger relationship to free-field behaviour in boys than in girls.* In our studies this is especially true for variables on amount and consistency in motor-activity and for play-activity measures.

DIFFERENCES BETWEEN OPTIMALITY-GROUPS IN BOYS
In *boys* significant differences between optimals and non-optimals were observed in each of the 6 experimental conditions, the most pronounced in the two conditions: 'for the second time alone in the empty room' and

Table 2. Free-field behaviour: motor- and visual activity. Optimal vs non-optimal groups. Differences between total scores on each of the variables are two-tailed tested (Mann-Whitney U test). Op and n.op indicate which group has highest score on a particular variable (*: no significant difference).

| | Boys ($N_{opt} = 15$; $N_{n,opt} = 23$) | | | | | | Girls ($N_{opt} = 20$; $N_{n,opt} = 14$) | | | | | |
| | No toys present | | | Toys present | | | No toys present | | | Toys present | | |
	With mother	Alone 1st time	Alone 2nd time	Blocks	Diff. toys	Non-mot. toy	With mother	Alone 1st time	Alone 2nd time	Blocks	Diff. toys	Non-mot. toy
Locomotion	*	*	*	*	*	n.op .05	*	*	*	*	*	*
Nr. of postures	n.op .02	n.op .09	n.op .01	n.op .03	*	n.op .08	*	*	*	n.op .08	*	*
Types of postures	n.op .001	n.op .06	n.op .01	n.op .05	*	n.op .01	*	*	*	n.op .09	*	*
Changes in movement patterns	*	n.op .10	n.op .10	*	*	n.op .09	*	*	*	*	*	*
Types of movement patterns	*	*	n.op .04	*	op .02	n.op .02	*	*	op .06	*	*	*
Additional movements	*	*	n.op .05	*	*	*	*	*	*	*	*	*
Movements toward one-way screen	*	*	*	*	op .10	*	n.op .03	*	*	*	*	*
Object manipulations	*	*	*	*	op .02	op .07	op .001	*	*	*	*	*
Manipulations of own body or clothes	*	*	*	*	n.op .08	op .08	*	*	*	*	*	op .05
Visual exploration of room	op .08	*	op .02	*	*	op .05	n.op .03	n.op .06	*	*	n.op .04	n.op .02

Table 3. Free-field behaviour: play-activity. Optimal vs non-optimal groups. See also legend to table 2.

	Boys ($N_{opt} = 15$; $N_{n,opt} = 23$)			Girls ($N_{opt} = 20$; $N_{n,opt} = 14$)		
	Blocks	Diff. toys	Non-motiv. toy	Blocks	Diff. toys	Non-motiv. toy
Play-activity level 1	*	*	n.op .03	*	*	*
,, ,, level 2	*	*	n.op .01	*	*	*
,, ,, level 3	*	*	*	*	*	*
,, ,, level 4	*	n.op .01	op .01	*	op .08	*
Changes in activity level	n.op .02	*	n.op .01	*	*	*
Longest activity duration	*	n.op .08	*	*	*	*
No play activity	n.op .05	*	*	op .05		op .06

'alone with one non-motivating toy' (see tables 2 and 3). In this last condition non-optimal boys show more changes in posture, in movement patterns and activity-level during playing than the optimal boys. Furthermore they show more low-level play-activity (as previously mentioned) than optimals in this non-motivating condition, whereas the last group is more involved in constructive play. As can be seen in the tables 2 and 3 no such differences between optimal and non-optimal boys were found in the preceding condition with a variety of toys, in which the non-optimal boys played even at a higher level than the optimals. *This finding may imply that in an environment with an (optimal!) variety of stimulating input boys with minor neurological signs (as our non-optimals are) can function quite well, whereas in conditions characterized by a lack of stimulating input the non-optimal boys drop to a lower level of activity and show less consistency in their motor and play activities than the optimals.*

The results of the boys obtained in the conditions: 'first and second time alone in the empty room' fit quite well with this supposition. This is illustrated in figure 2 for the variable: visual exploration of the room.

When for the first time alone, the non-optimal boys show a slight non-significant tendency to spend more time in visual exploration than the optimal boys. A remarkable change, however, takes place during the second time alone: the non-optimal boys show a clearcut drop in their exploration of the room, which is not observed in the optimals. The same drop although less pronounced is found in the non-optimal girls whereas again the optimals show only a slight non-significant difference in exploratory activity between these two situations. For both sexes the medium groups get results in between those of the optimals and the non-optimals. *It appears that non-optimal boys (and to a lesser extent non-optimal girls) are quicker 'satiated' by the environmental stimuli than optimals.* The non-optimal children need more variation of stimuli to remain interested in the environment.

DIFFERENCES BETWEEN OPTIMALITY-GROUPS IN GIRLS

As is shown in the tables 2 and 3 in *girls* differences between optimal and non-optimal groups are smaller and less consistent than in boys. Moreover associations between neurological score and behaviour manifest themselves in a different way. Only in the situation 'together with mother in the empty room', the first of the observation situations, are there clear-cut differences between non-optimal and optimal girls (tables 2 and 4).

In this situation non-optimal girls react much more to the one-way mirror than optimals, showing a lot of body movements while looking at the mirror. The optimal girls keep more in contact with the mother and show more manipulations of their own body and clothes than the non-optimals. It appears that the optimal girls feel less secure in this unfamiliar environment than the non-optimals. A trend in the same direction is observed in the non-motivating condition: here again the optimal girls tend to react more pass-

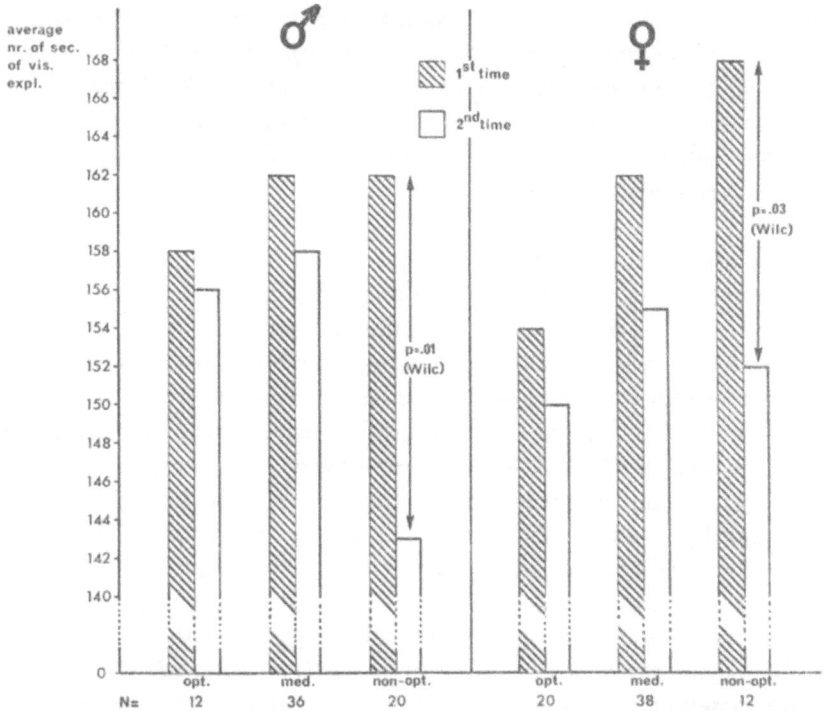

Fig. 2. Average time spent in visual exploration during the 1st and the 2nd time alone in the empty room. The drop in amount of visual exploration reaches significance only in the non-optimal groups (Wilcoxon two-tailed test).

Table 4. Free-field behaviour: contact with mother in an unfamiliar room. Optimal vs non-optimal groups. See also legend to table 2.

	Boys (N_{opt} = 15; $N_{n.opt}$ = 23)	(Girls N_{opt} = 20; $N_{n.opt}$ = 14)
Tactile contact with mother	n.op .05	*
Spatial ,, ,, ,,	*	opt .01
Visual ,, ,, ,,	*	*
Verbal ,, ,, ,,	*	opt .06

ively and support-seeking than the non-optimals, weeping more, showing more self-manipulations, less visual exploration and play-activity than the non-optimal girls. A short comment on these results.

The above data suggest a different relationship between neurological dysfunctions and free-field behaviour in boys than in girls. Behavioural variables, which discriminate between the neurologically optimals and non-optimals are quite different in both sex-groups. 'Motor inconsistency' and 'level of play-activity' only discriminate between the two groups of boys, but do not differentiate at all in the girls. On the other hand, 'contacting the mother' and 'manipulating the own body and clothes' only discriminate between the neurological groups in the girls. To clarify the meaning of these differences further analyses are necessary especially as to the composition of the neurological compound score in boys and girls and the interrelationship of the behavioural variables.

It is interesting to note that the variable 'locomotion' (= the number of blocks covered during an experimental condition) hardly discriminates between neurological optimality classes (only slight differences in boys were found in the non-motivating condition). Further analyses must demonstrate if possibly the variability in locomotion during an experimental condition will differentiate between our groups. Up till now our findings on this aspect of motor activity are in agreement with results of studies in which not the 'amount' but the 'consistency' and 'situational appropriateness' of the motor activity discriminated between children with and without neurological disorders (9, 10).

Finally I wish to point out briefly how the relationship between minor neurological symptoms and behaviour can be analysed in greater detail applying the optimality score.

To gain more insight in the significance of a specific neurological dysfunction for behaviour, complete neurological data must be available. Then the first step can be to classify the cases according to the *number* of minor neurological signs.

The analyses can proceed along the following lines:

First the behaviour can be compared in groups of children of which only one group shows a specific neurological symptom or dysfunction, whereas the groups are matched for the number of additional deviant findings. The results of such an analysis can shed some light on *the significance* for the behavioural aspects on which one focusses *of that particular neurological symptom*.

The next step can be the comparison of groups all of which show a particular neurological symptom whereas they differ as to the number of additional non-optimal signs. Such an analysis gives information on *the significance of these additional deviant signs*.

These ways of analyses represent only a starting point of how one can apply quantitative neurological data (such as optimality scores) to obtain insight in the association between specific neurological dysfunctions and behavioural variables.

This may be illustrated with a few results concerning the significance of choreiform dyskinesia for behaviour.

The conflicting findings on the implications of this neurological symptom for behaviour are due to differences between the samples of children observed by different investigators (children selected at random from a normal population, children who had already developed learning and/or behavioural disorders, children who visited an out-patient clinic etc.), and to the lack of a complete evaluation of the nervous functions in most studies. In general behavioural variables were only correlated with choreiform jerks in the fingers. It remained unknown whether other neurological deficits influenced the behavioural phenomena.

Following the strategy pointed out above we first compared the behaviour of groups of choreiform and non-choreiform children who were matched for the number of other non-optimal neurological signs. In the boys differences between these two groups were found, especially in the non-motivating condition. In this condition the choreiform boys showed more changes in activity level during playing and more changes in body posture than the non-choreiform boys. This result suggests that in boys choreiform dyskinesia is related to specific aspects of the 'free-field' behaviour. Such a relationship was not found in the girls.

Secondly we compared choreiform children who had a relatively high optimality score with choreiform children with a low optimality score. Again significant differences in behaviour were found in the boys.

In the non-motivating situation choreiform boys with high optimality scores showed less locomotion and a higher level of play-activity than choreiforms with low optimality scores.

Evidently, minor neurological signs which compose our optimality score relate to behaviour in a different way. For example: *choreiform dyskinesia* is in our group of boys associated with *inconsistency* in motor-activity and play-behaviour, whereas *other minor neurological signs* influence the level of play-activity and the *amount* of locomotion. Analyses of this kind give us a more refined picture of the relationships between minor neurological dysfunctions and behaviour, which can not be obtained when 'syncretic' concepts such as 'minimal brain dysfunction' are applied.

CONCLUDING REMARKS

In this paper some preliminary results were presented of observations of free-field behaviour in pre-school children, as they are related to neurological variables. Multivariate statistical analyses are in progress to study in greater detail the complicated interrelationships. Therefore I will confine myself here to a few remarks.

1. Literature on 'minimal brain damage' or 'minimal brain dysfunction' inevitably deals with *school age children* (between 6 and 13 years of age) *in whom learning and/or behavioural disorders have developed already*. In this follow-up study relationships between neurological findings and aspects of the free-field behaviour in differently structured laboratory settings could be shown in a group of *'clinically normal' pre-school children* who were *not selected on the basis of behavioural problems*. Refined techniques for the assessment of nervous functions and behaviour, as we have attempted to apply, may be relevant for the detection of children 'at risk' early enough to prevent them from developing more serious disturbances.

2. Concepts such as 'minimal brain dysfunction', if considered as 'clinical syndromes', which suggest a more or less 'fixed relationship' between behaviour and neurological signs, are unfit for research in this field. They suggest solutions which are not yet available. Concepts are necessary, which allow for a detailed analysis of relationships. Neurological optimality, containing only neurological items, seems to be such a concept.

3. The observation and analysis in descriptive terms of 'spontaneous' behaviour may be considered as a very useful method in the study of brain-behaviour relationships in younger children. One of the advantages of such observations is that one can focus on aspects of behaviour such as motor-inconsistency, fluctuations in level of activity, distractibility etc., which especially in younger children, may affect the results of psychometric tests, resulting in unreliable findings.

4. The results of this study illustrate that in the analysis of behaviour in relation to neurological findings in children the sex of the subjects must be taken into account: neurological signs have a different distribution in each

of the sexes; furthermore there is evidence from our data that the presence of neurological signs has stronger implications for behaviour in boys than in girls.

SUMMARY

In the course of a follow-up project, focussing on consequences of pre- and perinatal complications for the later development, the 'free-field' behaviour in a group of approx. 150 'clinically normal' pre-school children was systematically observed in differently structured laboratory-settings. Motor, visual and verbal behaviour were analysed from video-audio tapes.

According to results of a standardized neurological examination groups of children could be discriminated, which differed in the number of 'optimal' neurological signs. Some first data on behavioural differences between optimals and non-optimals are presented in this report.

Significant relationships between the neurological condition and aspects of behaviour are found in both sexes. They are stronger in boys than in girls.

Non-optimal boys show more fluctuations in motor-activity as a reaction to 'lack of sensory input' or 'lack of motivating toys' than optimal boys. In this last condition they play at a lower level than optimal boys, which is not the case in a condition in which a variety of motivating toys is available.

Non-optimal girls show less support seeking behaviour in a novel situation with mother than optimal girls.

Both non-optimal boys and girls show a clear-cut drop in visual exploration from the 1st to the 2nd time alone in the empty room, which is not found in the other groups.

Practical and methodological implications of the results are shortly discussed.

ACKNOWLEDGEMENTS

I am greatly indebted to Mrs H. Sanders and Mrs J. H. van Dijk for the analysis of the video-recordings and the coding of the data. Further my thanks are due to Prof. H. F. R. Prechtl, Dr Y. Akiyama and Dr P. Casaer for their help and criticism in the preparation of this paper and to Miss W. van Dijk, Miss G. Hindriks and Miss F. van der Velde for their assistance.

REFERENCES

1. Eisenberg, L., Psychiatric implications of brain damage in children. *Psychiat. Quart.* 1, 21 (1957).
2. Zimet, C. N. & Fishman, D. B., Psychological deficit in schizophrenia and brain damage. *Ann. Rev. Psychol.* 21, 113 (1970).
3. Touwen, B. C. L. & Prechtl, H. F. R., *The neurological examination of the child with minor nervous dysfunction.* Little club Clin. dev. Med., London 1971.
4. Hutt, C., Hutt, S. J. & Ounsted, C., The behaviour of children with and without upper CNS lesions. *Behaviour* 24, 246 (1965).
5. Kalverboer, A. F., Observation of exploratory behaviour of preschool children alone and in the presence of the mother. *Psychiat. Neurol. Neurochir.* 74, 43 (1971).
6. Stemmer, Chr. J., *Choreatiforme bewegingsonrust*, Groningen 1964.
7. Rutter, M., Graham, P. & Birch, H. G., Interrelation between the choreiform syndrome, reading disability and psychiatric disorder in 8 to 11 years old children. *Develop. Med. Child Neurol.* 8, 149 (1966).
8. Berkson, G., Stereotyped movements of mental defectives, part 5 (Ward behavior and its relation to an experimental task). *Am. J. Ment. Defic.* 69, 253 (1969).
9. Benton, A. L., Behavioral indices of brain injury in school children. *Child Develop.* 33, 199 (1962).
10. Schulman, J. L., Kaspar, J. C. & Throne, F. M., *Brain damage and behavior (a clinical experimental study)*. Springfield (Ill.) 1965.
11. Reed, H. B. C., Reitan, R. M. & Kløve, H., Influence of cerebral lesions on psychological test performances of older children. *J. Consult. Psychol.* 29, 247 (1965).

DISCUSSION

Roebers: Prof. Snijders has developed an intelligence test for children. This test may be extremely valuable also for children if brain-damaged. I should like to ask you if there is any experience with children with minimal brain damage.

Kalverboer: The Snijders-Oomen test is a non-verbal test consisting of four subtests (mosaic, visual memory, picture assembly and analogies) on visuo-motor functioning, visual memory, concrete and abstract reasoning. My own experiences with this test are with 'candidates' for a special school for children with learning and behavioural disorders, many of whom are considered as suffering from 'minor brain dysfunction'. These children show quite different 'test-profiles'. Relatively often, however, the visuo-motor functions are impaired, implying low scores on the mosaic subtest, while scores on the visual memory subtest are relatively high. Often the basis of the visuo-motor difficulties is the inability to structure the behaviour temporally and spatially. If the examiner presents to the children a certain 'strategy' e.g. by saying: 'start with copying the top line of the model, then take the second line and so on', they generally are able to do it. That was one experience. Many people feel that in children with minor brain dysfunction the whole 'test-profile' is less homogeneous than in normal children. However, the findings are quite contradictory. Reed (11) found that scores on verbal tests were often lower than on visuo-motor tests, while other authors found just the reverse. One of the things about tests such as the Snijders-Oomen test and many others, is that the way in which a child arrives at a solution is perhaps much more important than the final result. Therefore, tests which evaluate the methods by which the child arrives at a solution are needed.

Roebers: Yes, I agree with you. But I think it extremely important to follow up one test, the test one has used before. And I think this particular test seems to be a quite suitable test for a follow-up.

Kalverboer: I don't know. In a way I agree with Dr Freedman, when he said that we have to design our instruments and observational situations starting from the problems that we have. Well, Snijders started with the problem of how to evaluate intellectual abilities in deaf children. Later, norms were also developed for hearing children. Now it may happen that this instrument discriminates also between groups of a different neurological condition, although it has not been developed for this purpose. As long as no other instruments are available, they are useful. Better, however, are tests designed on the basis of theoretical considerations and empirical data concerning relationships between brain and behaviour, such as the Hallsteadt-Reitan-test.

Roebers: I have known children with the diagnosis minimal brain damage and I think the term minimal is somewhat dangerous. What is minimal? The term brain damage too. What is damage and who can prove that a child of which I only have anamnestic data was really minimally damaged or damaged at all? Some such children had choreatiform movements, and in some these choreatiform movements, the dyskinesia, disappeared after some years. There was improvement in motor function and disappearance of visible small dyskinesias and also all of these children had a significant improvement in IQ. Both in the total IQ and in the profile of this particular test I mentioned. So they had improvement of motor and psychological functions. But the greatest difficulty remained with arithmetics. That was the handicap for those children at school. And some of them had normal general IQ's but in arithmetics they were absolutely sub-normal and they stayed sub-normal.

Van Uden: Could you explain somewhat further what you mean by choreatiform motor behaviour.

Kalverboer: Well, choreatiform movements are in fact sudden jerks one can observe in the fingers, the arms, the trunk, the face and the tongue. They can be more or less generalized over the entire body and they are often thought to indicate a certain lability of the nervous system. There have been a lot of studies in which these signs were related to very complex behavioural difficulties. In my opinion such conclusions went too far. There are a lot of children with choreiform movements who do not show any behavioural difficulties. If we compare *choreatiform* children from a normal primary school (and there are quite a number of them there) with *non-choreatiform* children from a school for children with learning difficulties, we find that the behaviours generally attributed to choreiformity, occur much more frequently in the *non-choreatiform* children of the special school than in the *choreatiform* children of the normal primary school. So the relationship must be much more complex.

Van der Werff ten Bosch: I am worried about the term 'neurological optimality'. To what extent do you defeat your own purposes by taking a mixed bag of symptoms and signs that you collectively call symptoms of neurological optimality or non-optimality.

Kalverboer: I shall perhaps pass this question on to the earlier speaker (Touwen), but first I would like to say one thing. In my opinion the optimality-score is an operational concept, which is the starting-point for the analyses of brain-behaviour-relationships in these children with minor neurological dysfunctions. It is true that the most simple method one can use is simply adding up your signs. But that is only a starting-point. In psychology it is known from behavioural questionnaires that simply adding up item-scores is often the best procedure. It is quite good to start with a sort of overall measure, however crude it may seem, of the functions of the nervous system. It is possible, as I tried to stress in this presentation, to work with this concept. In subsequent analyses one can try to further define the behavioural and neurological characteristics of different sub-groups within the original optimal and non-optimal groups. I think, therefore, that optimality is a useful operational concept.

Van der Werff ten Bosch: This is like Dr Dobbing's work, isn't it. He would probably be the first to agree that this is comparable to the way he deals with the chemistry of the brain. I don't object to it, I was just wondering how you know where you can go from here, and this applies to the various speakers which have gone before.

Prechtl: I was actually expecting this question since this issue may be somewhat confusing. What has not been said is that, of course, if you want to treat a patient for convulsions you will not be terribly interested in his neurological optimality score but you will want to know exactly what the clinical symptoms are. On the other hand, very often children who are sent to the neurologist are referred back to the psychologist with the message that there is nothing wrong. Their reflexes were found to be all right and perhaps the EEG has been borderline. However, if you can then discriminate within this group a gradation of optimal functions with a detailed age specific neurological examination, I think this is clinically a very helpful step. In addition there is the problem of the relationship between obstetrical data on which I developed originally this optimality concept. You can see now in England the complete failure of 'at risk registers' which relied on counting up complications. You end with almost 60% of your population of new-borns falling into the at risk group, but, of course, nobody can handle this 60%. Instead, put the whole thing in reverse order, look up who are the babies who are the best off and who are the worst off according to the op-timality score. Then put your cutting point wherever it is meaningful. If you have in your national health service the capacity for dealing with say 12 or 17% of the newborns, well then you know which score is the cutting point for the 12th or 17th percentiles of the lowest range. This seems to be the solution to that problem. In addition, if you want to analyse the sequelae in the infant of, let's say, toxaemia of the mother or of foetal distress, or if you pull out a group of asphyxiated newborns and compare them with a control group you will end up with rather meaningless results, if you don't look very carefully at all the other items in the obstetrical history. But there are de-finitely clinical problems which can not be solved by this optimality score, which I have, of course, never intended.

Goldfoot: Should not other methods for the statistical analyses of the data be applied. I think multivariate statistics might be applicable in your work.

Kalverboer: I am glad that you ask this question. At the same time, I expect you are glad that I did not attempt to go into complicated statistical proce-dures during this 20 minute lecture. In this presentation I had to confine my-self to some very simple illustrations of my points. However, in fact several 'sophisticated' statistical methods were used. First we applied the so-called 'Zaehl-program' which gave us frequency-distributions per variable and scatterplots of relationships between different aspects of the behaviour we observed. This information is crucial for the interpretation of more abstract statistical measures such as correlation-coefficients, factor- or cluster-scores etc., which we calculated afterwards. In this presentation I confined myself to results obtained with simple statistical techniques on rather global aspects of the behaviour (namely total scores over the entire observation period). One refinement will be the analysis of differences in the temporal organisa-tion of the behaviour. How did behaviour change from minute to minute or from 10"-epoch to 10"-epoch? It needs no account that these are time-con-suming procedures, not fitted to discuss in this 20"-presentation, but essential in the analysis of these complex data.

GENETIC INFLUENCES ON DEVELOPMENT OF BEHAVIOR

D. G. FREEDMAN

Logically speaking, genes must influence *all* behavior, to some extent at least. Otherwise one is faced with the unacceptable concept of behavior which is independent of structure. Not only is this a logical position, but there is evidence for it as well. I refer here to a demonstrable trend in studies of twins, to wit, the greater the number of twins, the greater the number of behavioral items which are significantly more alike among the identical pairs (1). If one were to project this trend to an infinite number of twins, it would indeed appear that *all* differences in behavior could be related to variations in genotype.

Let us, therefore, start this paper by taking the position which Hebb (2) promulgated, that all behavior is 100% inherited and 100% acquired. (Indeed, in the behavior-genetic literature, no bio-statistician has yet been able to get rid of a residual Heredity by Environment factor.) This will serve to rid us of a host of pseudo-problems at the outset, and enable us to better concentrate on the presentation of data.

ONE, TWO, OR MANY GENES

Before we get to the data, a few words on what constitutes a demonstration of genetic cause or influence. Usually, when we talk of genetic influences on behavior, we are talking about the *difference* between two groups, e.g., between two inbred groups, or between groups of fraternal versus identical twins. Such studies usually demonstrate only that genetics is playing some kind of (unknown) role.

The classical Mendelian study, therefore, has much more scientific merit, for here we have the possibility of relating specific genes and specific behavior. Consequently, a number of pioneering behavior-geneticists have striven, through Mendelian studies of fruit flies, mice, and dogs to duplicate classical studies on structure. What have we learned from such studies?

As I read it, the problems are precisely those which faced the great geneticist Morgan in the 1920's. For example, while he knew the location of the single gene which caused white eyes in Drosophila, Morgan estimated that at least 50 unknown genes played a role in *normal* eye coloration. And so it was for every other trait: wing-veinlessness, a single gene; normal veination, probably hundreds of genes, and so on. Classical genetics has taught us precious little about normal structure or normal development.

The same situation holds for behavior. Phenylketonuria is the result of a single recessive gene which apparently causes an enzyme block, which in turn interferes with normal metabolism, which then results in mental deficiency. Other mental deficiencies may be traced to various chromosomal trisomies, and with each year new cause-effect relations are found between genetic anomaly and mental defect. The genetics of mental *efficiency*, on the other hand, are vastly complex, and hardly illuminated by the aforementioned work. Many more examples are available (3) and it would appear that Mendelian inheritance has been demonstrable only in defective structure or function. Traits which have proved phylogenetically adaptive are invariably polygenic, i.e., they have invariably accumulated a substantial number of supporting genes.

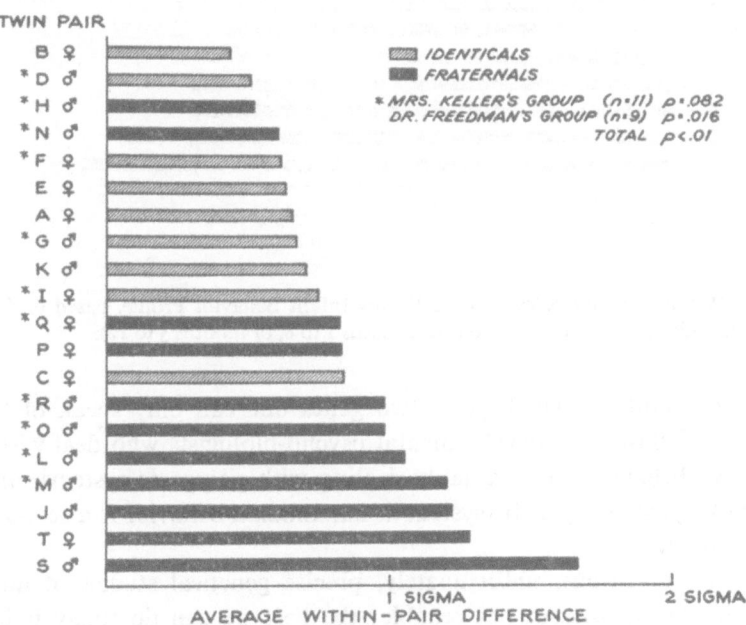

Fig. 1. Within-pair differences on the Bayley Mental and Motor Scales, based on 8-10 administrations over the first year of life. There were two investigators.

While some will argue against this position, perhaps as a matter of faith, we have yet to see a demonstration of a single gene which accounts for a substantial part of the variance in a normal behavioral trait (4). This generality holds as well for two-gene systems (my friend, Benson Ginsburg's (5) excellent work with audiogenic seizures in mice notwithstanding). And, as

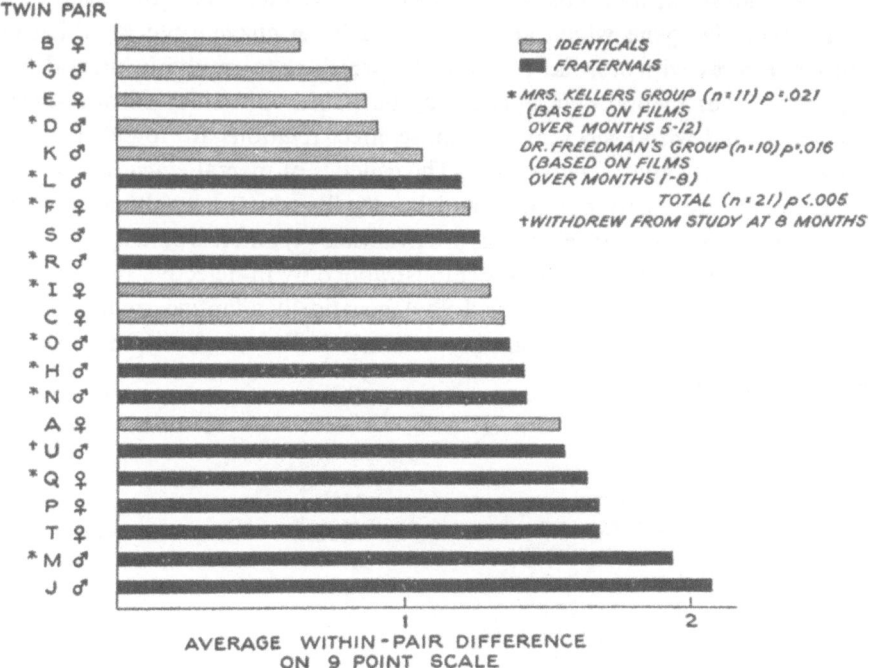

Fig. 2. Within-pair differences on the Bayley Infant Behavior Profile, based on 8 consecutive months of filmed behavior (either months 1 to 8, or months 5 to 12).

Crow has aptly stated, beyond two genes one can only speak of 'many' genes. It follows that developmental psycho-biologists who deal with nondefective behavior are invariably dealing with polygenic systems, and the search for a simple genetic system in mammalian behavior is a search for a will-o'-the-wisp.

For these reasons, unfortunately, precise genetical studies of adaptive behavior are at present not tenable; the best we can do today is impute genetic cause for the differences we find between our experimental groups. The rest of this paper is comprised of such data.

INDIVIDUAL GENETIC VARIATION IN HUMAN SOCIAL BEHAVIOR

Ever since Galton, demonstration of an hereditary basis for a behavioral trait has usually been via the twin-method, and considerable data are now available to the effect that identical twins score more alike than do same-sexed fraternals on a variety of measures, ranging from primary mental abilities to personality tests (6). The conclusion that heredity plays a role in these behaviors would seem incontrovertible, but certain difficulties with the twin-method, such as the possibility of more mutual imitation within identical pairs, has served to blunt these results.

Our own contribution to this area has been via investigations of *infant*-twins over the first year, i.e., before mutual imitation is a factor. We were nevertheless able to show that the results in infancy are of the same order as those found with older twins, a result which helps boost the validity of all studies on twins not reared apart.

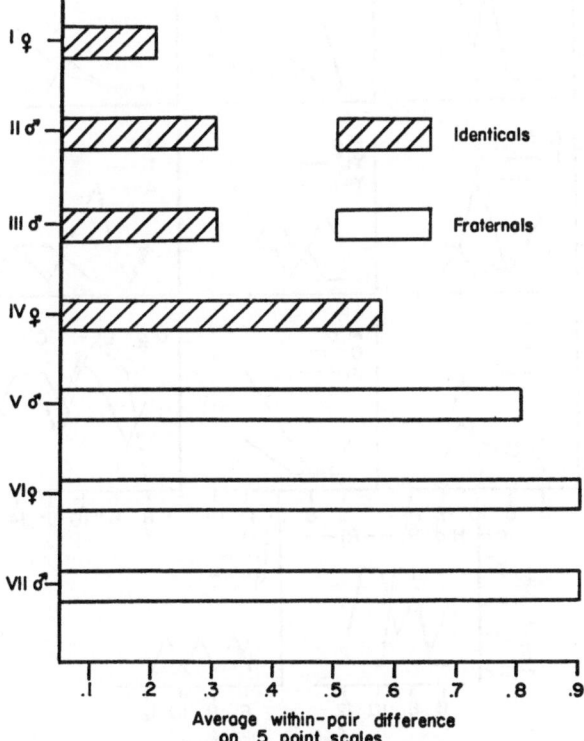

Fig. 3. Seven pairs of twins; attending, smiling and vocalizing to mother and to the experimenter were each scored separately on 5 point scales, and the scales averaged over the first four months of life. Average number of home visits was 10 (range 7-14).

As an example of our work, figures 1 and 2 represent intra-pair differences over the first year on the Bayley Mental and Motor Scales and the Bayley Infant Behavior Profile (7). On the Behavior Profile, a rating scale assessing infant personality, we were able to eliminate any 'halo' effect of one twin on the other by having each twin's *filmed behavior* rated by separate groups of judges. It is clear that identical twins were seen as substantially more alike than fraternals.

One scale on the Infant Behavior Profile, 'Social Interest' (in experimenter and in mother), was of particular interest to us (p <.005, identicals more alike over the first year). In order to assure ourselves of its correctness, we followed an additional four pairs of fraternal and three pairs of identical twins on a *weekly* basis, from birth through five months of age.[1] On the

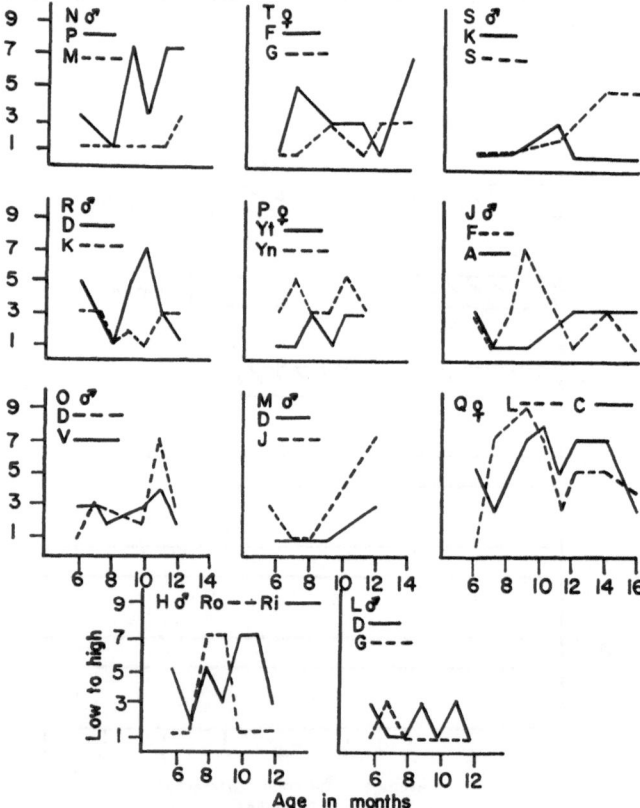

Fig. 4. Fear-reaction to the examiner. Fraternal twins exhibited quite different patterns.

1. This study was carried out by Nina A. Freedman and the author.

basis of a standardized routine in the homes, we noted the amount of smiling, vocalizing and attending to mother and to the experimenter over this period; in figure 3 we see that these results were in the same direction as the initial distributions and they provide further evidence that these basic ingredients of social relating have a demonstrable genetic component.

There is additional corroboration for this from a study at Harvard by Reppucci (8). Reppucci presented a series of visual stimuli to ten identicals and ten same-sexed fraternals at four months of age and found that the identicals were significantly more alike than the fraternals in amount of smiling to one of her stimuli, a 3-dimensional mask. Thus, it appears fair to say that the smiling response has proven a stable and readily demonstrable reflection of genotypic differences.

With regard to the fear of strangers, a good deal has been written about

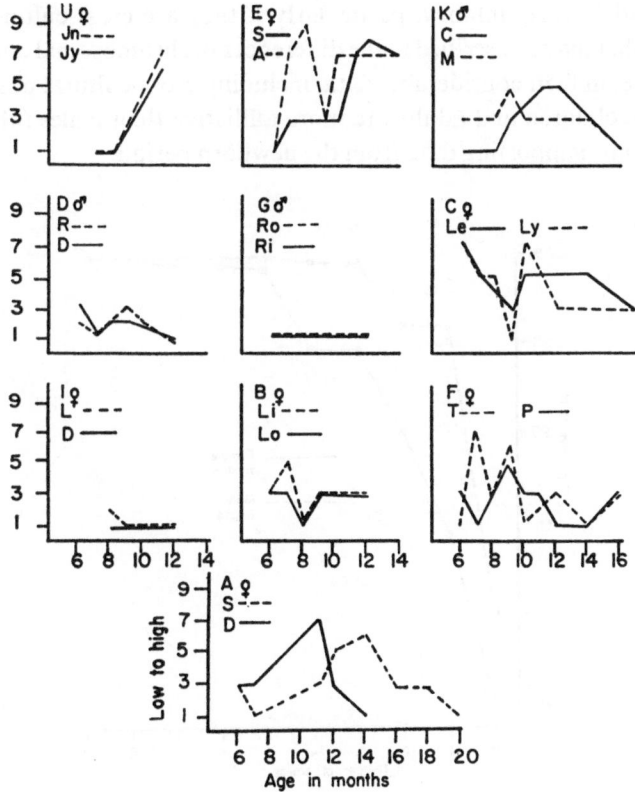

Fig. 5. Fear-reaction to the examiner. Identical twins. In half the pairs, both twins exhibited similar patterns.

the average age of appearance, but it is clear that averages help very little in accurate prediction to individual cases. Figures 4 and 5 represent the course of *fearfulness* from 6 to 12 months in each child in the study. Note that while about half the identical pairs are very similar in the course of these ratings, fraternals never are, nor do any *two genotypes exhibit a similar course*. The course of this behavior is as unique as a finger print.

SEX-DIFFERENCES. I. SOCIAL MODALITY
The study of sex-differences in infancy is a logical extension of behavior genetics.

Whereas one cannot specify exactly how the XY constitution yields maleness, we assume, as do most geneticists, that the XY takes the *entire* genome in the male direction, in part through the pervasive action of testosterone (Levine, this publication p. 285). Thus studies of male-female difference at birth and in early infancy, particularly if they are cross-cultural, should yield data that may be ascribed to the differences in chromosomal constitution.

There are, in fact, considerable data, including cross-cultural observations, that female children and adults are more affiliative than males (9). We have gathered some supporting data from the newborn period.

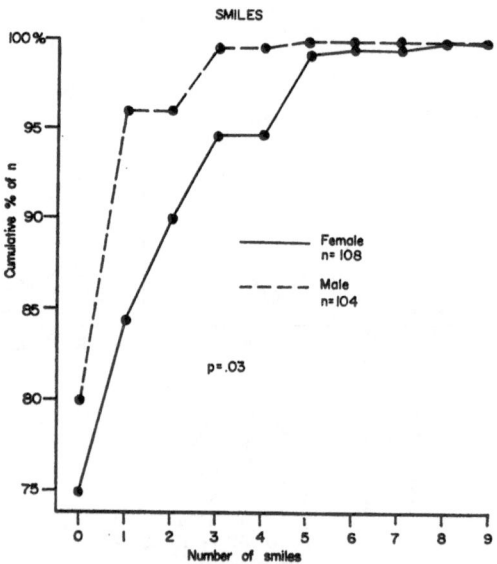

Fig. 6. Newborn females gave indications of a more affiliative orientation than males. On these graphs low scores accumulate on the left, high scores on the right.

In figure 6 we see that newborn girls smile with greater frequency than newborn boys (eyes-closed smiling). Korner (10) and Horowitz (11) have made similar observations. This suggests that girls are born with a lower threshold to smiling and, ergo, a stronger tendency towards affiliative encounter.[2] The experimental work of Lewis, Kagan, and Kalafat (12) with 6 month olds, appears to bear this out further. In figure 7 we see that

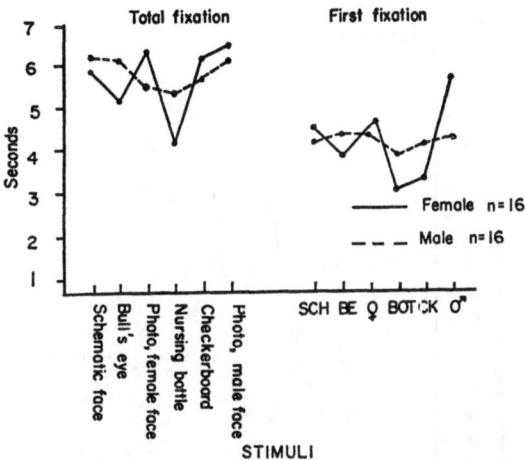

Fig. 7. Comparison of total fixation and first fixation by stimulus and sex (After Lewis, Kagan and Kalafat, 1966). Six-month old girls showed specific preferences for social objects (human faces), whereas boys payed indiscriminate attention to social and non-social stimuli.

whereas girls preferred to gaze at social objects, boys showed no such preference. In what appears to be a related finding, we found that girls were more sensitive than boys to strangers entering the home over the first year (Fig. 8).

Just beyond infancy boys start to assert their independence more frequently than girls, and many studies report greater temper outbursts in boys and a greater tendency for them to wander farther from the caretaker by the second year (13).

2. Since our twin studies had previously indicated that frequent newborn smilers tend to have lowered thresholds for later social-smiling as well, we wondered if this might also be true of the male-female differences. A little study by McLean (24) appears to point this way. Examining high school and college yearbook photos from 1900 until present, McLean found significantly more smiling among the females. Even when overall smiling was low, as in the depression years, approximately the same male-female differential was observed. Additionally there were but eleven smiling faces between 1900 and 1917 in the college yearbook, and all were female.

We also have considerable data on male-female differences in social organization from three to seven years (which parallel sex-differences among the terrestrial macaques), but that takes us beyond the limits of this paper. Let it suffice here to report that consistent differences in levels of aggression and social competition have now been observed over a wide variety of cultures.

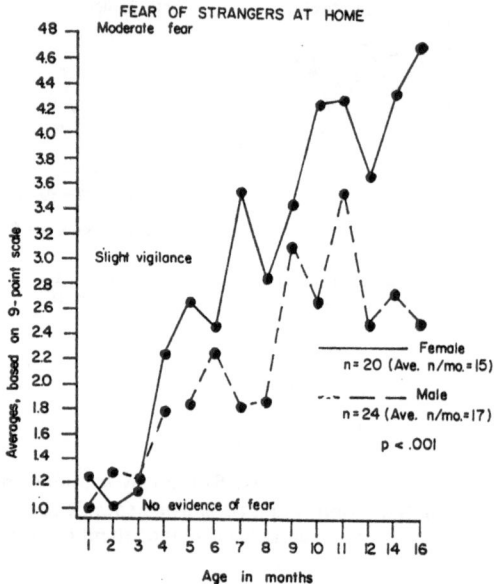

Fig. 8. Fearfulness of a stranger visiting at home. Boys and girls in longitudinal study of twins.

SEX-DIFFERENCES. 2. PREFERRED SENSE MODALITIES IN INFANCY
Sex-differences in preferred sensory modality have been rather widely noted. Boys of 4 months are equally attentive, visually and vocally, to persons and things (14). Their vocalizations, in fact, appear to be almost random and consequently correlate with nothing whatsoever in later development. Differences in girl's vocalizations on the other hand tend to be stable, and the vocalization frequency at 4-months correlates with the frequencies found later in the first year. Also, the relative precocity of the first words spoken by girls actually correlates significantly with adult IQ (15). Girls seem thus to be stable in their social vocalization habits from early infancy. As Kagan (14) has stated it, girls seem to have 'a disposition to express excitement through talking'.

Boys, on the other hand, as early as 10 weeks, show greater increments in learning to visual reinforcement, while girls do best (as we could now expect) under auditory reinforcement (16). Hull (17) has found that these two modalities continue to differentially affect the performance of boys and girls through 18 months of age, the span of her study. Further, a whole host of studies, summarized by Oetzel (13), point to the conclusion that males and females similarly differ in preferred modality throughout the life span: females usually do better at verbal and linguistic tasks, while males usually do better at visual-spacial tasks.

This should perhaps not be surprising given the affiliative nature of language acquisition and the mechanical nature of visual-spacial tasks, where objects must be imaginally rotated in space. It appears that males are simply more interested and more capable of taking apart and putting together toys, mechanical devices and other objects, throughout the life span. Further, in a study involving thousands of subjects, males actually *saw* better and in a number of other studies females have been found to actually *hear* better (reviewed in Garai & Scheinfeld, 9).[3] Probably related is

Table 1. Ethnic groups administered infant behavioral and neurological scales. The criterion for all but the Afro-American group was four grandparents of the same ethnic background as baby. Skin color alone was used as the criterion for Afro-Americans.

Ethnic Group	Place	Predominant S.E.C.	N	Tester(s)
Chinese-American (2nd through 5th generations)	San Francisco	Middle	24	D. G. Freedman N. Freedman
Japanese-American (3rd and 4th generation)	Hawaii	Middle	41	D. G. Freedman N. Freedman
Navajo	New Mexico, Arizona	Lower	36	D. G. Freedman N. Freedman
Afro-American	Chicago	Lower	84	J. Kuchner J. Durfee
African	Northern Nigeria	$\frac{1}{2}$ Lower (Public Hospital) $\frac{1}{2}$ Middle (Private Hospital)	22	D. G. Freedman
European-American (2nd through 4th generations)	San Francisco, Hawaii, Chicago	Middle	65	D. G. Freedman N. Freedman J. Kuchner

3. Differences in vision, however, are not the basis for the differences in mechanical ability. Burlingham and co-workers at the Hampstead Clinic in London have filmed a congenitally blind boy's rather amazing abilities with mechanical toys (contrasted with the exaggerated mechanical helplessness of a congenitally blind girl).

the fact that males are usually initially stimulated by the visual modality in courtship (23, 18), whereas females respond sexually primarily via touch (19). There is rather direct evidence, in fact, that females are born with a lower threshold to tactile stimulation than males in that Bell and Costello (20), in a well controlled study, found this in newborns.

INTER-GROUP VARIATION AMONG NEWBORNS

Even as genetic variation within any group accounts for much of the individual variation seen, a cornerstone of evolutionary theory is the fact that gene-pool differences arise between groups which have been somehow isolated from one another. It would, therefore, be extremely surprising to find

Table 2. Comparisons of potential co-variables.

	Chinese-American	European-American
Mean age and range in hours (N.S,)	32.75 (7-75)	33.27 (5-72)
Initial state (rated 0-6, from deep sleep to very alert) means (N.S.)	3.58	2.79
Distribution of sexes*	11 male, 13 female	11 male, 13 female
Mean birth weight in grams** (P = 0.05)	3,194.33	3,447.91
Mean Apgar*** rating at 5 min after birth (N.S.)	8.86	9.00
Mean hours of labour (N.S.)	6.08	5.77
Medication during labour****	16 received systemic drugs	13 received systemic drugs
	8 received only local anaesthetic or none	11 received only local anaesthetic or none
Mean age of mothers (N.S.)	26.70	26.66
Mean number of previous pregnancies (N.S.)	1.83	2.41
Hospital	16, Kaiser Hospital, San Francisco	20, Kaiser Hospital, S.F.
	5, Chinese Hospital, S.F.	4, Lying-in, Chicago
	3, U.C. Medical Center, S.F.	

* There was no significant interaction between race and sex.
** When weight is treated as a co-variable it does not affect ethnic differences.
*** A rating of viability; based on heart rate, colour, respiration, tonus, and crying. Optimal score is 10.
**** Although systemic drugs significantly lowered Apgar (P = 0.02), automatic walk (P = 0.02) and tonic deviation of the head (P = 0.02), statistical treatment indicates that these drug differences did not affect ethnic differences.

a lack of such variation among human groups which have histories of relative isolation one from the other. Conversely, fewer differences should characterize groups which have had ample opportunity for genetic exchange.

As a result of this reasoning, my wife and I embarked on a series of behavioral studies of newborns of various ethnic groups. Thus far we have tested within six ethnic groups, as listed on table 1. Because of limited space, we will detail only on the results of our first study, a comparison of 24 Chinese-American and 24 European-American newborns.

The Orientals were largely of Cantonese background, and the Caucasians largely of middle-European background. All families were middle class and the bulk were members of a pre-paid health plan (Kaiser Hospital, table 2). Table 2 summarizes the potentially important co-variables other than ethnic group, and we see that none could have accounted for the ethnic differences presented here.

Briefly, the behavior scales consisted of twenty-eight general behavioral items rated 1-9 and eighteen standard neurological signs, frequently used to screen for neural damage, rated 0-3. The twenty-five general items may be somewhat arbitrarily arranged into five categories as follows: 1. temperament – five items; 2. sensory development – three items; 3. autonomic and central nervous system maturity – eight items; 4. motor development – six items; 5. social interest and response – six items. As will be seen, any single item may overlap categories (e.g., lability of skin color can reflect temperament as well as autonomic maturity). *The manual to this test is presented in this volume* (p. 104).

All testing was done during September and October, 1968. Each test session lasted between 30 and 40 minutes. Testing was performed in the new-born nursery by the author's wife as the author watched, and scoring was done immediately afterwards in a room next to the nursery. Apart from a reliability sample which was marked independently, scoring depended on verbal agreement between the testers.[4]

4. As a reliability check, twenty-one cases have been scored independently by the author and Mrs Freedman over the various ethnic groups they have tested together. Only two items reported on in this chapter, *consolability* and *following the face-voice*, achieved a Pearson r of less than 0.65. The correlation in these items was 0.49 and 0.52 respectively due to the occurrence of large discrepancies in a few cases. These items were retained since they had achieved correlations above 0.90 on a previous reliability sample. Over-all, the average correlation was 0.82, the twenty-fifth percentile r = 0.88, and the seventy-fifth percentile r = 0.70.

We cannot leave the subject of reliability without stating Bock's (25) somewhat unorthodox but sensible view. He points out that, due to high variance, unreliable items would be unlikely to differentiate two comparison groups. The very fact that an item does so is *prima facie* evidence of its reliability.

A multivariate analysis of variance indicated that, on the basis of total performance, the two groups were decidedly different (p = .008). Further analysis indicated that the main loading came from the group of items measuring temperament, which seemed to tap excitability/imperturbability (p = .001). While the following discussion is based on mean ethnic differences on the distinguishing items, it should be emphasized that there was substantial overlap in range on all scales between the Chinese and Caucasian infants.

The European-American infants reached a peak of excitement sooner (rapidity of buildup, fig. 9) and wavered back and forth between states of contentment and upset (lability of states, fig. 10). They showed more facial and bodily reddening (Fig. 11), probably as a consequence. The Chinese-American infants were scored on the calmer and steadier side of these items. In an item called *defensive movements*, the tester placed a cloth firmly over the supine baby's face for a few seconds. While the typical European-American infant immediately struggled to remove the cloth by swiping with his hands and turning his face, the typical Chinese-American infant lay impassively, exhibiting few overt motor responses (Fig. 12). Similarly, when placed in the prone position, the Chinese infants frequently lay as placed,

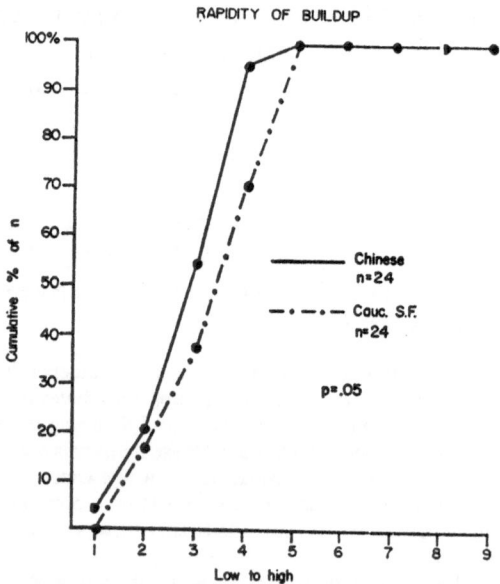

Fig. 9. Rapidity of build-up. A rating of how quickly the infant reaches a state of excitement from the initial sleep state.

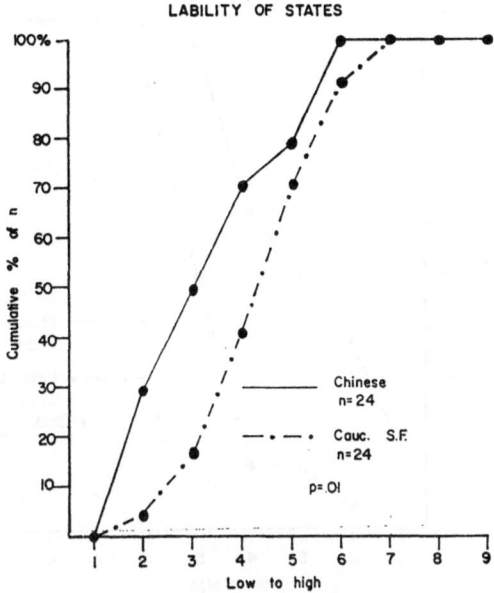

Fig. 10. Lability of states. A rating of number of state changes over the entire test.

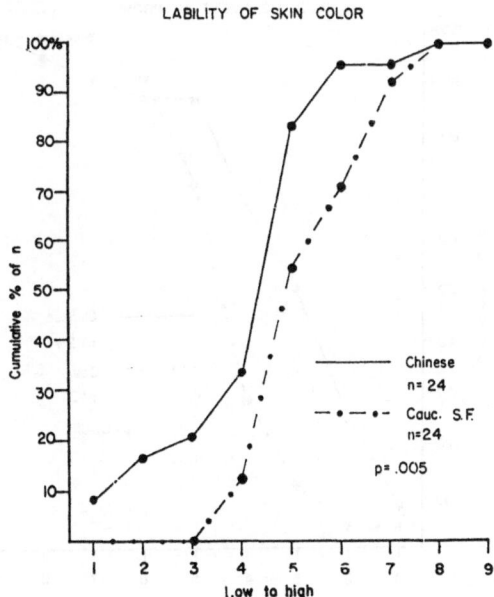

Fig. 11. Lability of skin color. A combined rating of number and strength of skin-color changes.

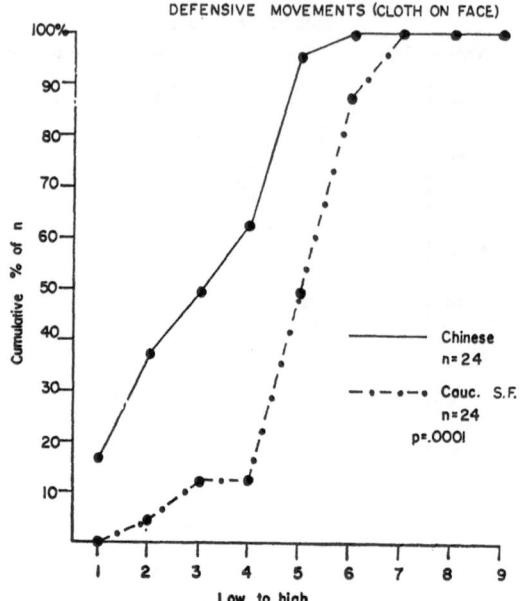

Fig. 12. Defensive movements. A cloth is placed firmly over the infant's nose, and the energy expended and the success of his attempts to remove it is rated.

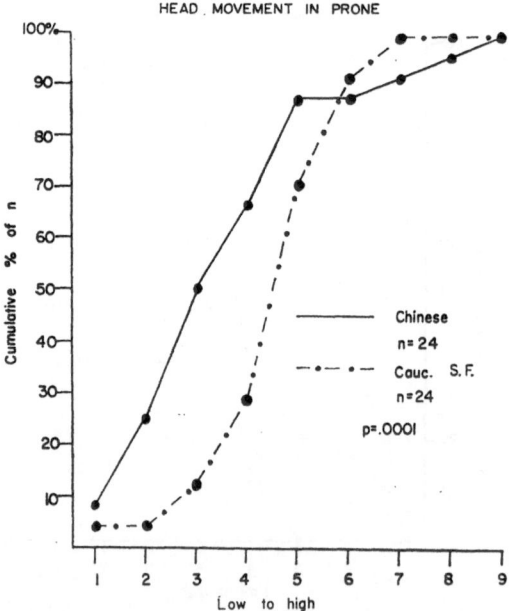

Fig. 13. Head lift. The infant is placed in the prone with hands at either side of the head, and the extent of head lift is then rated.

with face flat against the bedding, whereas the Caucasian infants either turned the face to one side or lifted the head (Fig. 13). Inasmuch as there was no difference between the groups in the ability to hold the head steady in the upright position (p = .91, pull to sit), this maintenance of the face in the bedding is taken as a further example of relative imperturbability or ready accommodation to external changes.[5] In an apparently related item, rate of

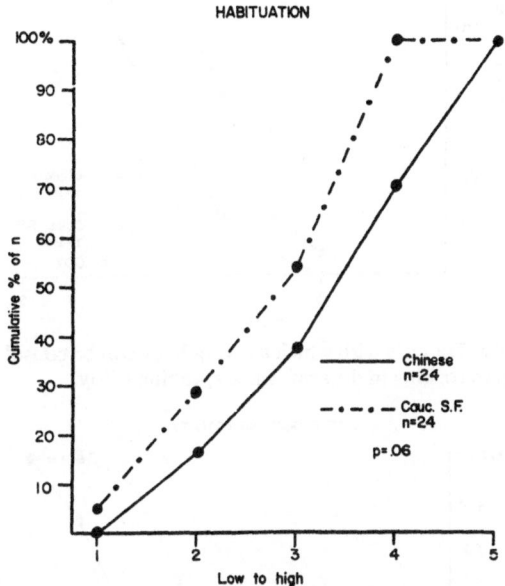

Fig. 14. Habituation. A pen light was shone on the eyes at about half second intervals, and the number of reactive blinks counted. When blinking ceased, the infant was said to be habituated.

habituation, a pen light was repeatedly shone on the infant's eyes, and the number of blinks counted until the infant no longer reacted (shuts-off). The Chinese infants tended to habituate more readily (Fig. 14).

There were no significant differences in amount of crying and, when picked up and consoled, both groups tended to stop crying. The Chinese infants were, however, often dramatically immediate in their cessation of crying when picked up and spoken to, and therefore drew extremely high

5. Another possible explanation for these differences in defensive reactions involves the obvious difference in nasal bone structure between Orientals and Caucasians. The average Caucasian newborn has a considerably more prominent nose. However, experimental occlusion of the nasal passages has yielded results similar to the above.

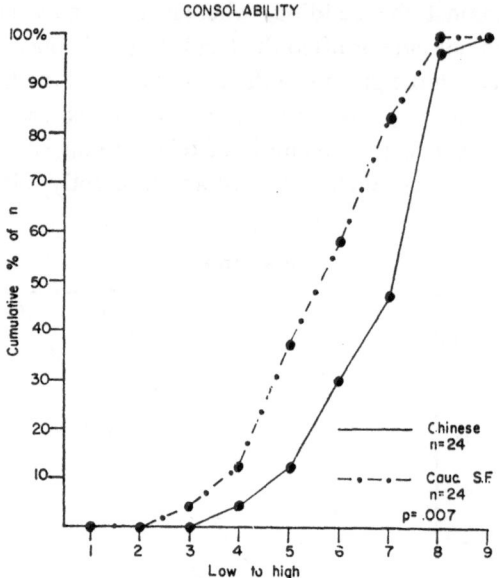

Fig. 15. Consolability. The ease with which a crying baby can be consoled, ranging from a hand on the stomach to rocking in the arms while speaking softly.

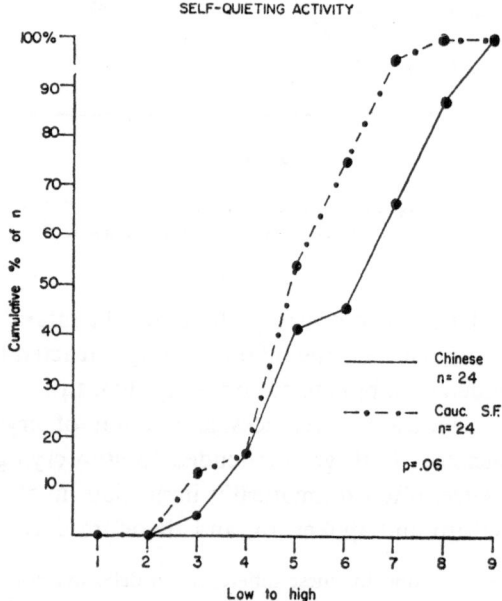

Fig. 16. Self-quieting ability. How readily, on the average, a crying baby ceases to cry without intervention.

ratings in consolability (Fig. 15). The Chinese infants also tended to stop crying sooner without soothing (self-quieting ability, fig. 16).

To summarize, the majority of items which differentiated the two groups fell into the category of temperament. The Chinese-American newborns tended to be less changeable, less perturbable, tended to habituate more readily, and tended to calm themselves or to be consoled more readily when upset. In other areas (sensory development, central nervous system maturity, motor development, social responsiveness), the two groups were essentially equal.

In general, we found that each of the six ethnic groups studied was unique in some respects, but that by and large similarities were much more prevalent than differences. This twofold truth – unique yet similar – is not at all surprising, given the facts that all are con-specifics and that there has been substantial geographical separation over long periods of time. Of the 48 items on the *Cambridge Newborn Behavioral and Neurological Scales* (see p. 104), 30 significantly differentiated ethnic groups at a probability of .05 or less and 9 of these items were significant at a probability of less than .0001.[6]

THE NAVAJO SAMPLE

The combined Oriental groups (Chinese, Japanese and Navajo) were compared with a larger Caucasian population on the same items first reported for Chinese vs. Caucasians, and the same contrasts persisted,[7] save for *lability of skin color* (Fig. 17); this deviation was largely due to the Navajo sample.[8]

The Navajo infants, in fact, exhibited two outstanding differences from all other groups, a tendency for the entire body to become red when excited

6. Inasmuch as the following basic items also significantly differentiated ethnic groups, they were statistically 'eliminated' from all our analyses: *weight, age of infant, Apgar rating, mother's age, number of previous pregnancies, length of labor and presence or absence of systemic medication.* All P values on graphs in this chapter were calculated with these co-variates eliminated.

7. Given the geographic proximity and numerous historical links between Japan and China, one would expect the least differences between these two groups which is, in fact, the case. The Navajo, an Athapaskan Indian sub-group, are also linked historically with these two modern Oriental groups. They descend from a migratory Asian people which came to rest in Northern Canada, before 200 B.C. Migrating into the area now the U.S. southwest by 1400 A.D., the Navajos mixed to some extent with the Pueblos and other established descendents of earlier Asian migrations. It is, thus, of great interest to find that Navajo newborns resemble the Chinese and Japanese neonates considerably more than they do the remaining groups.

8. It may be additionally noted that the combined Oriental group exhibited significantly less spontaneous activity than the Caucasians or Africans.

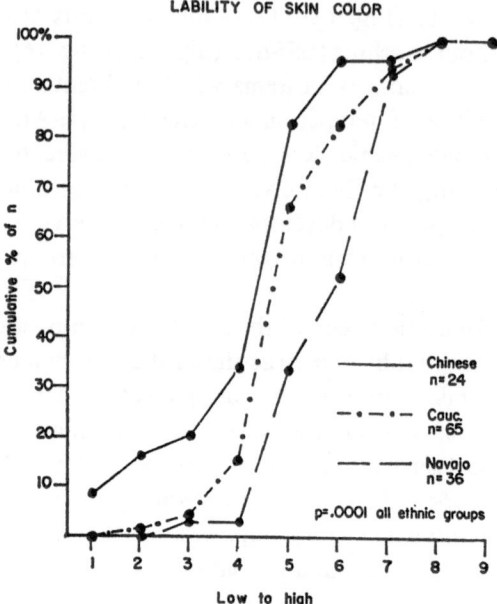

Fig. 17. The Navajo infants showed unusually high and persistent reddening of the skin when crying.

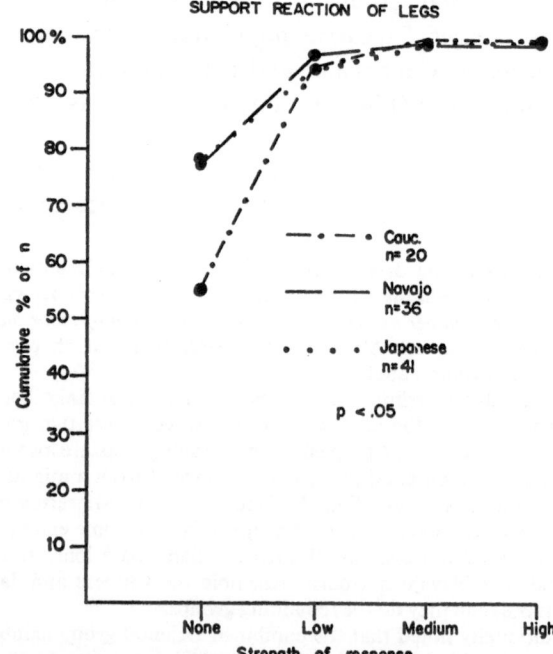

Fig. 18. Leg-support reaction. An infant is held under his arm pits with feet touching the table. Very few Navajo infants attempted to stiffen their legs to support the body, while among other groups this is an average reaction.

and to remain that way for much of the examination (Fig. 17), and a remarkable absence of any leg support reaction (Fig. 18), or automatic walk (Fig. 19). Finally, a related item, *passive movements of the lower limbs* (Fig. 20) reflects the lack of 'snapback' and the greater malleability of the lower limbs.[9]

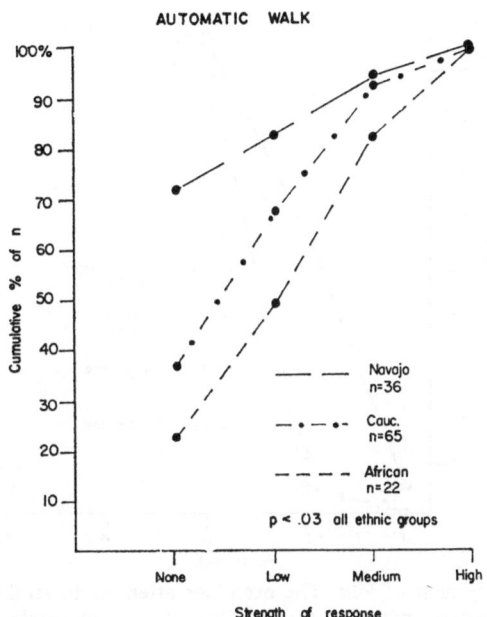

Fig. 19. Automatic walk. After the leg-support reaction, most infants proceed to take some steps. Again, Navajo infants were exceptional, and showed practically no stepping.

While there are no figures on the rate of motor maturation in Navajo infants, Dennis (21) reported that the average Hopi infant walked at $14\frac{1}{2}$ months; this is approximately $2\frac{1}{2}$ months later than the European-American average, and $3\frac{1}{2}$ to 4 months later than the African and Afro-American averages. Judging by the condition of the Navajo's lower limbs, we would predict similar later walking for them.

The question arose in the Dennis study, and remained unresolved, as to whether cradle-boarding of infants or gene-pool differences was the basis for the observed differences in norms. The six Pueblo Indian newborns we have

9. Highly malleable lower limbs may be related to the fact that 'congenital hip' is very common among the Navajos (U.S.P.H. report, 1969), possibly because of weak muscling around the hip joint.

tested were very similar to the Navajo, which supports the gene-pool
hypothesis for later walking, and tends to confirm Dennis's feelings that
cradle-boarding has little effect on motor behavior.

This brings up another commonly heard speculation, i.e., that the sub-
dued emotionality commonly observed in Navajo youngsters (22) is due to

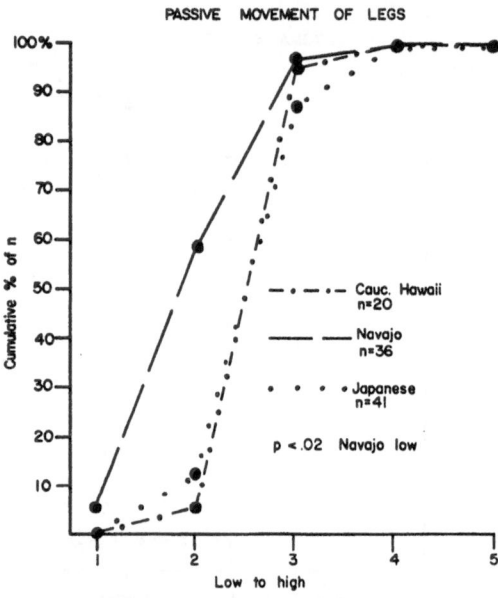

Fig. 20. Passive movement of legs. The examiner attempts to straighten and bend the
limbs, noting rigidity vs. malleability; the legs of Navajo newborns were extremely
flexible.

an infancy on the cradle-board. This frequently expressed notion, however,
seems to reverse the actual situation. It appears instead that Navajo babies
are particularly suited, physically and temperamentally, to the cradle-board
in that they are more likely to *permit it* than highly active and complaining
babies.

On the basis of such data, then, we have concluded that while it must
be true that different cultural practices differentially reward babies' behavior,
it is equally likely that biological predispositions effect what become the
cultural norms. The tendency to explain cultural differences in behavior
only in social-learning terms can no longer go unquestioned; it now appears
most reasonable to start with a holistic position in which man is fully
acknowledged as a bio-social being, a product of his ontogenetic history and
his phylogenetic past.

REFERENCES

1. Freedman, D. G., *Human infancy in evolutionary perspective*, Manuscript.
2. Hebb, D. O., Heredity and environment in mammalian behavior. *Brit. J. Anim. Behav.* 1, 319 (1953).
3. Fuller, J. L. & Thompson, W., *Behavior genetics*, New York 1961.
4. Scott, J. P. & Fuller, J. L., *Genetics and social behavior of the dog*, Chicago 1965.
5. Ginsburg, B. E., Genetic parameters in behaviour research. In: *Genetics and behavior* Hirsch, J. (ed.), New York 1968.
6. Vandenberg, S. G., *Hereditary factors in normal personality traits*. Research report from the Louisville Twin Study Child Development Unit, Department of Pediatrics, University of Louisville 1966.
7. Bayley, N., *Bayley scales of infant development*, New York 1970.
8. Reppucci, C., Hereditary influences upon distribution of attention in infancy. Unpublished doctoral dissertation. Harvard University 1968.
9. Garai, J. E. & Scheinfeld, A., Sex-differences in mental and behavioral traits. *Genet. Psychol. Monog.* 77, 169 (1968).
10. Korner, A. F., Neonatal startles, smiles, erections, and reflex sucks as related to state, sex, and individuality. *Child Devel.* 40, 1039 (1969).
11. Horowitz, F. D., Unpublished data. Department of Human Development, University of Kansas 1970.
12. Lewis, M., Kagan, J. & Kalafat, J., Patterns of fixation in the young infant. *Child Devel.* 37, 331 (1966).
13. Oetzel, R. M., Annotated bibliography. In: *The development of sex differences*, Maccoby, E. (ed.), Stanford 1966.
14. Kagan, J., *Change and continuity in infancy*, New York 1971.
15. Cameron, J., Livson, N. & Bayley, N., Infant vocalizations and their relationship to mature intelligence. *Science* 157, 331 (1967).
16. Watson, J. S., Operant conditioning of visual fixation in infants under visual and auditory reinforcement. *Develop. Psychol.* 1, 508 (1969).
17. Hull, E., Sex-differences in infant test performances. Unpublished research paper, Committee on Human Development, Chicago 1967.
18. Master, W. H. & Johnson, V. E., The sexual response cycles of the human male and female: comparative anatomy and physiology. In: *Sex and behavior*, Beach, F. A. (ed.), New York 1965.
19. Kinsey, A. C., *Sexual behavior in the human female*. The Institute for Sex Research, Indiana University. Philadelphia 1953.
20. Bell, R. Q. & Costello, N. S., Three tests for sex-differences in tactile sensitivity in the newborn. *Biol. Neonat.* 7, 335 (1964).
21. Dennis, W., *The Hopi child* New York 1940.
22. Kluckhohn C. & Leighton, D., *The Navajo*, Cambridge (Mass.) 1946.
23. Kinsey, A. C., Pomeroy, W. B. & Martin, C. E., *Sexual behavior in the human male*, Philadelphia 1948.
24. McLean, D., *Sex-correlated differences in human smiling behavior; a preliminary investigation*. Unpublished research paper, Committee on Human Development, Chicago 1970.
25. Bock, D., Personal communication 1970.

DISCUSSION

Casaer: Dr Freedman, what is the effect of body weight on the results in your studies? It has been shown by Michaelis *et al.* that small-fordates are less well performing than appropriate weight-for-age newborns in those items in which muscle mass is involved (Michaelis, R., Schulte, F. J. and Nolte, R., Motor behaviour of small for gestational age newborn infants. *J. Pediat.* 76, 208 (1970).

Freedman: There were significant differences in weight between most groups and so we had to do a statistical analysis in which weight was one of the co-variables that we eliminated. Thus we controlled for weight in all the graphs that you saw.

Casaer: But then there is another problem. If they were controlled for weight, and let's say they were not controlled for age because that may be very difficult in these genetically different groups, then it could be that some of your Caucasians were likely to be older (postmenstrual age) babies than the Navajos although they had comparable weights.

Freedman: They were indeed controlled for age as well, so that I don't think that would apply to our data. Besides, *none* of the Navajo exhibited full stepping.

Dobbing: Dean in Uganda has said many times and has commented many times on the apparent precocity, neurological precocity, of the new-born African child as compared with European children in Africa. A similar thing has been commented on many times by several Central-American and South-American authors. And I have sometimes wondered if that is true, whether this could be due to a slightly different timing of birth in relation to the growth of the brains. I was just wondering how this idea would fit in with your findings.

Freedman: Some of our African findings seem to bear out those described by Geber and Dean* in Uganda. The African babies hold their heads very erect. They frequently showed lordosis right after birth and if you pull an African baby up to sit, the head frequently is up and the back arched, and they may even look around. I have seen very few Oriental or Caucasian babies who could duplicate that. Almost invariably, if you pull these latter babies to a sit, they do so with a kyphotic, rounded back and wobbly head. Another thing that you find in African newborns from time to time is that when balanced prone on the palm of the hand one may elicit full body extension (the Wolf-Landau reflex) which you don't find in Caucasian babies for several weeks. Small wonder then that in Northern Nigeria a woman can put her newborn in a shawl on her back and walk off without worrying about the head flopping back and forth. Thus we are able to corroborate some of Geber's findings found among the Ganda in Uganda. However, unlike Geber, the precocity we observed is very specific for the motor system, and we did not find it in any of the other systems we measured. I would therefore not speak of a generalized precocity. With regard to gestation time, the best data I could find in Northern Nigeria indicated that gestation was the same as it is in Caucasian groups; such records however are bad everywhere.

Marshall: Can I just add to this: we have studied, in conjunction with Ashcroft, skeletal development in Jamaican negro-babies. They seemed to have the same gestation period as Caucasian babies but their skeletal maturity was advanced and remained ahead of the European population for about three years. So this is in keeping with an idea of general overall advancement of maturity rather than a specific one confined to one system. (Marshall, W. A., Ashcroft, M. T. and Bryan, G. Skeletal maturation of the hand and wrist in Jamaican children. *Hum. Biol.* 42, 419 (1970).

Van der Werff ten Bosch: Dr. Freedman, you have not suggested and perhaps you would not want to do this, that the cause of the differences that you find between the sub-species may not be due to genes but to the ante-natal environment.

Freedman: We have certainly thought about these alternate hypotheses, and the most frequently mentioned potential pre-natal causal factor is differential

* Geber, M. and Dean R. F. A., Precocious development in newborn African infants. *readings in infancy and childhood*, Brackbill and Thompson (eds.) New York (N.Y.) 1966.

diet. Without having checked this in detail, the main difference between the San Francisco Chinese and Caucasians is probably the starch staple, i.e., rice vs. bread. There was no difference in annual income, and each appears to consume comparable amounts of protein. Furthermore, where substantial socio-economic differences did occur within the Oriental group, i.e., the Chinese and Navajo, the newborns were nevertheless very similar and both groups differed in about the same way when compared to the Caucasian sample.

Van der Werff ten Bosch: I was not thinking of the diet. I was thinking of the temperamental differences between the mothers. Their responses to their own worries in life on the development of the adrenal system.

Freedman: You are suggesting that there may be some very mysterious prenatal mechanisms by which mothers transmit behavioral tendencies to their infants. Montagu* has reviewed this literature and finds good evidence only for rather straight forward effects, e.g., drugs that depress or speed up maternal heart rate do so to the fetal heart rate as well. Similarly prenatal anoxias or toxemias are connected with all sorts of behavioral disorders, but no one has yet demonstrated or even hypothesized a mechanism whereby normal temperamental differences may be transmitted from a mother to her fetus. I believe a more reasonable position to be that there are indeed gene-pool differences which yield different average temperaments. Mothers then proceed to either reinforce or change these behaviours. A student of mine, Joan Kuchner, is conducting a study within this general framework, and I believe it will be a most important study when completed. She is recording mother-infant interactions from birth thru four months of age among 30 mother-infant pairs, half of them Chinese-American, half European-American. Her first generalization, which she gives tentatively since the work is in progress, is that the mothers are not different, but that the babies are!

N.N.: It has been found that in the higher socio-economic levels of African mothers this precocity was less than in the lower socio-economic level. Did you find anything like that?

Freedman: No we did not. We did have the two groups, but we had small numbers in each group as you saw. We had only 22 in all and about half in

* Montagu, M. A., *Prenatal Influence*. Springfield, (Ill.) 1962.

the higher and half in the lower income classes. However, I have never seen the data to back the point you are making, although I've heard it frequently. If true, high infant mortality among the African poor must be an important selective factor to consider.

NON-GENETIC PRENATAL INFLUENCES ON PSYCHOLOGICAL DEVELOPMENT

J. JANS

INTRODUCTION

'Entwendet die Mutter während ihrer Schwangerschaft etwas, so kann das Kind dem Hang zum Stehlen sein ganzes Leben lang nicht Widerstehen'. Thus Pachinger (1) reports on ancient myths in Austria.

Although the content of many of these superstitious old wives' tales has long ago been put into proper perspective by the advance of a more rational approach and by scientific research, the possibility remains that 'in most areas of present-day scientific inquiry antecedents of varying antiquity can be found' (Joffe, 2). Not until we have disentangled a host of problematic relationships will we be able to achieve an approach really different from the present one which can be described as no more than a sophisticated version of the ideas of earlier centuries.

In psychological research, the field of prenatal development has been explored only in the most recent decades 'and an unambiguous experimental indication that a mother's psychological experiences during pregnancy could influence the behaviour of her offspring was not presented until the 1950s' (Joffe, 2). One reason for the emerging interest is perhaps the critical reassessment of the influence of environment on the development of behaviour. From this viewpoint the prenatal period of development is only to a certain degree a unique part of the environmental continuum. The overemphasis on pathological problems in studies on prenatal development and the resulting taboos concerning pregnancy are probably related to the ambivalent emphasis which the mother as an aetiological factor has acquired in the area of the mother-child relation.

METHODOLOGICAL PROBLEMS IN RESEARCH

The main reason for the fact that no more than a start has been made on the subject at hand are the methodological difficulties inherent in all human studies – as compared to animal studies. In his excellent analysis, Joffe (2) shows that the difficulties are by no means small; with the result that the view on the various non-genetic influences is rather blurred. 'If it is not clear whether offspring behavioral differences are due to prenatal, postnatal or genetic causes, it is unreasonable to claim reliability for substantive findings, which must therefore be proceeded by a methodological review' (2). A clear-cut experimental method of investigation is obviously impossible, seeing suspected causal factors can never be administered deliberately to pregnant women! A statistical epidemiological approach is mainly used, and up till now this has been predominantly retrospective. 'Actuarial surveys seek to establish the aetiology of some form of abnormality by producing correlations between one or more variables in pregnancy and some disorder in the child. They are not experimental; they start with an observed abnormality or disorder in infants or children and search their prenatal history for the presence in this group of a greater frequency of some particular variable than is found in the history of some contrasting groups of children' (2).

The results found by statistical epidemiological methods are open to some doubt for the following reasons.

a. Anamnestic data after an interim of two years or more are so unreliable that they should in fact be ignored (3). This applies to an even greater extent in the case of mothers with high anxiety during pregnancy (4).
b. There are many examples of unfortunate effects of biased sampling. Because pathological studies are usually concerned with specific clinically described groups, the generalized risk proclaimed in such studies is grossly exaggerated; in prospective studies one does indeed encounter a considerable reduction in the risk. This has been demonstrated for example by Tartakow in his study on rubella (5).
c. Because of the length of the period elapsing between pregnancy and the time of the investigation, it is not possible to check on the early postnatal situation. The far-reaching consequences of the postnatal situation in general has, however, been sufficiently established.
d. Only inconclusive differentiation can be made between complications of pregnancy and those of delivery.

All these aspects indicate that the actual significance of the detected relationships is as yet undecided.

Moreover, the non-experimental character of these human studies implies that they frequently suffer from the drawback common to correlational studies of not being able to demonstrate that the correlated variables are causally connected. Besides, the size of the correlations is often relatively small, so that a large portion of the total variance remains unexplained. 'This type of investigation is certainly not capable of separating out the contributions of genetic variables and those of postnatal factors' (2). Specifically, this might mean that there is no verification and no practical possibility of verifying the question whether the non-genetic prenatal influences and the supposedly connected behavioral aspects in the child are both dependent on more central genetic factors. This is also the case for the question whether foetal abnormality produces the maternal dysfunction. An example of the complexity of the influencing factors is provided by studies on the effects of smoking. 'The smoking may be considered as an index which characterizes smokers, but smoking per se is only incidental and not essential as a causal factor in the observed phenomena' (6). In spite of these better developed insights, Joffe still feels compelled to say: 'the statement that behavior is determined by a multitude of complexly interacting events is a widely recognized truism, but it is one that appears in most cases to receive little more than lip service when experiments are undertaken to the prenatal determinants of behavior' (7).

This probably means that Zitrin's (8) statement 'that definitive elucidation of the relationships between prenatal and paranatal complication and psychiatric disorders of children will probably have to await careful, long-term prospective investigations', will have to be extended to the whole area of research on the relation between non-genetic prenatal influences and subsequent human behavior. The problem also does not seem to have been resolved by the numerous longitudinal studies, as is borne out by many critical notes made on the matter. As Meili says 'Man hat mit der grossen Schaufel gegraben und nicht recht gewusst wo' (9).

PREGNANCY COMPLICATIONS – NEUROLOGICAL AND BEHAVIORAL DISORDERS

There are a large number of studies on the association of complications during pregnancy with neurological and behavioral disorders. An important contribution in this area has been made by the work of Pasamanick and associates. They assume a continuum of reproductive casualty, with the implication that if severe prenatal and perinatal complications produce foetal or neonatal death or considerable damage, less severe abnormal conditions, while not lethal, would produce a graded series of neuropsychiatric disorders. In retrospective studies they successively compared groups of children suffering from cerebral palsy, epilepsy, mental deficiency, behavioral disorders, reading disabilities, tics, and speech problems with control groups of children without these disorders. The object of the investigation was the relative frequency of pregnancy complications – mainly anoxic conditions due to various circumstances. The data were obtained from hospital records during pregnancy and delivery.

Broadly speaking, Pasamanick and associates indeed observed an increased frequency in the various groups as compared to the non-disturbed group. The differences are, however, so small that a wide margin for further questions remains. Compare, for example, the frequency percentages of persons with one or more maternal complications in the epilepsy investigation (10), with 27.7% for the epileptic group, as compared to 18.8% for the control group. An interesting contrast appears in the studies concerning the connection between pregnancy and obstetric complications and mental retardation by Pasamanick (11) and Stott (12) on the one hand and by Fairweather and Illsley (13) and Barker (14) on the other. The difference in the proportional occurrence of the complications in these studies is so surprising that Joffe makes the following remark on it: 'If all the investigations were accepted at face value, it would be necessary to conclude that complications of pregnancy produce an increased incidence of mentally retarded children in Baltimore and Bristol, but not in Aberdeen or Birmingham' (2). Pasamanick and associates indeed appear to have included more detailed complications, while Fairweather and Barker took greater account of social and educational factors in their analysis. The arbitrariness of approach is illustrated by the fact that 'Stott rejected the possibility that mothers of retardates neglected their infants and that this produced the ill health, on the grounds that 'the maternal instinct towards a young infant is normally so strong that only severe depression or near psychosis inhibits it'. (2)

In a recent investigation into the relation between pregnancy and birth complications (PBC) and disturbed behavior, McNeil and associates (15) obtained significant differences between the groups: seriously and moderately disturbed, and controls (who were not further specified), but the occurrence of PBCs appear to be quite high in the control group.

	% of Subjects with at least one PBC	Mean PBC per subject
Seriously disturbed	75	.91
Moderately disturbed	51.7	.83
Controls	39.3	.62

The difference in type of PBCs between the disturbed and the control group points in the direction of findings of many investigations: namely birth complications in contrast to pregnancy complications. Prediction on group membership by means of discriminant functional analysis of 16 mainly perinatal factors produces as percentage correct predictions:

Seriously disturbed	Moderately disturbed	Controls
60%	41.4%	81%
49.2%		

The conclusions of the authors are these:

- for the 50% correctly predicted of the disturbed, the hypothesis might be held that PBCs were a contributing cause of the children's disturbance;
- a certain number of the PBCs is likely to be irrelevant to behavioral disturbance as is shown by the fact that 39.3% of the controls had at least one PBC.

Following Pasamanick and Knoblock (16) we must consider the following questions.

First. Why is it that a large number of cases do not have a history of prenatal abnormalities? With respect to this we may point to the fact that certain disorders, in spite of their obvious polyaetiology are still categorized too strongly into one single group (e.g. reading retardation, 17). It is precisely the less serious extreme of Pasamanick's continuum that provides difficulties with respect to its differentiation from educational factors.

Second. Why is it that children in the control group who have a history of prenatal abnormalities do not exhibit the disorders? With respect to this, we must seriously take into account the possibility of spontaneous or therapeutically induced recovery (18).

To sum up, it may be said that a certain association is found between prenatal factors and postnatal behavior, but that there is insufficient evidence of causal relationships. It has not yet been demonstrated under what conditions complications themselves are necessary and sufficient for the effects to occur later in offspring behavior. The value of the approach has been greatly reduced by the fact that in the investigations too little weight has been given to postnatal social and educational factors.

MATERNAL EMOTIONALITY IN RELATION TO CHILD BIRTH COMPLICATIONS AND SUBSEQUENT NEONATAL BEHAVIOR

Causal connections laid between maternal emotionality, childbirth complications and subsequent neonatal behavior may resemble the connections made in the superstitious old wives' tales, so that there is naturally some reluctance to accept this approach. However, let us consider it in more detail.

'Although the evidence is by no means conclusive, the general consensus of the research thus far conducted is that psychological factors are associated in some way with various aspects of the maternity cycle, that early psychological assessment of pregnant women holds promise of being predictive of the course and outcome of pregnancy' (19).

In research on this subject, pregnancy rejection and anxiety occupy a central position. Obviously, these investigations are concerned with an extreme increase of anxiety, seeing that anxiety during pregnancy generally shows an increase, anyway, compared with the prenatal and postnatal condition (20).

Davids and De Vault (20) found that in two groups (equivalent as to age, IQ, etc.) of 25 women, the one group with delivery complications, the other without, significant differences in anxiety scores (using MAS and projective techniques) was obtained in the third trimestrial period of pregnancy. The group with the higher anxiety scores also showed a longer and more variable labor time. Although the authors emphasize that there was no information regarding causes or reasons underlying the higher anxiety scores in the abnormal group, they still suggest a causal relation between increased anxiety and complications: 'Such evidence is not abundant, but it is definite and highly suggestive that this is a very fertile field for further study'. Joffe (2) on the other hand states 'if the investigators' conclusion is intended to imply an aetiological relationship between anxiety and all these disorders, then a considerable amount of implausible biological guesswork is required. Consistent differences* between groups in anxiety scores would seem to argue more for a constitutional factor'. Grimm and Venet (19), however, found almost no correlations between any of the psychological and any of the physical variables of the mother. Besides such authors as Turner (22), Otinger and Simmons (23) and Grimm and Venet (19), Ferreira (24) also investigated the relation between emotional attitude in pregnant women and the reflection of this attitude in the newborn. Using the FHB scale, he found a small, but significant difference between the 28 mothers of deviant children and the 135 mothers of non-deviant children in his investigation. The validity

* i.e. those remaining even after childbirth (author's note).

of the FHB scale is, in his opinion, supported by a difference between primi-paras and multiparas. The degree of deviance of the newborns during the first five days of life was judged subjectively by nurses by means of such factors as amount of crying, amount of sleeping, degree of irritability, bowel movements and feeding behavior. Ferreira drew the conclusion: 'We find it reasonably safe to state that the influence of the emotional environment (the mother's attitude) upon behavior has its zero hour before birth'. Similar results have been found by Otinger and Simmons (23) for two groups with extremely high and low IPAT anxiety scores respectively, using objective measures of neonatal criteria. The following remarks however by Spencer and Kass (25) will serve to illustrate the complexity of the relation.

a. 'One possible interpretation of this relation is that the conditions leading to abnormalities occurring at or around delivery were already present, but not detected during the pregnancy when the anxiety scores were obtained. Thus, the forebodings of the women in the abnormal subgroup, based on realistic but vague signs of turbulence in the pregnancy, could have ele-vated their anxiety scores'.
b. 'The findings may be in part an artifact of social-class status, since the less well educated mothers scored higher on the FHB scale and it is known that the incidence of birth complications is greater among less well edu-cated subjects'.
c. On the basis of a dominance of male infants over female infants in the in-vestigated groups, 'it seems plausible that these findings, which show a relationship between anxiety or attitudes during pregnancy and post partem abnormalities, are in part a function of the sex of the infant'.

It is important at this point to consider the fact that the so-called pregnancy attitude is not a simple entity. From research by Schaefer and Mannheimer (26) and by Grimm and Venet (19) this attitude appears to be separable into two main factors: dependence, fears for self, fears for baby, depression and withdrawal, irritability and tension, lack of desire for pregnancy. At the same time it appears that satisfaction with husband and life in general is an important factor. In these more differentiated studies consistent relationships appear to exist between the attitudes during early or late pregnancy and postpartem. This was also confirmed in the investigation by Davids (27). It constitutes an observation of special significance in the problem of post-natal influences. 'Any conclusion about 'blood-borne anxieties' however, must be modified by the knowledge that mothers who are under stress when they are pregnant, may also continue to be anxious and emotionally upset after they have given birth' (28). Grimm and Venet (19) furthermore found no significant correlations between any of the psychological variables and either the Apgar rating or the new-born record.

It is necessary to consider briefly some of the criticism on the methodology used.

Firstly, let us consider the value of responses as perceived and reported by the mother on structured interviews. Among others, the response set and the understanding of the purport of the questions vary with intelligence.

Besides, one could justifiably ask whether the limited view of the attitudes obtained in this piece of research, resulting from economizing on time and personnel for the sake of a large sample, can in any way convey the essential basic structures. It can be doubted whether a sufficiently valid measure of the satisfaction with husband and life in general can be obtained by judgments on such statements as 'In running my home, my husband and I agree on who should do what job' (29).

Secondly, the fact that there were almost no grossly pathological conditions in the women may be important. 'Perhaps within the normal range, emotional factors, even if they are found to play a role in the development of pathology, are too minor an influence to be detectable' (19).

EFFECTS OF SENSORY STIMULATION OF THE FETUS ON LATER BEHAVIOR
In his review of Joffe's publication, Bench (30) makes an interesting statement: 'No attempt is made to consider work involving the effects of sensory stimulation of the fetus on later behavior'. Although he has to admit that not much work has been done until now in this field. Let us consider some research in these lines.

Sontag (31) and his coworkers at the Fels Institute have demonstrated experimentally an increase of fetal activity (movement and heart rate) as an index for fetal sensitivity to vibratory and auditory stimuli. An important related question is, what effect does higher or lower fetal activity have on neonatal behavior?

Richards and Newberry (32) and Richards and Nelson (33) found a positive relation between fetal activity and postnatal development: more active fetuses were subsequently more advanced in general development (as measured by the Gesell tests at 6 months). In a study by Bernard (34), however, no prenatal-postnatal relations were found, especially not after 6 months. Level of fetal activity may, it seems, be induced by traumatic emotional states of the mother. Sontag (31) reports that in the group he investigated over 10 years, there were eight women who, at a late stage of their pregnancy, went through a severe traumatic experience whereby the fetuses showed an immediate and profound increase of activity level. Children of such mothers showed, of course, no congenital defects. They were, however, in general irritable, hyperactive and tended to have frequent stools, while three of them had marked feeding problems. Turner (22) too reports similar findings – which have been alternatively described by other authors as congenital hypertonicity or vagogenic enterospasm and partly ascribed to a congenital imbalance of the autonomic nervous system. However, the evidence Turner found was so slight that she herself declares: 'I suppose the survey which I performed proves nothing'.

Considering these findings, one may ask what in fact is known about the establishment during pregnancy of a normal, positive, basic structure for subsequent postnatal behavior. The many longitudinal studies have taught us how methodologically difficult it apparently is to determine consistent relationships between neonatal and later behavior. Through the changes that are interwoven in such a complex way, the insight into the continuity of behavioral contents is obscured, especially with respect to the non-physiological aspects of behavior. Hence there has been a steadily growing interest over the past years in the more formal characteristics of behavior. Generally these comprise temperamental characteristics and response capability, which may further be differentiated into, for example, early learning and habituation, thresholds of responsiveness, attention span and persistence.

In many investigations it has been observed that with respect to these variables there are strong congenital individual differences (35). The term congenital is not specific as to whether or not these behavioral characteristics are under the control of genetic determinants. In this connection one could ask when and how under the influence of the activation of the various receptor systems, stimulus control in fetal behavior begins. Although a considerable amount is known about the general prenatal functional development as such, very little is known about the distinction between genetic and environmental effects and their specific role in determining the nature of this receptor aroused activity in the fetus. Studies on the significance of early experiences have up till now almost exclusively examined the postnatal situation. Exceptions to this have been the prenatal conditioning studies by Spelt (36) and some investigations about drug use, e.g. Stechler (37) and the above mentioned studies by Sontag and his co-workers.

Thus, there is reason to state in Carmichael's (38) words 'In any consideration of fetal psychology, therefore, special attention should be given to the facts of stimulus control of behavior'. At the same time, however, 'This is a field in which much active research and theoretical writing is in progress and anything asserted about it at one time must always be considered subject to change as additional scientific evidence is secured'. The nature of the specific individual environmental stimulation in contrast to the general ontogenetic development by the genetic code, is still an open question.

CONCLUSION

From the points raised above, it has appeared that sufficient arguments prevail to assume the presence of meaningful environmental factors in the prenatal condition. Though the old wives' tales have been corrected, still it would be incorrect to say that a fetus will maintain its integrity no matter what environmental contingencies might be imposed on the mother during pregnancy. However, true causal relationships of these influences, both in pathology and – more specifically – as regards positive development, will have to be determined in more detail by future research.

REFERENCES

1. Pachinger, A. M., *Die Mutterschaft in der Malerei und Graphik*, München 1906.
2. Joffe, J. M., *Prenatal determinants of behavior*, Oxford 1969.
3. Yarrow, M. R., Problems of methods in parent-child research. *Child Development* 34, 215 (1963).
4. Brekstadt, A., Factors influencing the reliability of anamnestic recall. *Child Development* 37, 603 (1966).
5. Tartakow, I. J., The teratogenicity of maternal rubella. *J. Pediat.* 66, 380 (1965).
6. Jerusalhmy, J., Mother's cigarette smoking and survival of infant. *Am. J. Obstet. Gynec.* 88, 505 (1964).
7. Joffe, J. M., Prenatal determinants of emotionality. *Ann. N.Y. Acad. Sc.* 668 (1969).
8. Zitrin, A., Ferber, P. & Cohen, D., Pre- and paranatal factors in mental disorders of children. *J. nerv. ment. Dis.* 139, 357 (1964).
9. Meili, R., Einige Gedanken zur longitudinalen Persönlichkeitsforschung. *Human Development* 8, 48 (1965).
10. Lilienfeld, A. M. & Pasamanick, B., The association of prenatal and paranatal factors with the development of cerebral palsy and epilepsy. *Am. J. Obstet. Gynec.* 70, 93 (1955).
11. Pasamanick, B. & Lilienfeld, A. M., Association of maternal and fetal factors with the development of mental deficiency. I. Abnormalities in the prenatal and paranatal periods. *J. Am. med. Ass.* 159, 155 (1955).
12. Stott, D. H., Physical and mental handicaps following a disturbed pregnancy. *Lancet* 1006 (1957).
13. Fairweather, D. V. I. & Illsley, R., Obstetric and social origins of mentally handicapped children. *Brit. J. prev. soc. Med.* 14, 149 (1960).
14. Barker, D. J. P., Low intelligence and obstetric complications *Brit. J. prev. soc. Med.* 20, 15 (1966).
15. McNeil, Th. F., Wiegerink, R. & Dozier, J. E., Pregnancy and birth complications

in the births of seriously, moderately, and mildly behaviorally disturbed children. *J. nerv. ment. Dis.* 151, 24 (1970).

16. Pasamanick, B. & Knobloch, H., Retrospective studies on the epidemiology of reproductive casualty; old and new. *Merill-Palmer Quart.* 12, 7 (1966).

17. Jans, J. S. M., De krisis in het onderzoek naar de leeszwakte. *Gawein* 13, 1 (1965).

18. Strengers, L., van der Zee, C. L. M., Jans, J. S. M. & Hettinga, I. E. M., Kanttekeningen bij praematuur geboren kinderen (1956-1965). In: *Klinische ervaringen in een algemeen ziekenhuis*, Nijmegen 1968.

19. Grimm, E. R. & Venet, W. R., The relationship of emotional adjustments and attitudes to the course and outcome of pregnancy. *Psychosom. Med.* 28, 34 (1966).

20. Davids, A., De Vault, S. & Talmadge, M., Anxiety, pregnancy and childbirth abnormalities. *J. cons. Psychol.* 25, 74 (1961).

21. Davids, A. & De Vault, S., Maternal anxiety during pregnancy and childbirth abnormalities. *Psychosom. Med.* 24, 464 (1962).

22. Turner, E. K., The syndrome in the infant resulting from maternal emotional tension during pregnancy. *Med. J. Australia* 1, 221 (1956).

23. Ottinger, D. R. & Simmons, J. E., Behavior of human neonates and prenatal maternal anxiety. *Psychol. Rep.* 14, 391 (1964).

24. Ferreira, A. J., The pregnant mother's emotional attitude and its reflection upon the newborn. *Amer. J. Orthopsychiat.* 30, 553 (1960).

25. Spencer, Th. D. & Kass, N. (eds.), *Perspectives in child psychology*, New York 1970.

26. Schaefer, E. S. & Mannheimer, H., *Dimensions of perinatal adjustment*. (Paper read at Eastern Psychol. Ass., 1960).

27. Davids, A. & Holden, R. H., Consistency of maternal attitudes and personality from pregnancy to eight months following childbirth. *Devel. Psychol.*, 2, 364 (1970).

28. Mussen, P. H., Conger, J. J. & Kagan, J., *Child development and personality III*, New York 1969.

29. Gerets, J. P., *Een vergeten waarheidscriterium*. Unpubl. Doct. Scr. Nijmegen 1968.

30. Bench, J., Review: prenatal determinants of behavior by Joffe. *Brit. J. Psychol.* 61, 130 (1970).

31. Sontag, L. W., Implications of fetal behavior and environment for adult personalities. *Ann. N.Y. Acad. Sci.* 134, 782 (1966).

32. Richards, T. W. & Newbery, H., Studies in fetal behavior: III. Can performance on test items at six months postnatally be predicted on the basis of fetal activity? *Child Development* 9, 79 (1938).

33. Richards, T. W. & Nelson, V. L., Studies in mental development: II. Analysis of abilities tested at the age of six months by the Gesell Schedule. *J. genet. Psychol.* 52, 327 (1938).

34. Bernard, J., Prediction from human fetal measures. *Child Development* 35, 1243 (1964).

35. Stevenson, H. W., Hess, E. H. & Rheingold, H. L. (eds.), *Early behavior*, New York 1967.

36. Spelt, D. K., Conditioned responses in the human fetus in utero. *J. Exp. Psychot.* 38, 338 (1948).

37. Stechler, G., New-born attention as affected by medication during labor. *Science* 144, 315 (1964).

38. Mussen, P. H. (ed.), *Carmichael's manual of child psychology III*, New York 1970.

COMMENT

R. ADER

The organizers of the conference have been kind enough to invite me to make some comments, so I thought I would supplement what Dr Jans has said using illustrations from research on animals. The vast majority of these studies on humans have been retrospective in nature and, although provocative, are limited by the problems entailed in such methodologies. Dr Jans has made a number of very relevant points for determining the effects of prenatal factors, particularly in emphasizing the interaction and effects of the postnatal environment, maternal factors, and the subsequent social environment. I would like to show you some data on these very points derived, not from a retrospective approach, but from animal experiments in which it has been possible to actually manipulate the prenatal environment, to control for the postnatal effects of maternal factors, and demonstrate differences in development, behavior, and ultimate susceptibility to somatic disease.

Under usual laboratory conditions, rats maintained under a 12-hour light-dark regimen evidence a 24-hour rhythm in adrenocortical function between 21 and 25 days of age [1]. If, however, rats are handled prenatally, i.e., if pregnant females are subjected to 3 minutes of handling each day throughout the period of gestation and the offspring of these and nonhandled controls are fostered to nonhandled animals at parturition, the development of adrenocortical rhythmicity is accelerated [2]. These data are shown in figure 1. Further, there is an accelerated maturation of behavioural function. As can be seen in figure 2, the 24-hour activity rhythm characteristic of the rat is observed earlier in the offspring of handled as compared with nonmanipulated mothers.

Figure 3 provides an example of the interaction between prenatal maternal stimulation and the subsequent social conditions under which the offspring are maintained. Here, again, the offspring of handled and nonhandled mothers were fostered to nonhandled females at parturition. After weaning half of each population was caged individually and half was caged in groups. Differences in susceptibility to experimentally-induced gastric lesions as a function of prenatal maternal handling were observed only within the individually-housed population.

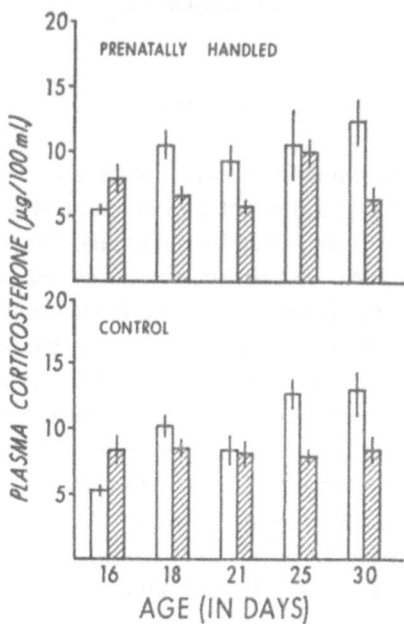

Fig. 1. Development of the 24-hour adrenocortical rhythm as a function of prenatal maternal handling (light bars = values obtained 2 hr. before the onset of darkness; hatched bars = values obtained 2 hr. before the onset of light; vertical lines = standard error of the mean). From Ader and Deitchman (2).

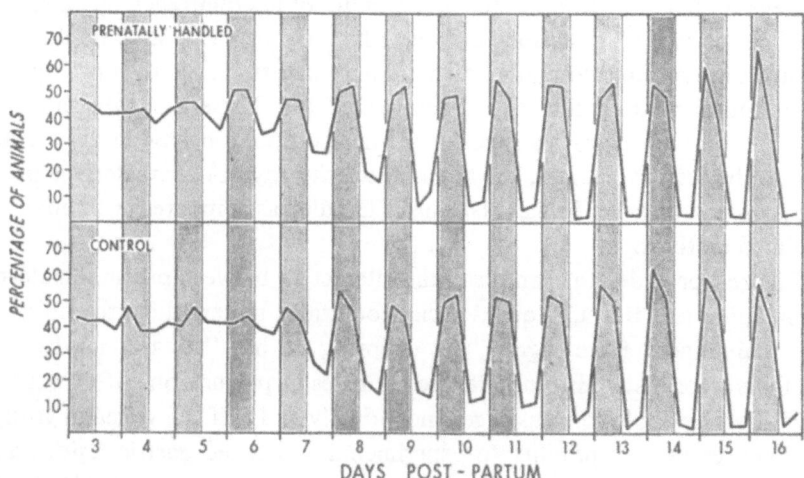

Fig. 2. Development of the 24-hour activity rhythm as a function of prenatal maternal handling of the rat. The values represent the mean percentage of animals per litter engaged in some motor activity during direct observation periods conducted in the light (light areas) and in the dark (shaded areas). From Ader and Deitchman (2).

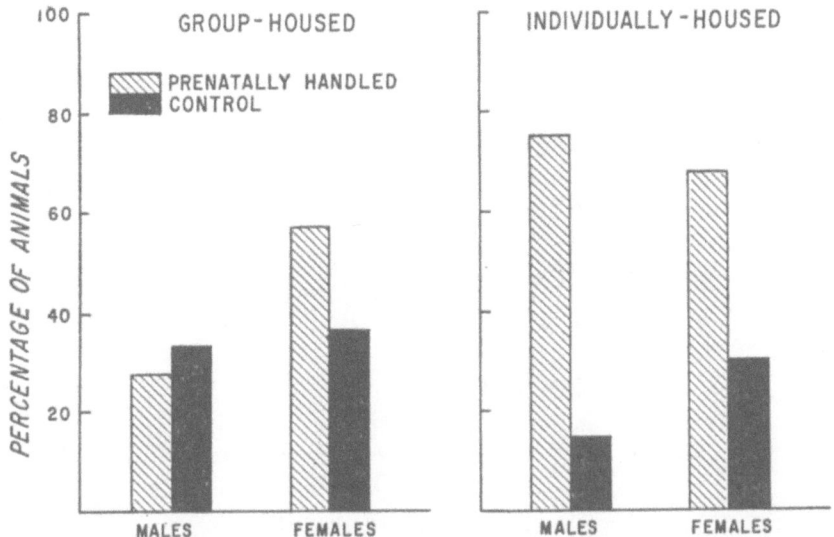

Fig. 3. Effects of prenatal maternal handling on the percentage of animals developing gastric erosions following 6 hours of physical restraint. From Ader and Plaut (4).

For several years now experimenters have been studying the behavioural effects of prenatal maternal x-irradiation. Recently we were led to ask if x-irradiation experienced during pregnancy could influence the postnatal maternal behavior of these animals and to what extent might such an effect account for the behavioral consequences of fetal irradiation. Rats were irradiated (200 R) or sham irradiated on day 16 of pregnancy. At birth the population was divided such that irradiated and nonirradiated females reared litters of fetally irradiated or nonirradiated pups in cages designed to automatically monitor the time that lactating females spend with their litters (3). These cages did uncover a difference in the maternal behavior of animals as a function of whole body x-irradiation (Fig. 4). Animals irradiated during pregnancy spent significantly less time with their pups than animals that were not irradiated – irrespective of whether or not the pups were irradiated during fetal life. Figure 5 contains the data from a reaction-to-handling procedure used to reflect differences in emotional reactivity in the rat. Irradiation during fetal life did not influence subsequent emotional reactivity, but rats reared by irradiated mothers were significantly less reactive than rats reared by control mothers. Similarly, the response to whole body x-irradiation administered when these animals were adults was not influenced by whether animals were irradiated during fetal life, but by

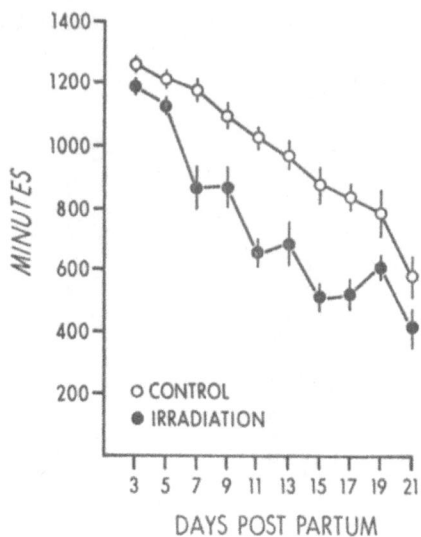

Fig. 4. Mean time spent with the litter by rats irradiated or sham irradiated on day 16 of pregnancy. From Ader and Deitchman (5).

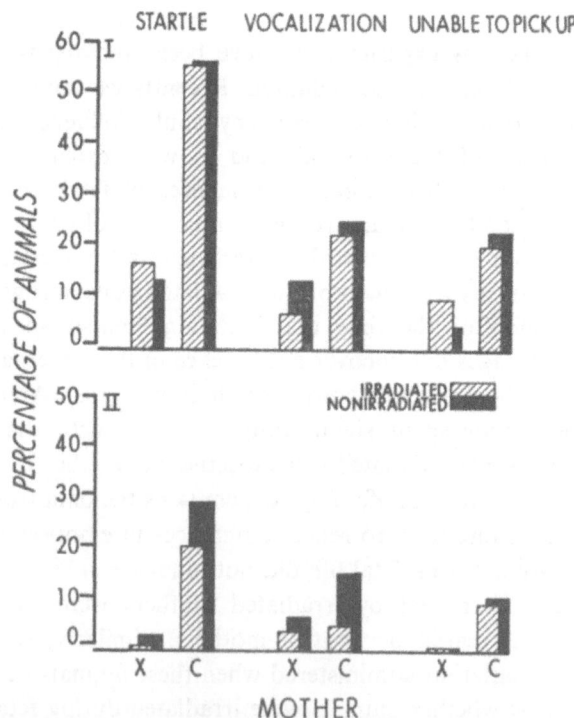

Fig. 5. Emotional reactivity in prenatally irradiated and non-irradiated rats reared by irradiated or nonirradiated foster mothers.

whether they were reared by an irradiated or a nonirradiated mother. Whereas 100% of the animals reared by control mothers survived, there was a 50% mortality among the prenatally irradiated and control animals reared by irradiated mothers.

Although the experimental analysis of prenatal effects is a complex affair, these prospective studies on animals provide ample evidence that prenatal factors are capable of modifying behavioral and physiologic development as well as subsequent psychophysiologic function.

REFERENCES

1. Ader, R., Early experiences accelerate maturation of the 24-hour adrenocortical rhythm. *Science* 163, 1225 (1969).
2. Ader, R. & Deitchman, R., Effects of prenatal maternal handling on the maturation of rhythmic processes. *J. comp. physiol. Psychol.* 71, 492 (1970).
3. Grota, L. J. & Ader, R., Continuous recording of maternal behaviour in *Rattus norvegicus*. *Anim. Behav.* 17, 722 (1969).
4. Ader, R. & Plaut, S. M., Effects of prenatal maternal handling and differential housing on offspring emotionality, plasma corticosterone levels, and susceptibility to gastric erosions. *Psychosom. Med.* 30, 277 (1968).
5. Ader, R. & Deitchman, R., Prenatal maternal X-irradiation: maternal behavior in irradiated and nonirradiated rats and subsequent emotional reactivity and susceptibility to X-irradiation in the offspring. (Unpublished data).

CONGENITAL DEAFNESS AND DISTURBED
PSYCHOMOTOR DEVELOPMENT

A. M. J. VAN UDEN

INTRODUCTION. A CYBERNETIC DEFINITION OF DEAFNESS

Deafness (congenital deafness) is defined here cybernetically, as a hearing loss such that the patient cannot hear his own voice and the other sound-giving effects of his own body without a hearing aid. Concerning the hearing of one's own voice, the following curve of deafness has been described by Von Békésy (1):

Hz.	125	250	500	1000	2000	4000	
dB.	50	60	90	90	90	80	(I.S.O.)

This curve coincides with another definition of deafness: those children are called 'deaf' who will not, even with the best possible equipment and training, be able to understand speech mainly by hearing (2). This inadequate auditory perception of the sound-giving effects of their own body movements may cause some motor difficulties such as:

1. a shuffling gait with accompanying bad postures;
2. difficulties in blowing, including of the nose; i.e. in the control of breathing;
3. backwardness in developing speed of movements (3), which – apart from other causes such as overprotection and so on – may also be due to the longer reaction time to visual than to auditory stimuli (Brills, 1949, in Myklebust, 3).

CONGENITAL DEAFNESS AND EURHYTHMIA

It is thought that eurhythmia, i.e. the ability to execute, imitate, and re-member rhythmic movements, develops in a baby with normal hearing by auditory control: the child sucks, babbles, claps his hands, shakes his cradle and so on, and perceives auditorily the sound-giving effects of his own move-ments. Most of these movements are not visually perceptible, but their sound-giving effects are perceived almost continuously, at least from 0.7 years of age (4).

We applied a test of eurhythmia (5) in three groups of children, 3.6 through 6.5 years of age, by tapping on a table and saying 'baba' in different rhythmic patterns, and obtained the following results (maximum score 40):

A. Congenitally deaf, n = 36: 27.71 ± 8.11
B. Hearing losses between 75 and 85 dB (including children with progressive deafness), n = 14: 32.66 ± 4.21
C. Children with normal hearing, n = 11: 39.66 ± 0.51

$$A < B \qquad t = 2.1244 \qquad p < 0.05$$
$$B < C \qquad t = 2.7175 \qquad p < 0.02$$

We thus found a significant backwardness of deaf children with respect to eurhythmia. This is in agreement with daily experience. This backwardness can be corrected, however, in a cybernetic way. In a pilot study done in two groups of deaf children, we found (5, 6) that melodies played on 'blow-organs' with electronic amplification by the children themselves (group I) were recognized better than the same melodies played to them by another person (group II). Moreover, the first group showed spontaneous rhythmic movements of the trunk and the arms during the recognition task, the second group not at all.

EUPRAXIA AND EURHYTHMIA IN CONGENITALLY DEAF CHILDREN

We constructed a test for eupraxia (7). This test measures the speed of finding arms and legs and the fingers, for intransitive movements. We found a significant and high correlation between this eupraxia and eurhythmia as measured by these tests. Both are correlated with speech-reading and with memory for spoken sentences (8), in the following way:

Matrix of correlations. Prelingually deaf children, n = 60, aged 10,0–17,11 yrs.

	Eurhythmia	Speech-reading	Memory for sentences	Mental age
Eupraxia	0.85 (p < 1%)	0.76 (p < 1%)	0.62 (p < 1%)	0.14 (NS)
Eurhythmia	———	0.77 (p < 1%)	0.67 (p < 1%)	0.20 (NS)
Speech-reading		———	0.77 (p < 1%)	0.32 (p < 2%)
Memory for sentences			———	0.49 (p < 1%)

DYSPRAXIA AND DYSRHYTHMIA

On the basis of these findings, we could predict difficulties in teaching young
deaf children to lipread and talk as well as in auditory training.

*It should be stressed that all deaf children, including the deafest, can and
should be trained auditorily and in vibration-feeling as an aid to lip-reading* (9).

When deaf children are found to score below the 25th percentile rank of the
tests for eupraxia and eurhythmia, within the population of deaf children
of the mental ages 3.6–5.6, typical difficulties in speech can be expected
(with related difficulties in speech-reading and auditory training):

a. perseverations of phonemes, e.g. lomonade;
b. inversions of phonemes, e.g. milonade;
c. cut-offs, e.g. limade;
d. difficulties in short-term memory, i.e. a continuous demolition of the
   words and phrases when the child is requested to repeat them by heart,
   e.g. (5 times) lemonade, lomade, lomo, lamo, lo...

We measured this last finding by counting the total loss of phonemes within
these five repetitions:

Loss of phonemes in a speech memory test:

Deaf children < 25th perc. rank	83% ± 19	
Deaf children > 25th „ „	27% ± 21	t = 6.2500 p < 1%

This disturbance is a kind of dyspraxia of speech, or 'motor-dysphasia'
(10, 11). All this can also happen in children with high intelligence.

Methods of teaching to talk should be adapted to such children. Programs
for training have been developed or are in various stages of development
in our Institute on the basis of our findings, for training in eurhythmia (12),
control of the body scheme, serial successive memory, and integration of
movements with graphic symbols.

The number of deaf children in our Institute who show this multiple
handicap of deafness and 'motor-dysphasia' amounts to 20-25 per cent of
the prelingually deaf.

Only in exceptional cases is the disturbance so severe that means of communication other than the oral kind should be included, e.g. speech and
finger-spelling, purely dactylologic communication, or in some cases sign
language.

A TYPICAL PROFILE OF LEARNING APTITUDE IN DEAF CHILDREN
WITH DYSPRAXIA, INCLUDED DYSRHYTHMIA

The Nebraska non-verbal test of learning aptitude (13) was applied to two groups of 16 deaf children aged 4.6–9.6, one composed of dyspractics and the other of eupractics. These groups were matched according to age, deafness, and non-verbal intelligence (Performance IQ).

	Eupractics (n = 16)		Dyspractics (n = 16)		t	Significance
Chronological age:	7.11 ±	1.6	7.2 ±	2.4	0.0300	NS
Performance IQ:	103 ±	8.74	107 ±	11	1.0282	NS
Learning age:	7.6 ±	2.4	7.8 ±	1.8	0.1170	NS
Eupraxia:	101 ±	13.41	48 ±	18.26	9.0750	p < 1%
Eurhythmia:	117 ±	41.78	40 ±	16.69	6.7662	p < 1%
Speech-reading:	49.18 ±	21.14	15.17 ±	13.32	6.320	p < 1%

The Hiskey-Nebraska test (13) for these ages comprises 8 subtests.

1. Imitation and memory of Bead Patterns.
2. Memory for Colours.
3. Picture Identification.
4. Picture Association: the child is requested to find the correct picture according to some relation, e.g. (in pictures):

flying airplane	flying bird	?

The child has to fill in the picture of a flying kite.
5. Paper Folding: the child has to remember and imitate a series of paper-folding movements.
6. Visual Attention Span: the child has to remember series of pictures presented simultaneously.
7. Block-Patterns.
8. Completion of Drawings.

For each subtest, the rough scores are converted into an 'age', here in months. The median age of these 8 'ages' is the 'Learning Age'. The other 'ages' are scattered around this 'Learning Age'. We calculated the means of the 'ages' of the subtests of both groups separately around an assumed figure of 96 months, to permit comparison of the two groups. The results are plotted in two bar-diagrams (see fig. 1), the length of the bars indicating the deviation from the median age ('Learning Age').

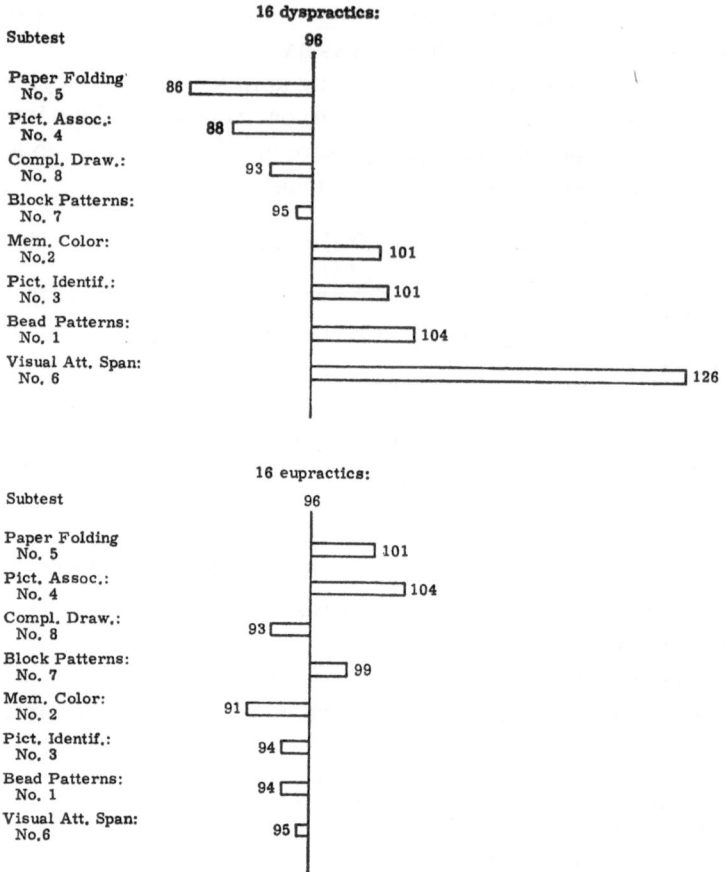

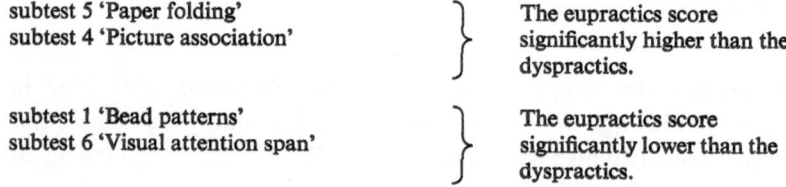

Fig. I. Profile of the learning aptitude according to the Hiskey-Nebraska Test (11). The lengths of the bars indicate the deviation from the average 'Learning Age'.

The difference between the two groups is significant in:

subtest 5 'Paper folding'
subtest 4 'Picture association'
} The eupractics score significantly higher than the dyspractics.

subtest 1 'Bead patterns'
subtest 6 'Visual attention span'
} The eupractics score significantly lower than the dyspractics.

The hyperplasia of the Visual Attention Span (subtest no. 6) is very striking. These dyspractic deaf children generally have a very good memory for simultaneous unrelated visual data. On the one hand this offers a stepping-

stone for their treatment: an educational development via the 'graphic con-
versation', i.e. using their strong side as a compensatory factor. On the other
hand these children seem to be 'absorbed' into a kind of 'visual-image-
thinking', a direct 'visualizing behaviour'. In connection with this, they
underdevelop insight into the invisible relations between pictures (subtest 4)
and have many difficulties with successive memory (subtest 5) too.

The profile of the dyspractic deaf children is significant with respect to:
subtest 'Attention Span' [6] in contrast to all other subtests; subtest 'Bead
Patterns' [1] and subtest 'Picture Identification' [3] in contrast to 'Paper
Folding' [5] and 'Picture Association' [3].
      The profile of the eupractic deaf children is only significantly prominent
for:
      Picture Association [4] – one of the weak sides of the dyspractic deaf child-
ren – in contrast to 'Memory Color' [2], 'Picture Identification' [3], 'Bead
Patterns' [1], and 'Visual Attention Span' [6].

CONCLUSIONS
There seems to be some relation between motor development and cognitive
development, mediately by means of speech and language, and perhaps also
immediately: Myklebust (3) found deaf children to rely more than hearing
children on trial-and-error manipulation in solving the problems of a
complex form-board. This was a task in which speech and language did not
seem to be involved.
      We have not yet applied our test of eupraxia to hearing children, but
Myklebust (3) found not-multiply-handicapped deaf children behind normal hearing in the 'Railwalking Test' of Heath (12), which measures the
integration of body movements 'governed' as a single unit (14). This seems to
indicate a backwardness in eupraxia, related to the backwardness in eurhythmia found by us. This double but not unrelated backwardness may include a
hyperplastic, uncoded, visual behaviour as found in the backwardness of
deaf as compared to hearing children in Picture Association (13), Picture
Analogies (15), Picture Arrangement and Digit Symbol (16).
      Auditory deprivation seems to be connected with specific disturbances
in motoric and cognitive behaviour. This calls for special programs of basic
training in eurhythmia, eupraxia, serial successive memory, integration of
motor behaviour (including speech) and of movement and symbol.
      There is, however, no reason for pessimism in view of the results shown by
many well educated deaf children with respect to the purely oral way of com-

munication and thinking. On the contrary, improvement of the educational programs may lead to a better-balanced integration of the deaf into the world of the hearing.

SUMMARY

A retardation in the development of eurhythmia in deaf children as compared to children with various degrees of partial hearing, is considered on the basis of a cybernetic definition of deafness.

A correlation was found between eupraxia and eurhythmia. Its implications for teaching deaf children to talk are explained. This problem is enhanced by disturbances of dyspraxia and dysrhythmia in a rather large percentage of deaf children. These children have been found to show a typical profile of learning aptitude.

An outline is given for a program of training which is basic for a purely oral method.

REFERENCES

1. Békésy, G. von, The structure of the middle ear and hearing of one's own voice by bone conduction. *J. Acoust. Soc. Am. 21*, 217 (1949).
2. Davis H. & Silverman, S., *Hearing and deafness*, St. Louis 1970.
3. Myklebust, H. R., *The psychology of deafness*, New York 1964.
4. Downs, M., Early identification (of hearing loss) and principles of management. In: *Proc. int. conf. oral educ.*, Washington 1967.
5. Van Uden, A. M. J., Inleidende proef met blaasorgeltjes. *T. Doofstommenonderw. 25*, 32 (1955).
6. Van Uden, A. M. J., Instructing prelingually deaf children by rhythm of bodily movements and of sounds, by oral mime and general bodily expression, – its possibilities and difficulties. In: *Proc. int. congr. educ. of the deaf*, Washington 1963.
7. Van Uden, A. M. J., *Eupraxie en spraak*, St Michielsgestel 1970.
8. Van Uden, A. M. J., *A world of language for deaf children*, Rotterdam 1970.
9. Van Uden, A. M. J., Het verstaan der spraak. In: *Jaarverslag Instituut voor Doven*, St Michielsgestel 1962.
10. Prick, J. J. G. & Van der Waals, H. G., *Nederlands handboek der psychiatrie, deel I en III*, Arnhem, 1958, 1965.
11. Luchsinger, R. & Arnold, G. E., *Lehrbuch der Sprech- und Stimmheilkunde*, Wien 1970.
12. Van Uden, A. M. J., Der Rhythmus bei der Hörerziehung gehörloser Kinder. Theorie und Praxis, besonders bei der Hausspracherziehung und im Kindergarten. In: *Arbeitstagung für Hörerziehung 1968-1969*, Erlangen 1971.
13. Hiskey, M. S., *Hiskey Nebraska test of learning aptitude*, Nebraska 1966.
14. Cratty, B. J., *Movement behavior and motor learning*, Philadelphia 1964.
15. Snijders, J. Th. & Snijders-Oomen, A. W. M., *Niet-verbaal intelligentieonderzoek van horenden en doofstommen*, Groningen 1961.
16. Murphy, L. J. & Murphy, K. P., in: *Educational guidance and the deaf child*, Ewing, A. W. G. (ed.), Manchester 1957.

DISCUSSION

Wensink: Did you differentiate between different kinds of congenital deafness? We are working with spastic children which are also deaf.

Van Uden: We have in our institute not so many spastic children. Only a very few, because these are mostly not quite deaf. You find them more in the schools for partially hearing. We have some of them. These spastic children have choreatiform movements, spastic movements and so on, sometimes, but not always dyspraxic disturbances. Dyspraxia occurs in almost all children deafened by maternal rubella, and in children with the Usher-syndrome, i.e. in children with deafness and retinitis pigmentosa.

Roebers: I have some experience with rhesus incompatibility. Children who are deaf and have serious motor-disturbances. It is very curious that they show, as you said, very good results with picture memory. But they have nearly all bad results with the so-called Knox' cube test. That is a test, also a short-term memory test, in which they need to comply some more acting, memory and movement together.

Van Uden: I found the same. I have not mentioned that, but I found the same difference, a significant difference between the groups by means of the Knox' cube test. The test is as follows. The child has four cubes before him and I arrange some structure, some pattern for the child by tapping the cubes e.g. 1-3-2-4. The child has to imitate me. If you compare that with, say, drawing in the Benton-test, you may find children with very high scores in the latter test and very low scores in the Knox' cube test. This is the same as I have given in that profile of learning aptitude.

Roebers: It is quite interesting that you get similar results for some children with a motor disturbance only.

Van Uden: The same results. Yes.

Levine: Is it possible to differentiate the retardation you see in these children, to distinguish between the consequences of the essential sensory deprivation and other neurological deficits which may be associated with deafness?

Van Uden: I found that dyspraxia in all kinds of children. Also in children with hereditary deafness. What is the reason? As a psychologist I cannot say the child has dyspraxia and thus there must be some neurological disturbance. I don't know. That is not my job.

Akiyama: The aspect of motor deficits in deaf children is very intriguing and I wonder if you have any experience with infants that are congenitally deaf. I have not had much experience, but as I recall the gross motor aspect of infants who are deaf but do not have other neurological deficits, appear to mature normally up to a certain point and the only major deficit is their babbling and onset of speech. I wonder if you or anyone else have any comments or any experience regarding this aspect of infant.

Van Uden: Congenitally deaf children babble also. But their babbling deteriorates very soon. In one year already the babbling is reduced to some vocalization and the first to get lost are the consonants, leaving A, O and so on. The point is to treat the child so that this babbling continues, and bring that babbling to speech. We have only a few children which we have known from ages of 4, 5 and 6 months; these were almost completely silent in the cradle, silent babies. And afterwards I found some of them had very serious dyspraxia. Some children had dyspraxia in such a degree that they could not learn to talk. And they had to learn finger spelling. Some of them had to learn signing too. This is the experience I have. The second point is: there is a big difference between the gross movement control and the fine movement control. I have found that the fine movement control of the fingers is much more correlated with speech than the gross movement control.

EFFECTS OF CONGENITAL BLINDNESS ON DEVELOPMENT OF BEHAVIOUR

M. W. VAN HOF

In the seventeenth century the philosopher Locke in his *Essay concerning human understanding* (1) posed the question as to whether visual identification of shapes would be possible in man born blind and made to see at adult age. Nowadays there are many reports on patients operated on for congenital cataract and other causes of early blindness (2, 3, 4, 5). The answer to Locke's question is that immediately after surgery objects which can be recognized by touch cannot be identified by way of the visual system. A long period of training is required before the patients are able to make use, if ever, of the visual system.

At first sight these observations seem to support the importance of sensory rather than genetic factors in the development of the complicated neuronal network by which patterns are analysed. However, it could also be that initially the wiring diagram of the visual system develops but thereafter disintegrates due to disuse.

Considerations of this nature have stimulated a great deal of research on the visual system in animals raised in darkness or raised with closed eyelids. In this article a survey of some of these studies will be given.

The best known behavioural experiments on the effect of light deprivation are those by Riesen (6, 7) on chimpanzees. This author found that chimpanzees reared in darkness till the age of 16 months showed more or less the same symptoms as human patients after surgery for congenital cataract. The animals for instance did not recognize the feeding bottle. If an object was brought slowly towards the face no behavioural response was elicited until the object made contact with the face. In normally illuminated surroundings only partial recovery took place.

Many studies have been carried out in kittens raised in darkness. Unfortunately some studies were done on animals raised under normal illumination conditions but with one eye sutured, other studies were done on animals raised in complete darkness.

Baxter (8) studied cats which had been raised in continuous darkness from before eye opening to approximately 1 year of age. A variety of tests was used: visual placing, jumping, following movements of the eyes and others. According to this author all animals recovered in 30 days or less after leaving the darkroom. In our experience (unpublished data) even in animals which are allowed to play several hours per day it takes several months before visually guided behavior becomes normal.

Wiesel and Hubel (9) studied kittens in which the lids of one eye were closed for the first 3 months of life. Thereafter the deprived eye was opened and the other one sutured. 'Visual placing never returned. When put on the floor to roam freely, the animal would at times avoid large obstacles, but at other times would collide with them. It seldom avoided small objects such as chair legs. Placed on a chair, it would slide down, feeling its way with its forepaws. If the good eye was uncovered, the kitten would promptly jump to the floor.'

Eighteen months were allowed for recovery in some animals. Unfortunately these results are only in partial agreement with the findings of Ganz and Fitch (10), who described severe visual deficits in monocularly reared cats but only some of those defects were found to be permanent. In all animals the visual placing reaction developed after opening the deprived eye and suturing the experienced eye. In the same study the ability to discriminate horizontal vs. vertical rectangles was studied. None of the monocularly deprived animals was able to learn this task. In a pilot study in our laboratory we found that cats reared in darkness for 4 months after birth are very well able to discriminate vertical vs. horizontal striations. Immediately after leaving the darkroom the animals showed the same symptoms as those described by Baxter (8). At the age of five months training was started in a discrimination box described previously (11, 12). Five out of six dark-raised animals learned to discriminate vertical vs. horizontal striations. However, as figure 1 shows, the results of the five animals that learned this task were not as good as those of four normally raised cats of the same age. This difference was not present in prolonged training with 45° vs. 135° striations. More studies will be necessary to find out whether the discrepancies between Ganz's results and ours are simply due to differences of experimental set-ups or to differences between monocularly and binocularly deprived cats.

Dews and Wiesel (13) varied the age of suturing the eyelids and the duration of deprivation. When the cats were a year old visual acuity of the deprived eye was tested by means of a behavioural technique. It was found that eyelid closure dimished visual acuity only when applied between 1 and 4 months after birth.

Blakemore and Cooper (14) raised kittens till the age of 5 months in an environment in which only horizontal or vertical contours were present.

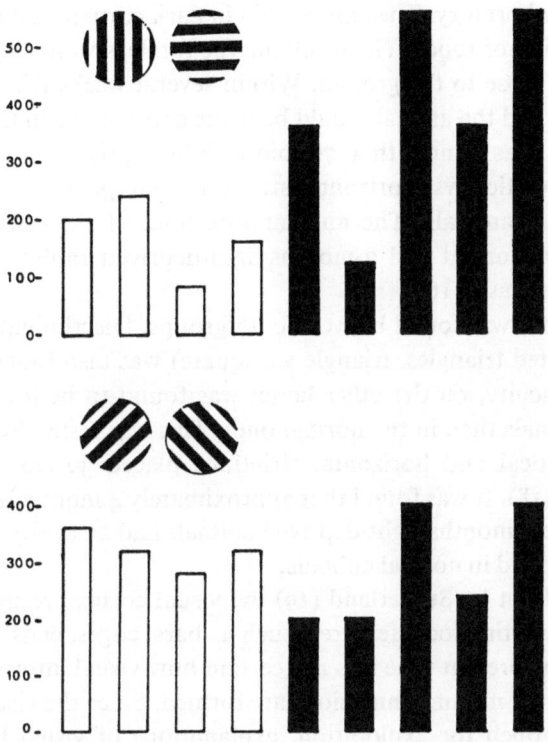

Fig. 1. Five-months old dark-raised (black bars) and normal cats (white bars) were trained to discriminate vertical vs. horizontal and 45° vs. 135° striations. Bar height indicates the number of pattern exposures offered before a score of 90 percent or better was reached.

Some of the deficits in these animals were permanent. The cats which had experienced only horizontal contours were blind for vertical contours and vice versa.

Summarizing one can conclude that these heterogeneous results in the cat clearly show that light deprivation causes visual defects. Only some of these defects are permanent. Some controversy exists as to the permanency of certain specific defects. In monocularly blinded animals a well defined critical period has been found. In our opinion the descriptions of the behavioural effects of light deprivation are not consistent enough to conclude that monocularly deprived cats (after covering the normal eye) are more impaired than animals reared in complete darkness.

Rabbits raised in darkness for 7 months after birth also show an abnormal behaviour after leaving the darkroom (15). This was confirmed in a recent study in our laboratory. The animals hid in dark corners and did not react to the presentation of food. When walking the forelegs were widely spread and the head was close to the ground. Within several weeks their behaviour became normal and the animals could be made cooperative in the training box. After this it was found that 7-months-light-deprived rabbits learned to discriminate vertical vs. horizontal striations and 45° vs. 135° ones equally fast as normal animals. The angular threshold of tilt discrimination was determined in normal and 7-months-light-deprived rabbits, in the way as described previously (16).

No difference was found between both groups. Discrimination of different shapes (inverted triangles, triangle vs. square) was also found to be normal (17). Visual acuity, on the other hand, was found to be lower in the light-deprived animals than in the normal ones. This was tested by decreasing the width of vertical and horizontal striations placed 30 cm in front of the training box (18). It was found that approximately 4 months after leaving the darkroom the 7-months-light-deprived animals had an acuity of about 36' instead of 20' found in normal animals.

As pointed out by Sutherland (19) the visual cortex presumably acts as a processor extracting local features (such as bars, edges, ends) from the input picture. At the present time it is not certain how visual information is stored and where visuo-motor connections are formed. Since the visual cortex is the highest level open for exploration, explanations of visual behaviour after light deprivation in neurobiological terms are inevitably incomplete.

In several species the development of the retina has been studied by means of the electroretinogram. In animals born with immature eyes and closed eyelids, like cats and rabbits, the electroretinogram develops during the first weeks after birth, more or less parallel with the morphological maturation of the retina. In spite of light deprivation the electroretinogram in cats (20) and rabbits (21) develops during the first weeks after birth. In the guinea-pig the retina develops during the intra-uterine period. These animals are born with open eyelids and are able to see (22). The electroretinogram is fully developed after birth (23).

Counting the number of ganglion cells it has been shown by Chow et al. (24) that light deprivation for more than 7 months is accompanied by the disappearance of a large percentage of the ganglion cells in the retina of the chimpanzee. This phenomenon was not found in dark-reared cats and rats (25). The inner plexiform layer of dark-reared cats was found to be thinner than in normals by Weiskrantz (26). In light-deprived rabbits abnormal enzyme concentrations are found (27), whereas the amount of RNA is reduced in ganglion cells as well as in cells of the outer and inner nuclear layer of light-deprived chimpanzees, cats and rats (28).

Electroretinographic studies have shown that a prolonged stay in darkness reduces the b-wave in dark-reared cats (29, 10) and guinea-pigs (30). A few days' exposure to light normalizes the electroretinogram. No investigations are available as to whether the biochemical changes disappear at the same rate as recovery of the electroretinogram. The rabbit's retinogram is remarkably resistant to light deprivation (21): b-wave reduction is almost absent after seven months of darkness.

As to the circuitry of the interneuronal connections in the retina these data allow very few definite conclusions. Since a severe loss of ganglion cells occurs in the chimpanzee it seems a likely assumption that this is at least partially responsible for the abnormal behaviour after light deprivation. In other species the situation is not clear. The fact that light deprivation has a reversible effect on the electroretinogram of cats and guinea-pigs and almost no effect on that of the rabbit, suggests that in those animals the retina is not affected by dark-rearing. However, the only generally accepted fact about the b-wave of the electroretinogram is that it is generated in the bipolar layer. A normal b-wave does not necessarily imply that the interneuronal wiring diagram is normally developed.

Single units in the visual cortex of 8- and 16-day old, visually inexperienced, cats have essentially the same response patterns as simple and complex units in the cortex of adult cats (31). The majority of the cells are driven by both eyes. This means that the visual cortex of the cat develops to a great extent without sensory stimulation. So far it has not been studied whether hypercomplex cells (32) are also present in young kittens.

Suturing the lids of one eye after birth causes morphological changes of those cells in the geniculate body which are connected with the deprived eye. A considerable reduction of the cell volume is found (33). In spite of this the electrical response to sensory stimuli changes very little. The response pattern of cortical cells, on the other hand, is altered: only very few cells can be driven from the deprived eye after an eyelid closure of 3 months. No changes are found in adult cats after a similar period of eye closure. By systematically varying the period of lid closure the susceptibility of those cortical cells to monocular deprivation has been determined (34). This period coincides with that found behaviourally (13). After 3 months monocular light deprivation, exposure to light for more than a year causes little recovery of the electrical reactions.

Binocular postnatal light deprivation decreases the cross-sectional areas of all cells in the geniculate bodies. The changes in the visual cortex were different from those after monocular deprivation. More than half of the cells reacted normally, the others were unresponsive or had lost the specificity for oriented lines (32). No recovery studies were done.

Hirsch and Spinelli (35) described that in the visual cortex of cats, raised with one eye viewing horizontal lines and one eye viewing vertical lines, only horizontally and vertically oriented receptive fields are found. All fields were monocularly driven. As described before, Blakemore and Cooper (14) raised cats in an environment with horizontal and vertical stripes. The orientation of most of the cortical receptive fields were parallel with the stripes the animal had experienced.

From the electrophysiological studies in the cat it follows that the inter-neuronal connections of the visual cortex are mainly determined innately. The connections can be modified by binocular and monocular deprivation as well as by raising the animals in an environment with only horizontal and vertical contrasts. Each of these conditions leads to characteristic changes of the electrophysiological responses of the cortical cell population.

Very few electrophysiological studies have been done in light-deprived rabbits. Recording visual evoked responses (V.E.R.) Bonaventura et al. (36) found that under normal circumstances a surface-negative wave can be recorded from the visual cortex at the age of 8 days. The initial surface positive component of the V.E.R. appears between the 10th and 12th day after birth, whereas the amplitude increases till the age of 2 months. In rabbits reared in darkness the surface negative wave can also be recorded from the 8th day. The initial surface positive component, on the other hand, is retarded and does not appear before the 17th day. The amplitude increases till the 21st day and decreases thereafter. The same authors found that when the rabbits were brought into an illuminated surrounding, the evoked responses recovered. In a pilot study (Kobayashi and Van Hof, in press) we found that after 7 months light deprivation the V.E.R. recovers. As figure 2 shows, the amplitude of the first positive deflection and of the positive-negative wave are both reduced in 7-months-light-deprived rabbits. After an additional exposure of one month the surface positive wave is of normal size, whereas the positive-negative deflection is in the normal range after 2 months. An interesting coincidence is that 7-months-light-deprived rabbits became cooperative in the training box more than one month after leaving the darkroom (48 ± 5 days, instead of 22 ± 1, 5 days in normal animals).

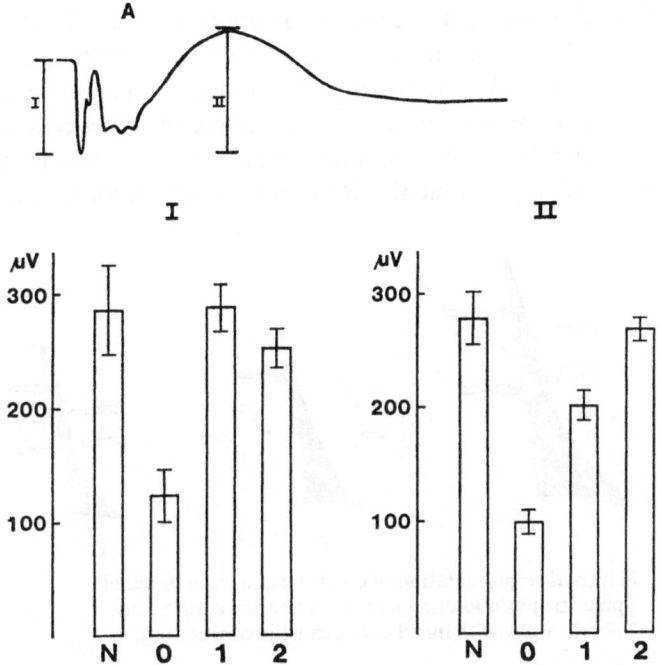

Fig. 2. A Visual Evoked Response determined by averaging the response to 100 flashes.
I.   Average amplitude and standard error of first cortical positive deflection in 4 groups
     of rabbits:
     N: normal animals;
     O: 7-months-light-deprived animals
         immediately after leaving the dark room;
     1.   7-months-light-deprived animals
         one month after leaving the dark room;
     2.   7-months-light-deprived animals
         2 months after leaving the dark room.
II. Average negative-positive difference and standard error in the same groups of
     animals.

Although these V.E.R. results need further confirmation they suggest that also in the rabbit initial development is followed by disintegration due to disuse. The V.E.R. and behavioural studies show that at least partial recovery takes place after additional light deprivation in 7-months-light-deprived rabbits.

In numerous reports it has been shown that morphological changes occur in the visual cortex. Coleman and Riesen (37) have shown that the length of the dendritic tree is reduced in neurons of the visual cortex in light-deprived cats, whereas Valverde (38) and Ruiz-Marcos and Valverde (39) found the number of dendritic spines to be reduced in light-deprived mice. Spine deformities have also been found in 30-days-light-deprived rabbits (40). Unfortunately it is not yet known as to whether the number of spines is reduced from the beginning of development or that the number of spines reduces after an initial normal development. The interpretation of spine loss is still speculative. One possibility is that the interneuronal connections are disrupted

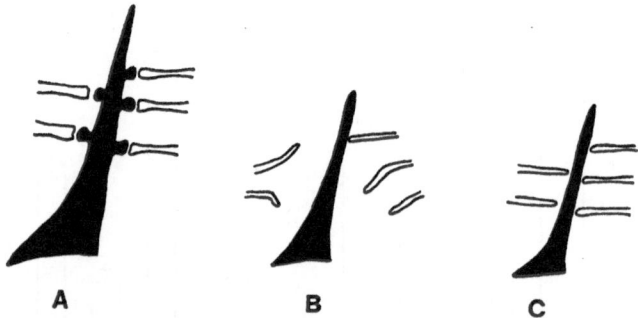

Fig. 3. A. Schematic representation of dendritic and axon terminals.
        B. Spine atrophy and disrupted exo- dendritic connections.
        C. Spine atrophy with intact exo- dendritic connections.

(Fig. 3B). The other possibility is that spine atrophy is an indication of reversible or irreversible unconductivity of the synapses (Fig. 3C). The loss of reactivity of cortical units after light deprivation can be explained by both possibilities. Fifkova (41) found the number of synaptic contacts to be reduced in light-deprived rats. This shows that disintegration of the wiring diagram occurs (3B) but it does not exclude the possibility shown in figure 3C.

The results obtained so far suggest that light deprivation will prove to be an important tool in future research on genetic and sensory factors in brain development. To me the most important problem in light deprivation research is the concept of the 'critical period'. If this concept is true with respect to the development of intra-neuronal circuitry the following must be explained:

1. the beginning of the critical period, i.e. the vanishing insensitivity of the early developing nervous system;

2. the end of the critical period, i.e. the nature of the consolidation process trailing early development;
3. eventual recovery after light deprivation.

REFERENCES

1. Locke, J., *Essay concerning human understanding*. 1690.
2. Gregory, R. L. & Wallace, J. G., Recovery from early blindness. *Exp. Psychol. Soc. Monograph* 2 (1963).
3. London, I. D., A Russian report on the postoperative newly seeing. *Amer. J. Psychol.* 73, 478 (1960).
4. Valvo, A., Behaviour patterns and visual rehabilitation after early and long-lasting blindness. *Am. J. Ophthalm.* 65, 19 (1968).
5. Von Senden, M., *Raum- und Gestaltauffassung bei operierten Blindgeborenen vor und nach der Operation*. Leipzig 1932.
6. Riesen, A. H., The development of visual perception in man and chimpanzee. *Science* 106, 107 (1947).
7. Riesen, A. H., Arrested vision. *Scientific Am.* 2 (1950).
8. Baxter, B. L., Effect of visual deprivation during postnatal maturation of the electroencephalogram of the cat. *Exp. Neurol.* 14, 224 (1966).
9a. Wiesel, T. N. & Hubel, D. H., Comparison of the effects of unilateral and bilateral eye closure on cortical unit responses in kittens. *J. Neurophysiol.* 28, 1029 (1965).
9b. Wiesel, T. N. & Hubel, D. H. Extent of recovery from the effects of visual deprivation in kittens. *J. Neurophysiol.* 28, 1060 (1965).
10. Ganz, L., Fitch, M. & Sattenberg, J. A., The selective effect of visual deprivation
11. Van Hof, M. W., Discrimination between striated patterns of different orientation in the rabbit. *Vision Res.* 6, 89 (1966).
12. Van Hof, M. W., Mechanisms of orientation discrimination. *Exp. Neurol.* 28, 494 (1970).
13. Dews, P. B. & Wiesel, T. N., Consequences of monocular deprivation on visual behaviour in kittens. *J. Physiol.* 206, 437 (1970).
14. Blakemoore, C. & Cooper, G. F., Development of the brain depends on the visual
15. Goodman, L., Effect of total absence of function on the optic system of rabbits. *Am. J. Physiol.* 100, 46 (1931).
16. Van Hof, M. W. & Wiersma, C. A. G., The angular threshold of discrimination for striated patterns of different orientation in the rabbit. *Vision Res.* 7, 265 (1967).
17. Kobayashi, K. & van Hof, M. W., Shape discrimination in normal and light de-
18. Van Hof, M. W., Visual acuity in the rabbit. *Vision Res.* 7, 749 (1967).
19. Sutherland, N. S., Outlines of a theory of visual pattern recognition in animals and man. *Proc. Roy. Soc. B.* 171, 297 (1968).
20. Zetterström, B., The effect of light on the appearance and development of the electroretinogram in newborn kittens. *Acta Physiol. Scand.* 35, 272 (1955).
21. Reuter, J. H. & Van Hof, M. W., The postnatal development of the ERG in rabbits reared in darkness. *Proc. 7th ISCERG symp.* 29 (1969).
22. Hess, H., Imprinting, *Science* 130, 133 (1959).
23. Bornschein, H., Zur postnatalen Entwicklung der Netzhautfunktion. *Wiener Klin. Wochenschrift* 71, 956 (1959).
24. Chow, K. L., Riesen, A. H. & Newell, F. W., Degeneration of retinal ganglion cells in infant chimpanzees reared in darkness. *J. comp. Neurol.* 107, 27 (1957).

25. Riesen, A. H., Effect of stimulus deprivation on the development and atrophy of the visual sensory system. *Am. J. Orthopsychiatry* 30, 23 (1960).
26. Weiskrantz, L., Sensory deprivation and the cat's optic nervous system. *Nature* 181, 1047 (1958).
27. Schimke, R. T., Effects of prolonged light deprivation on the development of retinal enzymes in the rabbit. *J. Biol. Chem.* 234, 700 (1959).
28. Rasch, E., Swift, H., Riesen, A. H. & Chow, K. L., Altered structure and composition of retinal cells in dark-reared mammals. *Exp. Cell Res.* 25, 348 (1961).
29. Baxter, B. & Riesen, A., Electroretinogram of the visually deprived cat. *Science* 134, 1626 (1961).
30. Legein, C. P. J. J. M. M. & Van Hof, M. W., The effect of light deprivation on the electro retinogram of the guinea pig. *Pflügers Arch.* 318, 1 (1970).
31. Hubel, D. H. & Wiesel, T. N., Receptive fields of cells in striate cortex of very young visually inexperienced kittens. *J. Neurophysiol.* 26, 994 (1963).
32. Hubel, D. H. & Wiesel, T. N., Receptive fields and functional architecture in two nonstriate visual areas (18 and 19) of the cat. *J. Neurophysiol.* 28, 229 (1965).
33a. Wiesel, T. N. & Hubel, D. H., Effects of visual deprivation on morphology and physiology of cells in the cat's lateral geniculate body. *J. Neurophysiol.* 26, 978 (1963).
33b. Wiesel, T. N. & Hubel, D. H., Single-cell responses in striate cortex of kittens deprived of vision in one eye. *J. Neurophysiol.* 26, 1003 (1963).
34. Hubel, D. H. & Wiesel, T. N., The period of susceptibility to the physiological effects of unilateral eye closure in kittens. *J. Physiol.* 206, 419 (1970).
35. Hirsch, H. V. B. & Spinelli, D. N., Visual experience modifies distribution of horizontally and vertically oriented receptive fields in cats. *Science* 1968, 869 (1970).
36. Bonaventure, N., Goswamy, S. & Karli, P., Maturation des potentiels ERG et évoqués visuels chez le lapin élevé dans des conditions naturelles d'éclairement ambiant. *C. R. Soc. Biol.* 161, 689 (1967).
37. Coleman, P. D. & Riesen, A. H., Environmental effects on cortical dendritic fields. *J. Anat.* 102, 363 (1968).
38. Valverde, F., Apical dendritic spines of visual cortex and light deprivation in the mouse. *Exp. Brain Res.* 3, 337 (1967).
39. Ruiz-Marcos, A. & Valverde, F., The temporal evolution of the distribution of dendritic spines in the visual cortex of normal and dark raised mice. *Exp. Brain. Res.* 8, 284 (1969).
40. Globus, A. & Scheibel, A. B., The effect of visual deprivation on cortical neurons: a Golgi study. *Exp. Neurol.* 19, 331 (1967).
41. Fifkova, E., The effect of monocular deprivation on the synaptic contacts of the visual cortex. *J. Neurobiol.* 1, 285 (1970).

DISCUSSION

Freedman: I just want to comment on your use of the term 'light-deprived animal'. What is in fact deprivation may be different in different species. The rodents you spoke about are all dark adapted animals. The chimpanzee is not. It sleeps at night. One would therefore expect different 'wiring diagrams' in these two groups, and different thresholds for pathological effects.

Van Hof: As far as I know the only clear-cut species differences with respect to light deprivation have been found at the retinal level. In the chimpanzee light deprivation leads to ganglion cell degeneration (24)* whereas this phenomenon does not occur in the cat's retina (25). The effect of light deprivation on the b-wave also differs among species. The guinea-pig's b-wave reduces already after 3 months light deprivation (30). In the rabbit, on the other hand, a 7-months' period of darkness has hardly any effect on the b-wave (21). To me it seems unlikely that species differences can be explained by the fact that the rodents I spoke about are 'dark-adapted' animals. On the average the locomotor activity of the rabbit during the day is certainly not less than during the night (Van Hof-Van Duin, to be published in Documenta Ophthalmologica).

Widdowson: Another species difference is that some animals are born with their eyes open and the human baby is one of these. He opens his eyes in the darkness, whereas other animals like the kitten and the rabbit, which you used, don't open their eyes till some time after birth, so that their first experience when they open their eyes is light.

Van Hof: Retinal development in the rabbit occurs during the first weeks after birth, whereas the guinea-pig is born with a mature retina. Whether the eye-lids are opened in darkness or in light seems irrelevant. The cat, the rabbit and the guinea-pig open their eyes in a period in which light deprivation has no effect on the retina.

* See references of previous article.

Baum: What are your criticisms of the Hubel and Wiesel experiment that you mentioned?

Van Hof: I do not criticize the experiments but the interpretation which one quite often finds in the literature.

1. Hubel and Wiesel's findings strongly support the view that the visual cortex is pre-wired. However, a certain caution is desirable since hyper-complex cells have not been studied so far in young visually inexperienced kittens.

2. A pre-wired visual cortex does not necessarily mean that the whole visual system is pre-wired. According to Sutherland the retina, the geniculate body and the visual cortex act as preprocessor, whereas pattern recognition, perceptual learning, visual memory is probably mediated by other, ill-defined, structures in the brain. The fact that the visual cortex is pre-wired does by no means prove that this also holds for those areas.

Akiyama: In infants, or in children with amblyopia ex anopsia, I believe if the defect is not corrected at a 'critical' or 'vulnerable' period, they can lose the vision of that particular eye. But yet I would imagine that they are still receiving light in that defective eye. Do you have any comments on what might be wrong here as to the permanent loss of vision in terms of the 'circuit' or 'wiring diagram' of the brain despite the fact that they have gotten light in their eyes?

Van Hof: This is different from light deprivation. In relation to amblyopia the most important studies are presumably those by Hubel and Wiesel on the effects of artificial squint (J. Neurophysiol., 28, 1041, 1965). They found that in young kittens several months after cutting the medial rectus of one eye, the recordings from single units were normal. However, the number of binocularly driven cells was strongly reduced. In this way it becomes understandable that the output of one eye only is processed in the brain.

THE INFLUENCE OF EMOTIONAL DEPRIVATION
ON GROWTH AND BEHAVIOUR

W. CROUGHS

THE INSTITUTIONAL SYNDROME

The first studies of emotional deprivation concerned children living in an institution (1-7). Spitz and Wolf (7) studied children in a foundling home where the infants lived in cubicles up to 15 to 18 months of age, completely separated from each other. Their visual radius and locomotion were extremely restricted. During their first few months these infants were breastfed by their mothers. Permanent separation from the mother took place predominantly in the sixth month. After removal of the mother, many of these children developed a syndrome that the authors called anaclitic depression. Beginning with apprehension, sadness, and weeping, the syndrome continued into rejection, withdrawal, loss of appetite, refusal to eat, loss of weight, loss of interest in the outside world, stereotyped movements, dejection, retardation, and finally a condition that could only be described as stuporous. In spite of the fact that hygiene and precautions against contagion were impeccable, the children showed marked susceptibility to infection and illness of every kind. During a follow-up period of two years this group showed a mortality of 37 per cent. Of 21 surviving children still at the institution, only 2 fell within the height range of a normal two-year-old child (6). Only 5 out of 21 were able to walk unassisted. Mental and speech development were extremely retarded. The authors also studied another institution where the infants were less isolated and were cared for by their mothers (delinquent girls). In a number of cases the mother was temporarily removed somewhere between the sixth and eighth month. Some of these children also developed the syndrome of anaclitic depression. After restoration of the love object following approximately three months of absence, the syndrome disappeared. This was in contrast to the cases of longer-lasting separation in the foundling home, where intervention was no longer effective and the syndrome appeared to become irreversible. During a follow-up period of one year not a single child died and motor and mental development were within normal limits. As regards the aetiology of the syndrome, Durfee and Wolf (1), who performed an investigation of institutional care of infants in 1933, already stressed two important factors that were responsible for the psychological injury suffered by these infants: lack of stimulation and absence of the mother. Spitz and Wolf (7) also stressed the importance of free locomotion in the second half-year of life, which they considered to be the most vulnerable age. At that age, motor activity can be used for an attempt to seek replacement for the lost love object. Moreover, it can be argued that in the syndrome of anaclitic depression the acute separation of mother and child is more harmful than mere absence of the mother.

The remote effects of institutional care on personality structure have been extensively studied (8-15). Lowrey (8) described aggressiveness, feeding difficulties (refusal, slow eating, voracity), enuresis, speech and language defects, attention-demanding behaviour, shyness and sensitiveness, in 28 children who had been institutionalized for the first three years of their lives. In contrast, three children institutionalized after two years of age for shorter periods did not present these personality and behaviour patterns. Goldfarb (11-15) compared children who had been institutionalized during the first three years of life, at which time they were transferred to foster-homes, with children whose life experience had been in foster-homes from early infancy. At the ages of six, eight, and twelve years, the children with institutional experience showed mental test results and language development consistently below those of the foster-home children. He concluded that extreme psychological deprivation in infancy produces a lag in mental growth which is maintained even under new conditions of enriched stimulation. Studies of older institutional children (16, 17) have strongly stressed the relationship between emotional adjustment and linear growth. However, inadequate caloric intake ('loss of appetite, refusal to eat') and frequent infections are part of the picture of anaclitic depression and cannot be ruled out as equally important factors interfering with growth in these infants. Subsequent to the institutional studies, reports have been published describing growth failure and psychological injury in infants (non-organic failure to thrive) and children (deprivation dwarfism) living in their own families (18-25).

NON-ORGANIC FAILURE TO THRIVE IN INFANTS

According to Elmer, Gregg and Ellison (26), 5 per cent of the infant admissions in 1966 to Children's Hospital in Pittsburgh were infants with non-organic failure to thrive. The major complaints indicated by the parents were failure to gain weight or develop motor skills, feeding difficulties, vomiting,

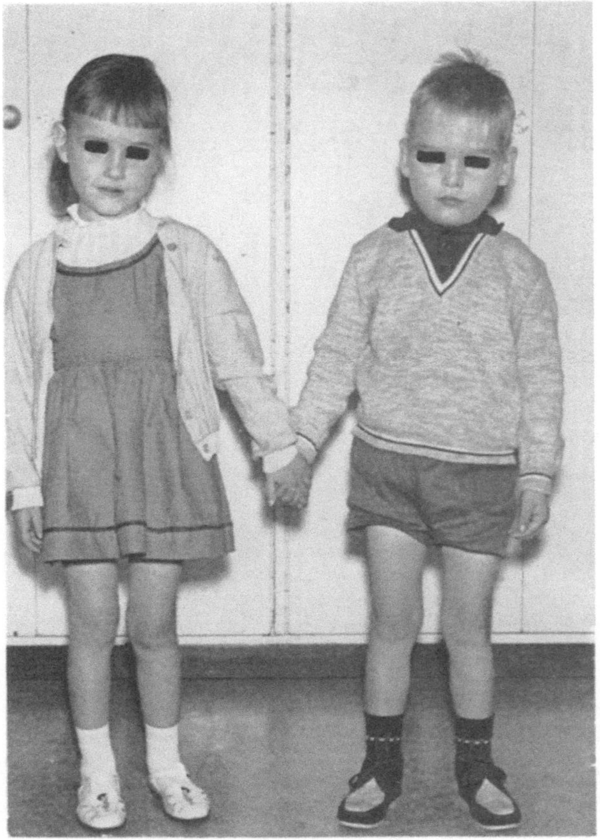

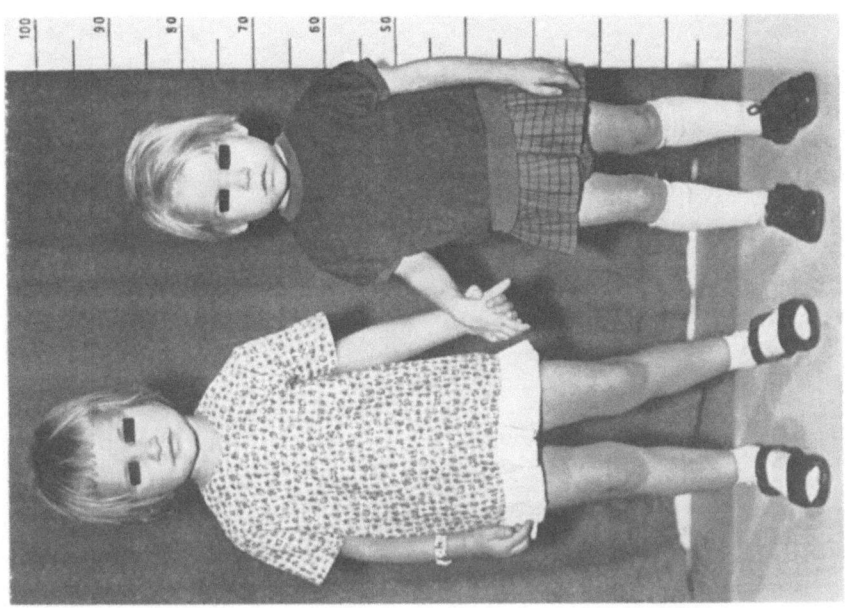

Fig. 6. Girl B (right in the picture), aged 4 years and 8 months, before admission to hospital, with her younger sister, aged 3

Fig. 1. Twinpair A, age 6 years and 5 months, before admission to hospital, see Croughs and Fedder (38).

diarrhoea, constipation, and excessive crying. Clinically, the children often showed watchfulness, minimal smiling, infantile posture (27), and developmental lags. Some were irritable and difficult to comfort, others tended to be quiet, undemanding, and withdrawn. Physical examination revealed pale, malnourished infants with loss of subcutaneous tissue and muscle mass. An organic diagnosis could not be established despite extensive laboratory investigations. The forms of deprivation described in these infants cover the whole spectrum of quantitatively and qualitatively insufficient mothering, socio-economic and emotional deprivation, poverty, unemployment, ignorance, overfatigue, quick succession of pregnancies, chronic disease, apathy, depression, mental retardation, anxiety, scrupulousness, seriously disturbed marital relations, etc. To quote Elmer et al. (26): 'Some form of maternal unavailability, whether through depression, fatigue or preoccupation, is probably responsible for initial failure to thrive.'

There are several ways in which these different forms of deprivation might interfere with growth in these infants. As Patton and Gardner (21, 22) have discussed, actual failure to provide the child with adequate nutrients and calories must be considered first. Whitten, Pettit and Fischoff (28) have given evidence that in a group of mainly quantitatively deprived infants, failure to gain weight was caused primarily by undereating. This might not be surprising, because factors often present in these families, such as poverty, ignorance, apathy, fatigue, and preoccupation, all carry the serious risk of failure to provide sufficient food.

Secondly, a reduction in appetite and vomiting undoubtedly play a role in many of these infants presenting feeding problems.

Thirdly, in these infants intestinal motility might be altered and absorption diminished by emotional factors. However, since the intestines are vulnerable in infancy, defective absorption and secondary intestinal atrophy might equally well be caused by enteric infections and/or wrong feeding habits. Balance studies quantifying absorption of nitrogen and fat are generally lacking.

Fourthly, emotional factors might directly influence endocrine regulation of growth. Both overproduction of corticosteroids and deficiency of growth hormone have been postulated (18, 21, 29). Endocrine function studies in infants with failure to thrive are also lacking.

In addition, a genetic factor cannot be ruled out in at least some of these infants with so-called 'non-organic' failure to thrive, because birth weight was below average in the great majority of reported cases of failure to thrive in full-term infants.

Follow-up studies of infants with failure to thrive have been performed
by several authors (26, 30, 31). Elmer *et al.* (26) re-examined 15 children with
early failure to thrive, after they had reached ages of from 3 years 3 months
to 11 years 7 months. Height and weight were below the normal range in
more than half of their children. Only a third functioned normally mentally,
the majority showing some degree of mental retardation. The majority of
school-age children showed behavioural disturbances and were maladjusted
at school. The authors concluded that except for a lack of physical deformities, their group of failure-to-thrive children functioned almost as poorly
as a group of abused children (32). In contrast, for 40 children with hospital
records of failure to thrive in infancy studied by Glaser *et al.* (30) at an
average age of 4½ years, height and weight were within the normal range in
about 60 per cent, IQ was normal in 85 per cent, retarded intelligence being
found in 6 out of the 40 children. Projective testing of the older children revealed no consistent pattern of emotional disturbance or personality configuration. The great difference in prognostic outcome between these two
studies can only be explained on the basis of the heterogeneity of aetiological
factors of non-organic failure to thrive, ranging from minor adaptational
disturbances between mother and child to complete rejection.

DEPRIVATION DWARFISM

In 1967, two groups of authors (24, 25) called attention to a syndrome of
'emotional deprivation and growth retardation simulating idiopathic hypopituitarism' (24) or, more briefly, 'deprivation dwarfism' (25). Growth
failure in these children most typically developed after a variable period of
adequate growth in infancy. They showed disturbances of behaviour including polydipsia, polyphagia, stealing food, eating from garbage cans,
shyness, sensitiveness, retarded speech, temper tantrums, sleep problems,
encopresis, and enuresis. According to the history, the children often ate
two or three times as much as their siblings, who generally were of normal
height. Some gorged themselves. A number had a history of foul-smelling
stools. Emotional disorders in the parents were invariably present, and the
child seemed to be selected and made the target for rejection and sometimes
even physical abuse, whereas the other siblings sometimes gave evidence of
overprotection. When removed from home, the children showed considerable catch-up growth. Powell *et al.* (33) found evidence of decreased secretion
of growth hormone and ACTH in the majority of their patients. After removal
from home, release of growth hormone rapidly returned to normal, con-
comitantly with catch-up growth. Return of ACTH secretion was less rapid.

Deprivation dwarfism probably represents one segment of the spectrum of the battered child syndrome. It might be mentioned here that only in part of the group of battered children is the experience of deprivation accompanied by growth retardation. Is their growth failure mainly psychosomatic or are these children underfed as well as hated by their parents and are growth failure and growth hormone deficiency entirely secondary to malnutrition? As already mentioned, Whitten *et al.* (28) have shown that in a group of mainly quantitatively deprived infants the dietary histories were unreliable and growth failure was secondary to undereating. However, children with deprivation dwarfism usually are not mainly quantitatively deprived, but may come from rather compulsive, neat families where deprivation is often more qualitative. Contrary to the situation in the infants studied by Whitten *et al.* (28), provision of calories during the period of

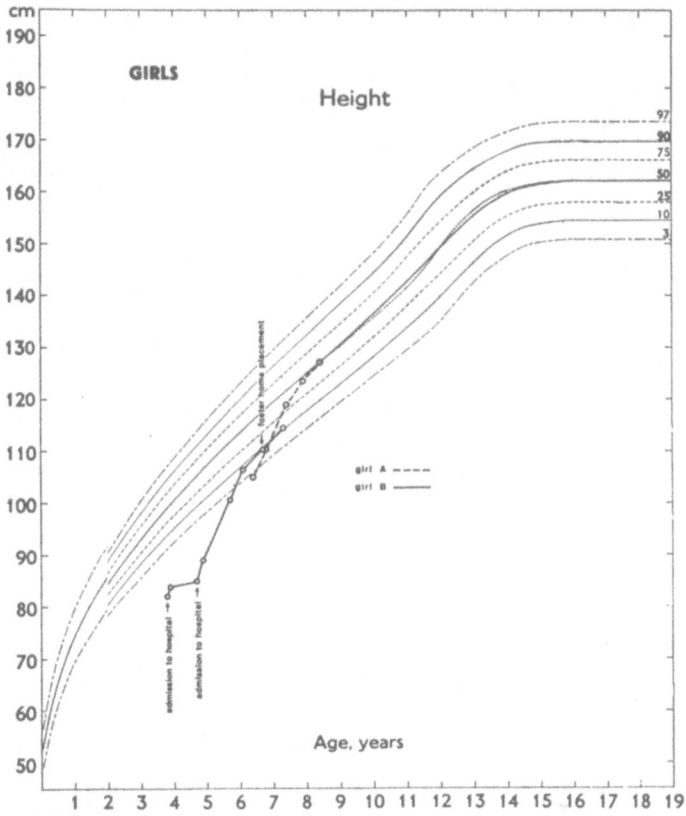

Fig. 2. Increase in height of girls A and B.

greatest caloric demands must have been sufficient, as is proved by the normal growth in infancy of children with deprivation dwarfism. Moreover, recent investigations (34-37) have shown that in malnutrition, growth hormone secretion is not deficient but increased. Therefore, the documented growth hormone deficiency in these children cannot be secondary to malnutriton.

Our patients, the rejected twinpair boy and girl A (Figs. 1-5) might be examples of predominantly psychosomatically induced growth failure (38). Early growth was normal (weight of the boy at 6 months of age: 8400 g, 75th percentile for Dutch children (39), weight of the girl at 6 months of age: 8320 g, 75-90th percentile for Dutch children). When removed from home at the age of 6 years and 5 months, there were no physical or laboratory signs of malnutrition and intestinal absorption of nitrogen and fat was normal.

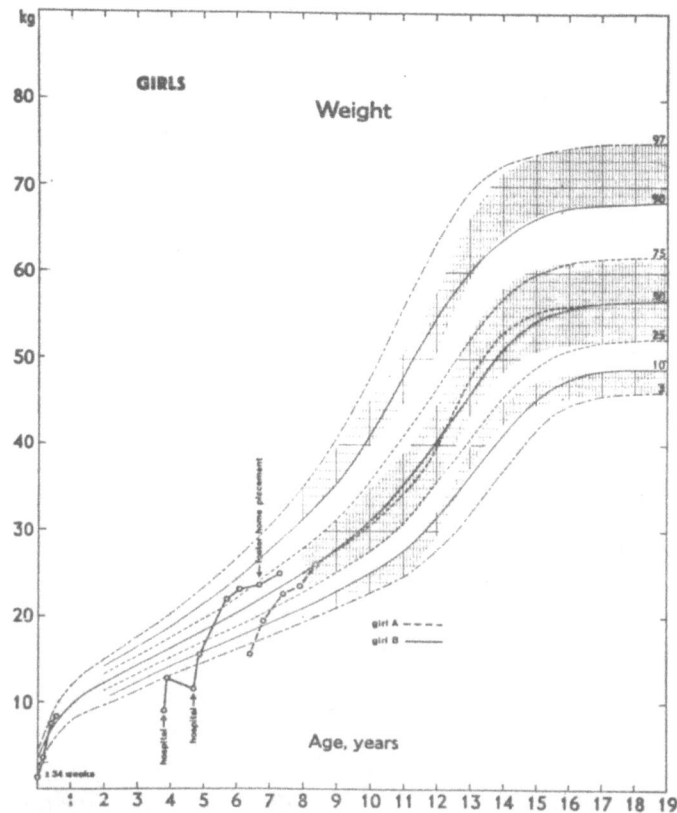

Fig. 3. Increase in weight of girls A and B.

Skinfold thickness over triceps was augmented in both children (boy: 10 mm, 75-90th percentile according to Tanner and Whitehouse (40), girl: 12 mm, 75-90th percentile), which is in accordance with growth hormone deficiency. According to Keet *et al.* (41), skinfold thickness is a reliable and objective measure of suboptimal nutrition, skinfolds in malnourished children

Table 1. Comparison of growth data of the boy A, before removal from home, with his younger brother, not rejected by the parents.

	Boy A	Younger brother
Chron. age (yrs)	6 5/12	4 10/12
Height (cm)	101.9	104.0
Weight (kg)	15.3	15.3
Triceps skinfold (mm)	10	6

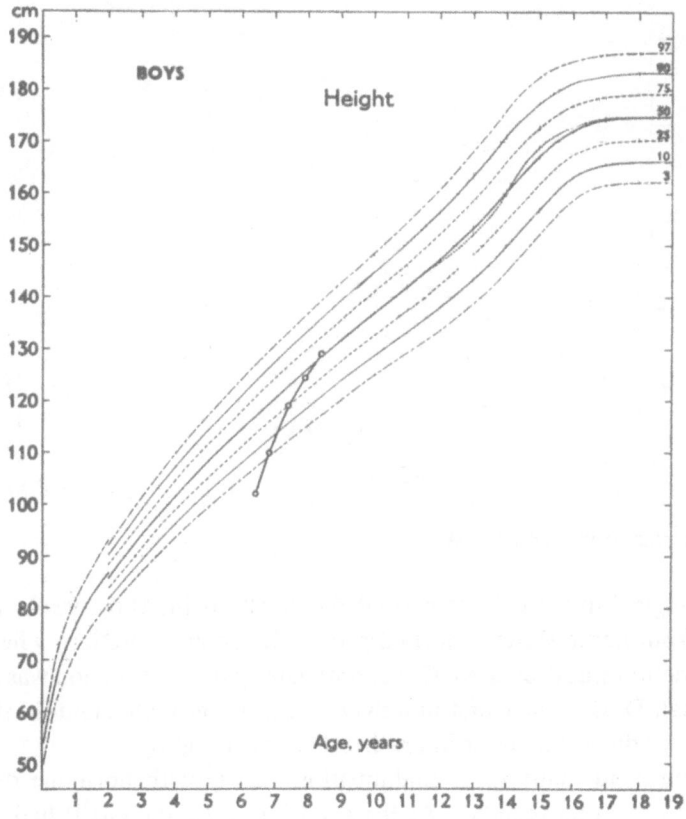

Fig. 4. Increase in height of boy A.

being usually below the 10th percentile and mostly far below the 3rd percentile. Comparison of growth data of the boy A before removal from home with his younger brother (Table 1), not rejected by the parents, provided additional evidence against malnutrition as the cause of growth failure. En-

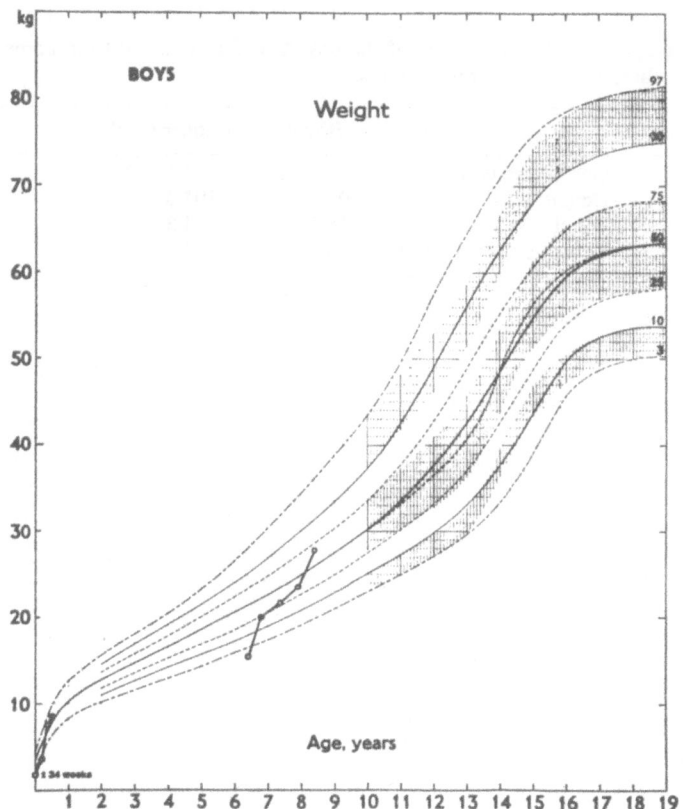

Fig. 5. Increase in weight of boy A.

docrinological investigations carried out in the twins three weeks after removal from home showed normal growth hormone secretion, whereas adrenal function was decreased. One month later, adrenal function was restored to normal. During their first months of catch-up growth, skinfold thickness over triceps did not increase but rather decreased slightly.

Of course, in many cases malnutrition and growth hormone deficiency could be operating together. At the age of 3 years, the girl B had a period with markedly foul-smelling stools and rapid weight loss, probably mediated by enteric infection leading to her first hospital admission, when she showed a protuberant abdomen and clinical signs of suboptimal nutrition. At the age of 4 8/12 years (Fig. 6, opp. p. 273) she was removed permanently from her home and spent 2 years in a hospital, after which she was placed in a foster-home where she is living happily now. Eight weeks after removal from home, growth hormone secretion was normal and adrenal function decreased.

The prognosis of height growth after removal from home seems favourable in these children, growth retardation being accompanied by a proportional retardation of bone age.

The ultimate effects of the rejection experience on emotional and intellectual development seem very much more deleterious. However, as Goldfarb (14) has already pointed out, these rejected children seem to be more accessible to therapy than the children showing the classical institutional syndrome. Rejected children are children in conflict and not necessarily quite unstimulated, undeveloped children. During the first year of hospital treatment, the girl B showed an intellectual catch-up from IQ 84 (Binet-Norden) to 99. But emotionally too she showed a slowly growing capacity to form ties, a growth process which is still progressing in the warm environment of her foster-family. There seems to be hope for her future.

The problem of emotional deprivation in children living in their families is increasing in importance. Knowledge of the syndromes of deprivation is essential for recognition and early treatment.

The author expresses his gratitude for advice and correction of the manuscript to Dr J. Fernandes, Department of Pediatrics, University of Rotterdam, and to Dr K. J. de Haas, Andover, Massachussetts.

REFERENCES

1. Durfee, H. & Wolf, K., Anstaltspflege und Entwicklung im ersten Lebensjahr. *Zeitschr. Kinderforschung* 42, 3 (1933).
2. Gesell, A. & Amatruda, T., Environmental retardation. *Developmental diagnosis.* New-York 1941.
3. Bakwin, H., Loneliness in infants. *Amer. J. Dis. Child.* 63, 30 (1942).
4. Bakwin, H., Emotional deprivation in infants. *J. Pediat.* 35, 512 (1949).
5. Spitz, R. A., Hospitalism. *Psychoanal. Stud. Child* 1, 53 (1945).
6. Spitz, R. A., Hospitalism. A follow-up report on investigation described in Vol. I, 1945. *Psychoanal. Stud. Child* 2, 113 (1946).
7. Spitz, R. A. & Wolf, K., Anaclitic depression. *Psychoanal. Stud. Child* 2, 313 (1946).
8. Lowrey, L. G., Personality distortion and early institutional care. *Am. J. Orthopsychiat.* 10, 576 (1940).

9. Bowlby, J., The influence of early environment in the development of neurosis and neurotic character. *Int. J. Psychoanal.* 21, 1 (1940).
10. Bowlby, J., *Maternal care and mental health.* World Health Organisation monograph series, Geneva 1952.
11. Goldfarb, W., The effects of early institutional care on adolescent personality. *J. Exp. Educ.* 12, 2 (1943).
12. Goldfarb, W., The effects of early institutional care on adolescent personality (Graphic Rorschach data). *Child Developm.* 14, 4 (1943).
13. Goldfarb, W., The effects of early institutional care on adolescent personality. *Am. J. Orthopsychiat.* 14, 3 (1944).
14. Goldfarb, W., Psychological privation in infancy and subsequent adjustment. *Am. J. Orthopsychiat.* 15, 247 (1945).
15. Goldfarb, W., Effects of psychological deprivation in infancy and subsequent stimulation. *Am. J. Psychiat.* 102, 18 (1945).
16. Fried, R. & Mayer, M. F., Socio-emotional factors accounting for growth failure in children in an institution. *J. Pediat.* 33, 444 (1948).
17. Widdowson, E. M., Mental contentment and physical growth. *Lancet* I, 1316 (1951).
18. Talbot, N. B., Sobel, E. H., Burke, B. S., Lindemann, E. & Kaufman, S. H., Dwarfism in healthy children: its possible relation to emotional, nutritional and endocrine disturbance. *New Engl. J. Med.* 236, 783 (1947).
19. Coleman, R. W. & Provence, S., Emotional retardation (hospitalism) in infants living in families. *Pediatrics* 19, 285 (1957).
20. Elmer, E., Failure to thrive. Role of the mother. *Pediatrics* 25, 717 (1960).
21. Patton, R. G. & Gardner, L. I., Influence of family environment on growth; the syndrome of maternal deprivation. *Pediatrics* 30, 957 (1962).
22. Patton, R. G. & Gardner, L. I., *Growth failure in maternal deprivation.* Springfield (Ill.) 1963.
23. Leonard, M. F., Rhymes, J. P. & Solnit, A. J., Failure to thrive in infants. *Amer. J. Dis. Child.* III, 600 (1966).
24. Powell, G. F., Brasel. J. A. & Blizzard, R. M., Emotional deprivation and growth retardation simulating idiopathic hypopituitarism. I. Clinical evaluation of the syndrome. *New. Engl. J. Med.* 276, 1270 (1967).
25. Silver, H. K. & Finkelstein, M., Deprivation dwarfism. *J. Pediat.* 70, 317 (1967).
26. Elmer, E., Gregg, E. S. & Ellison, P., Late results of failure to thrive syndrome. *Clin. Ped.* 8, 584 (1969).
27. Krieger, I. & Sargent, D. A., A postural sign in the sensory deprivation syndrome in infants. *J. Pediat.* 70, 332 (1967).
28. Whitten, Ch. F., Pettit, M. G. & Fischoff, F., Evidence that growth failure from maternal deprivation is secondary to undereating. *J. Amer. med. Ass.* 209, 1675 (1969).
29. Blodgett, F. M., Growth retardation related to maternal deprivation. In: *Modern perspectives in child development.* Solnit, A. J. & Provence, S. A. (eds.), New-York 1963.
30. Glaser, H. H., Heagarty, M. C., Bullard, D. M. & Pivchik, E. C., Physical and psychological development of children with early failure to thrive. *J. Pediat.* 73, 690 (1968).
31. Shaheen, E., Alexander, D., Tuskowsky, M. & Barbero, G., Failure to thrive – a retrospective profile. *Clin. Ped.* 7, 255 (1968).
32. Elmer, E. & Gregg, G. S., Developmental characteristics of abused children. *Pediatrics* 40, 596 (1967).
33. Powell, G. F., Brasel, J. A., Raiti, S. & Blizzard, R. S., Emotional deprivation and growth retardation simulating idopathic hypopituitarism. II. Endocrinologic evaluation of the syndrome. *New Engl. J. Med.* 276, 1276 (1967).

34. Pimstone, B. L. Wittman W., Hansen, J. D. L. & Murray, P., Growth hormone and kwashiorkor. *Lancet* II, 779 (1966).
35. Pimstone, B. L., Barbezat, G., Hansen, J. D. L. & Murray, P., Studies on growth hormone secretion in protein-calorie malnutrition. *Amer. J. Clin. Nutr.* 21, 482 (1968).
36. Graham, G. G., Cordano, A., Blizzard, R. M. & Cheek, D. B., Infantile malnutrition: changes in body composition during rehabilitation. *Pediat. Res.* 3, 579 (1969).
37. Milner, R. D. G., Hormonal and metabolic interrelationships in malnutrition. *Pediat. Res.* 4, 213 (1970).
38. Croughs, W. & Fedder, J. J., Psychogene groeistoornis en battered child syndroom bij drie kinderen. *Ned. T. Geneesk.* 114, 672 (1970).
39. Van Wieringen, J. C., Wafelbakker, F., Verbrugge, H. P. & de Haas, J. H., *Groeidiagrammen Nederland 1965*. Groningen 1968.
40. Tanner, J. M. & Whitehouse, R. H., Standards for subcutaneous fat in British children. *Brit. med. J.* I, 446 (1962).
41. Keet, M. P., Hansen, J. D. L. & Truswell, A. S., Are skinfold measurements of value in the assessment of suboptimal nutrition in young children? *Pediatrics* 45, 965 (1970).

DISCUSSION

Polman: You mentioned functional disorders in the endocrine system. Almost the same disorders can be seen in girls with anorexia nervosa. Don't you agree?

Croughs: I am not quite sure because, as far as I know, girls with anorexia nervosa don't have a decreased growth hormone secretion.

Huyberechts: I would like to know which group of muscles are especially affected in cases of emotional deprivation.

Croughs: I don't know. You can only say that if these children have augmented subcutaneous tissue then they must have less muscle. This is also what you see clinically, but you have to make many photographs if you want to measure this precisely. From a clinical point of view you have this wonderful thing, this skinfold caliper. Then you can find that the skinfold thickness of these children is augmented; and because their weight for height is not augmented, this proves, like in real hypopituitary children, that their muscle tissue must have decreased. But I have not done real body composition studies.

Wensink: I understood that one of your patients stayed in hospital for two years. What kind of treatment did she receive?

Croughs: I see that the child psychiatrist, who has taken special care of the psychiatric treatment of these children, is just coming in.

Fedder: In the child psychiatric clinic we tried to enable the children to establish new ties with adult people and with children. And this process took a rather long time, sometimes more than one year. When they first came into the ward they were very anxious about opening doors, about entering a room, about meeting unknown people; these caused reactions of fear and anxiety. Another interesting point was that we were obliged to expose these children to visits by their parents. Such visits caused great anxiety and tension in the children, which often lasted for several days. It was interesting too that they had abnormal reactions when they saw their parents. The parents might be bringing new clothes and presents for them and the children said 'well, we don't need it, we already have clothes, no thank you, take it home, please'. After a long time they grew more normal in their contacts with adults and with children. The mentally deficient one of the twins (IQ 80) did not have nearly as much difficulty to establish new contacts as the girl with normal intelligence. The mentally deficient boy could be transferred to a therapeutic foster-home much sooner than the normal girl of this pair of twins.

NEUROENDOCRINE FACTORS AND THE ONTOGENY
OF BEHAVIOR

S. LEVINE*

During recent years there has been a growing body of evidence which indicates the important influence of endocrine processes upon the ontogeny
of physiological and behavioral systems. Although the major evidence of the
influence of hormones during very sensitive periods in development upon
later behavior comes primarily from manipulations of gonadal hormones
early in development, there is now new evidence which also indicates that
manipulation of the pituitary-adrenal system pre- and postnatally may also
have profound effects upon later neuroendocrine processes. The evidence on
the influence of gonadal hormones on determination of sexuality, both behaviorally and physiologically, is now well documented. The basic hypothesis
developed by Professor Harris (1) and the late Professor W. C. Young (2)
states that hormones acting on the central nervous system during fetal and
neonatal life organize the sexually undifferentiated brain with regard to
patterns of gonadotropin secretion in sexual behavior. Specifically, this
hypothesis states first that androgens acting on the central nervous system
during critical periods in development are responsible for the programming
of male patterns of gonadotropin secretion and sex behavior in much the
same way that they determine the development of anatomical sexual characteristics. Second, during adult life gonadal hormones activate the sexually
differentiated brain and elicit the responses that were programmed earlier.
Third, an additional component of the process of sexual differentiation is to
render the tissues which are responsive to gonadal hormones differentially
sensitive in the male and the female. Illustrative of this latter aspect of
sexual differentiation is a phenomenon observed in normal adult rats. If a
normal adult male is castrated and given large replacement doses of estrogen,
rudimentary and partial female lordosis behavior will be facilitated, but in
the normal castrate female, minute quantities of estrogen will facilitate

* This study was supported by USPHS Research Scientist Award 1-K05-MH-19936 from the
National Institute of Mental Health and also by the Leslie Fund, Chicago.

complete sexual behavior. Further, if the male which is showing rudimentary sexual behavior is given doses of progesterone, no further elaboration of sexual behavior is observed. However, the female given estrogen alone and then given progesterone will show further facilitation of sexual behavior. Thus the capacity of both estrogen and estrogen plus progesterone to elicit lordosis behavior is much greater in the female than in the normal adult castrate male.

In a recent experiment in collaboration with Dr Julian Davidson (3) we observed that progesterone facilitates the appearance of female sex behavior (lordosis) in neonatally castrated males where it failed to facilitate sexual behavior in males castrated after the critical period. It should be noted that this differential sensitivity to hormones is observed very early in postnatal life. If the neonatally castrated rat is given sesame oil during infancy the amount of female sexual behavior induced by a small dose of estrogen and progesterone does not differ from that observed in a normal castrate female. However, if androgen is given to the neonatal castrate or the neonatal female rat within 96 to 127 hours after birth, an interesting phenomenon occurs. The lower doses of androgen do not abolish the sexual receptivity of the female but the receptivity is abolished in the castrated male given the same amount of testosterone at the same time. Thus it appears that already within the early stage of development there exists a differential sensitivity to the androgen in the male (4). The mechanisms whereby this differential sensitivity occurs early in development are obscure. It may be a function of some prenatal priming with testosterone in the male which may render the brain more sensitive to postnatal testosterone.

Thus far the notion of differential tissue sensitivity to hormones has been inferred primarily from the behavior elicited by the hormone in the adult animal, but there exist models in peripheral tissues which indicate the same phenomenon more precisely.

We have studied the cornified papillae on the surface of the penis (5). These papillae are androgen-dependent tissues, so when the male is castrated in adulthood they atrophy within three weeks to the point where they are no longer observable. However, they will reappear after a course of androgen treatment. If the male is castrated neonatally, these cornified papillae are absent in the adult, but if these adult males are now given testosterone the response of the penile tissue to androgen is markedly diminished. If however the neonatally castrated male has been given testosterone in infancy, its response to androgen in adulthood is markedly different from that of controls given no androgen, and it shows a marked, almost normal response to the androgen in terms of the appearance of cornified papillae in adulthood. Parenthetically, administration of estrogen to the neonatally castrated rat further diminishes the response to androgen in adulthood.

We have so far assumed that the function of gonadal hormones in infancy is to organize the central nervous system with regard to neuroendocrine function in patterns of behavior. Although we have focussed primarily on reproductive behavior, numerous reports in the literature have indicated that there are sex differences in non-sexual behavior. There are striking differences in activity patterns between males and females (6). Activity patterns of females closely parallel estrous cycle activity and during the estrous phase of the cycle females show high peaks of activity. In contrast, the males show no apparent activity cycle and the overall levels of activity are markedly lower.

Professor Harris (1) observed that female activity cycles can be mimicked in the neonatally castrated animal by an ovarian transplant in adulthood. Thus, before transplantation of the ovary to the anterior chamber of the eye the neonatally castrated rat shows a low level of random activity. However, the appearance of the corpora lutea in the transplanted ovary marks the onset of female activity cycles which are indistinguishable from those of the normal female. During this period the neonatally castrated rat with the transplanted ovary also becomes sexually receptive on a cyclic basis.

Recently we have investigated (7) the effects of androgen on pain-induced aggressive behavior (8). Males and females differed reliably in the amount of aggressive behavior elicited by shock, with males fighting significantly more than females. Further, if males are castrated at weaning their aggressive behavior is reduced, but not quite to the level seen in the normal females. However, when they receive replacement treatment with testosterone propionate these males show significant increases in aggressive behavior equivalent to that observed in normal males. But in male rats castrated neonatally aggressive behavior is suppressed and further supramaximal doses of androgen given to the adult organism do not cause the increase in aggressive behavior seen in the weanling castrates. Thus again we have an example of the maintenance of feminine patterns of behavior when the newborn male is castrated. Further, there appears in these experiments that property of central nervous system organization which has been observed throughout the experiments discussed so far in this paper, namely that the female central nervous system is differentially responsive to androgen and that many behaviors which are elicited by androgen in normal males are generally incapable of appearing on androgen stimulation in the normal female or its equivalent, the neonatally castrated male.

Examination of the developmental pattern of the testis as first described by Hooker (9) and Niemi and Ikonen (10) indicates that during the late prenatal periods and for a brief period of time postnatally, the fetal and neonatal testes exhibit a high degree of activity. There is an active population of Leydig cells and recently Resko, Feder and Goy (11) have clearly isolated both testosterone and androstenedione from the testes and plasma of the newborn rat. However, after this brief period of activity, the testes become very quiescent and there is very little Leydig cell production; in terms of androgen production the testes do not become active again until just before puberty. Thus one can infer that this period of high androgen activity is biologically essential for sexual differentiation.

A number of years ago we began to study development of the adrenal, both in terms of spontaneous activity and in the development of the response to stress. The essence of our findings (12) was that adrenal activity is extremely high in terms of both plasma and adrenal concentrations of corticosterone in the newborn rat. There is also a clear and definitive response to administration of exogenous ACTH. However, after this initial period activity decreases markedly and the animal becomes unresponsive to ACTH, remaining unresponsive until approximately 15 to 18 days of age. At that time the animal also becomes responsive to stress. Failure of the adrenal to respond to ACTH does not appear to be a defect in the adrenal per se, for studies by M. X. Zarrow and V. H. Denenberg (unpublished) have shown that if the newborn rat is primed with ACTH an active response to ACTH continues as long as the adrenal remains stimulated. Apparently the newborn pituitary-adrenal system behaves similarly to that of the hypophysectomized animal, and if the adrenal is deprived of ACTH stimulation it becomes insensitive to ACTH given later.

We have recently concluded an extensive study of the development of the adrenal in terms of both plasma and adrenal corticosterone and pituitary and circulating ACTH (13). We felt that it was necessary to describe the total development of the system throughout the prenatal period. During the very early prenatal period there is a high concentration of corticosterone in the adrenal and ACTH can be detected by a biossay modified from that reported by Rerup and Hedner (14). However, there is a period of marked quiescence during which the plasma and adrenal concentrations of corticosterone are reduced and no ACTH is detectable in the plasma, although there is detectable ACTH in the pituitary. Pituitary ACTH increases markedly between six and nine days of age. Adrenal corticosterone concentrations and plasma ACTH again appear at approximately 12 days of age and by 15 days of age the system seems to be totally active. What is interesting about this pattern is its resemblance to the developmental pattern of the male gonads. Thus, there appears to be an initial period of high activity. This period seems to commence late prenatally, approximately 18 days after a conception, and it continues for a short time after birth. It then appears to become relatively quiescent and does not reappear again until later in the development of the organism.

The question then is, what is the relevance of these particular high values of circulating corticosterone, both late prenatally and during the early postnatal period, for subsequent functioning of the organism?

In response to this question we have conducted a series of studies in collaboration with Karmela Milkovic and Justin Joffe in which we have attempted to manipulate the fetal pituitary-adrenocortical system by various treatments to the pregnant female. We chose to manipulate adrenocortical systems fetally, because of the difficulties that are encountered, by giving injections of corticoids to newborn rats postnatally. In the studies by Shawn Schapiro (15) and others it was found that postnatal injections of cortisol produced marked inhibition of growth, runting, and often led to death. These toxic effects may indeed be dose-dependent, but it is also difficult to assess the fate of the adrenocortical hormone, given peripherally to the newborn. For these studies that are to be described two major procedures are used, 1. adrenalectomy of the female prior to the onset of pregnancy and 2. the implantation of a mammatropic tumor (MtT) which produces excessively high ACTH, leading to extensive hypertrophy in the pregnant female and large, excessive amounts of adrenal corticoids being secreted. We have demonstrated that adrenalectomized females maintained on saline cycle normally become pregnant and have no difficulty delivering offspring (16). The effects on the neonatal adrenal of these two procedures are almost diametrically opposed. Adrenalectomy of the female produces in the offspring an hypertrophy of the neonatal adrenal with elevations in the concentration of corticosterone in the adrenal. The mammatropic tumor produces a marked suppression of neonatal adrenal weight and a reduction in the concentration of adrenal corticosterone. However, plasma levels of corticosterone are elevated in the fetus of both preparations.

In most of these experiments conducted on the offspring of prenatally treated animals, the offspring are fostered to normal females immediately after birth so that any of the effects observed, both in later behavior and later activity of the pituitary-adrenal system, are assumed to be functions of the prenatal manipulations. The influence of manipulation of prenatal adreno-cortical activity by means of altering the maternal fetal adrenocortical rela-tionships is seen in a number of parameters in the adult organism. First, the adrenocortical response of the adult offspring of adrenalectomized and MTT treated females is significantly different from that of normal controls (see fig. 1). In the MTT treated animals there is a significant depression of

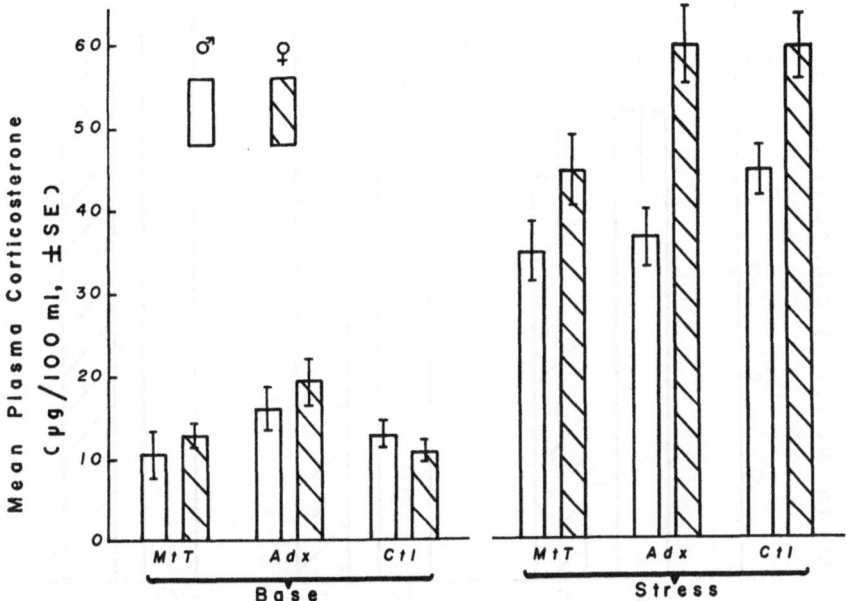

Fig. 1. Plasma corticoid values in rats whose mothers have been implanted with a mamma-tropic tumor, adrenalectomized, and control. The columns represent the mean and the vertical lines represent the standard error of the mean.

adrenocortical activity in the adult animal, in both male and female. In the adrenalectomized animal the male is affected but there is no significant effect upon the female offspring. Similarly, we see the same pattern occurring in the capacity of the animal to learn a shuttlebox avoidance response.

The shuttlebox avoidance response requires the animal to learn when a signal appears, in this instance a low level of noise and light, that this signal indicates that within a period of time shock will be presented in the compart-ment that the animal is standing. If the animal crosses during the period that the light and noise are on but before the shock, this is considered an avoidance response. If the animal crosses a barrier when the shock is already on, this is considered an escape response (Fig. 2). The MTT treated animals show a significant suppression in the number of conditioned avoidance responses made, as compared with controls. This occurs, again, in both male and

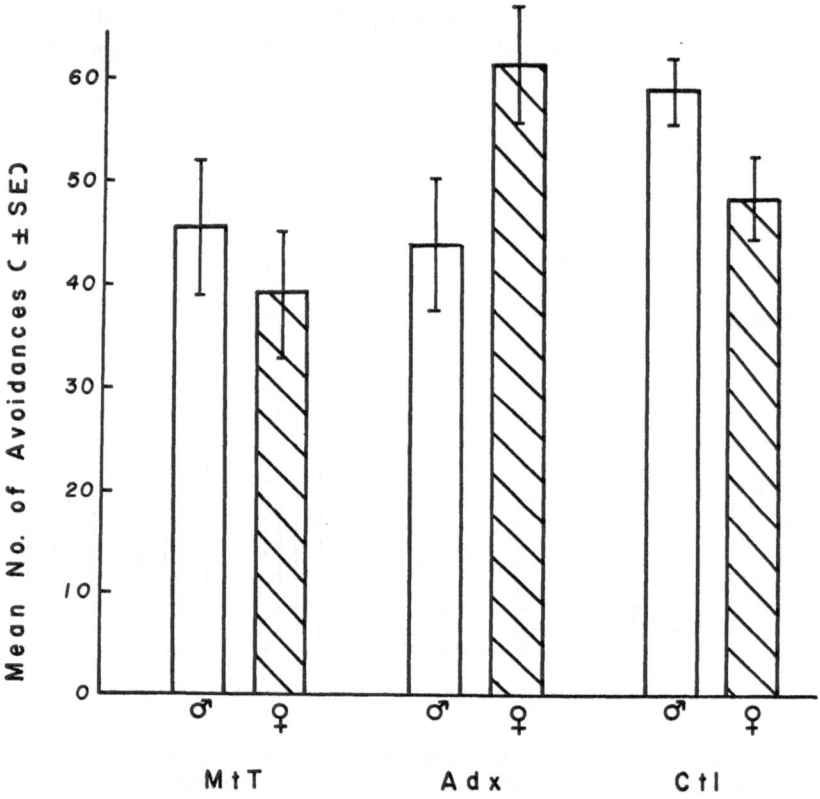

Fig. 2. Comparison of avoidance learning between rats whose mothers have been implanted with a mammatropic tumor, adrenalectomized, and control. The columns represent the mean and the vertical lines represent the standard error of the mean.

female, whereas in the animals of adrenalectomized mothers, the suppression again shows up in the male but does not appear to be there in the female. If we view these procedures as a continuum the MTT treated offspring are inundated with excessively high amounts of corticoids during fetal life as a consequence of the high corticoid output of the mother which has been demonstrated to cross the placental barrier. In the offspring of adrenalectomized animals, as a consequence of the absence of the normally occurring feedback control by maternal steroids, the animal's own adrenal becomes more active and therefore puts out greater amounts of corticosterone during the fetal period. The fact that both male and female are affected in the MTT treated group, whereas only the male is affected in the adrenalectomized group, would indicate that there may indeed be a differential sensitivity to corticosterone between male and female offspring. In the case of the MTT treated animals the amount of adrenocortical hormones secreted may exceed the threshold, thus affecting both sexes. Whereas in the case of the offspring of adrenalectomized females, the animal's own endogenous hormone may not be sufficient to reach threshold levels of the female.

This differential sensitivity to hormones between male and female is not a new phenomenon and has already been reported for the gonadal hormones. Thus, as described earlier, small amounts of androgen given to the female do not suppress female sexual responsivity; on the other hand, the same doses of androgen given to the neonatal castrate appear to suppress female receptivity completely.

In a subsequent experiment we compared the open-field behavior of offspring of adrenalectomized females with controls. These data are seen in

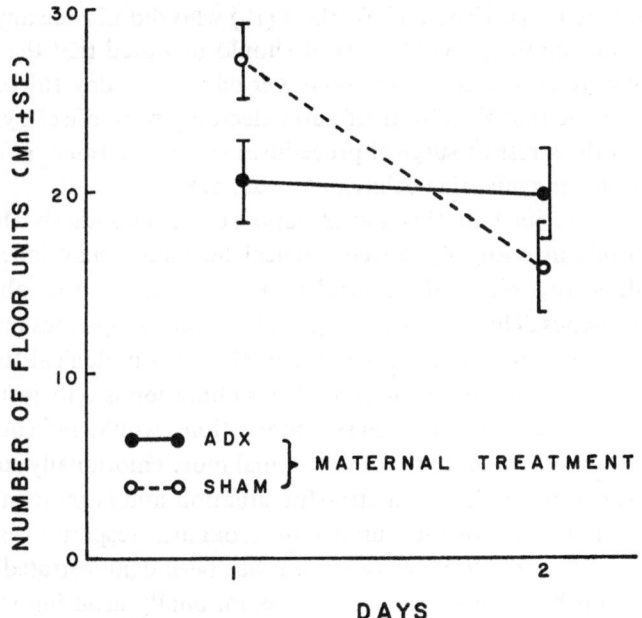

Fig. 3. Mean activity in the open field for offspring of adrenalectomized and sham mothers. The vertical lines represent the standard error of the mean.

figure 3. What these data indicate is that there is a marked change between day 1 and day 2 of open-field testing in normal animals. This is a pattern which has been observed on numerous occasions: on day 1 the normal animal tends to be highly active, whereas on day 2 considerably less activity is observed. This has been interpreted by Denenberg, Brumaghim, Haltmeyer & Zarrow (17) as indicating that the high level of activity on day 1 represents escape activity, but inasmuch as the animal cannot escape the situation, it then develops a highly emotional response and becomes immobile (freezes). In contrast, however, the adrenalectomized animal shows a more stable behavior between day 1 and 2, showing essentially no change. These results are very similar to those which have been seen in animals that have been handled in infancy insofar as they tend to show a greater stability over days, which has been interpreted as indicating less emotionality and therefore less freezing behavior. One can make a similar interpretation of the behavior of the offspring of adrenalectomized females and hypothesize that increases in adrenocortical activity during sensitive periods in development significantly alter those systems which are involved in the expression of emotionality as measured by the open field.

Although these data are at variance with those which have been reported in the literature by Havlena and Werboff (18) who did not see any effects of adrenalectomizing the gravid female, it should be noted that the females in their study were adrenalectomized on either day $10\frac{1}{2}$ or day $16\frac{1}{2}$ of gestation and it is possible that the effects of adrenalectomy were offset by effects resulting from the stress of surgical procedures since gestational stress itself is capable of affecting offspring behavior (19, 20, 21).

The data described in this paper support the hypothesis that during critical periods in ontogeny, adrenocortical hormones may indeed have a similar role in organizing the central nervous system as was observed for gonadal hormones. Thus, by increasing the levels of endogenous hormones in the fetal rat, we markedly alter a number of psychobiological functions in adulthood. The extent and the nature of this alteration is only just in the exploratory stage, yet the preliminary observations would indicate that the nature of the effects ought to make the animal more emotionally stable. Thus the organism responds less to a stressful situation and is more stable in its behavior. A reduction in the number of avoidance responses can also be viewed within the same framework since it has been demonstrated that there is a continuum between the intensity of emotionally arousing stimuli and learning ability in the shuttlebox avoidance situation. As one increases the shock intensity, learning becomes better in the avoidance situation up to a critical point when too high an intense shock leads to a decrement in avoidance conditioning. Further, animals that are handled neonatally show poor avoidance learning under conditions of high shock intensity in the avoidance situation.

This area of investigation however is now at about the same point where the study of developmental influences of gonadal hormones was about ten years ago. There are a multitude of questions yet to be answered but it appears that this is indeed a fruitful area of investigation.

REFERENCES

1. Harris, G. W., Sex hormones, brain development and brain function. *Endocrinology* 166, 627 (1964).
2. Young, W. C., The hormones and mating behavior. In: *Sex and internal secretions,* W. C. Young (ed.), Baltimore 1961.
3. Davidson, J. M. & Levine, S., Progesterone and heterotypical sexual behaviour in male rats. *J. Endocr.* 44, 129 (1969).
4. Mullins, R. F., Jr. & Levine, S., Hormonal determinants during infancy of adult sexual behavior in the male rat. *Physiol. Behav.* 3, 339 (1968).
5. Mullins, R. F., Jr. & Levine, S., Differential sensitization of penile tissue by sexual hormones in newborn rats. *Communs. Behav. Biol.* 3, Part A, 1 (1969).
6. Richter, C. P., The effect of early gonadectomy on the gross body activity of rats. *Endocrinology* 17, 445 (1933).
7. Conner, R. L. & Levine, S., *Hormonal influences on aggressive behavior,* Garattini, S. & Sigg, E. B., (eds.), Excerpta Medica, Amsterdam 1969.
8. Ulrich, R. E. & Azrin, N. H., Reflexive fighting in response to aversive stimulation. *J. exp. Analysis Behav.* 5, 511 (1962).
9. Hooker, C. W., The biology of the interstitial cells of the testis. *Recent Prog. Horm. Res.* 3, 173 (1948).
10. Niemi, M. & Ikonen, M., Histochemistry of the Leydig cells in the postnatal prepubertal testis of the rat. *Endocrinology* 72, 443 (1963).
11. Resko, J. A., Feder, H. H. & Goy, R. W., Androgen concentrations in plasma and testis of developing rats. *J. Endocr.* 40, 485 (1968).
12. Levine, S., Glick, D. & Nakane, P. K., Adrenal and plasma corticosterone and vitamin A in rat adrenal glands during postnatal development. *Endocrinology* 80, 910 (1967).
13. Levine, S., The pituitary-adrenal system and the developing brain. In: *Progress in brain research, Vol. 32, Pituitary, adrenal and the brain,* Wied, D. de & Weijnen, J. A. W. M., (eds.), Amsterdam 1970.
14. Rerup, C. & Hedner, P., The assay of corticotrophin in mice. *Acta endocr., Copenh.* 44, 237 (1963).
15. Schapiro, S., Some physiological, biochemical, and behavioral consequences of neonatal hormone administration: cortisol and thyroxine. *Gen. Comp. Endocr.* 10, 214 (1968).
16. Thoman, E. B., Sproul, M., Seeler, B. & Levine, S., Lactation suppresses adrenal corticosteroid activity and aggressiveness in rats. *J. comp. physiol. Psychol.* 70, 364 (1970).

17. Denenberg, V. H., Brumaghim, J. T., Haltmeyer, G. C. & Zarrow, M. X., Increased adrenocortical activity in the neonatal rat following handling. *Endocrinology* 81, 1047 (1967).
18. Havlena, J. & Werboff, J., Adrenalectomy of the pregnant rat and behavior of the offspring. *Psychol. Rep.* 12, 348 (1963).
19. Thompson, W. R., Influence of prenatal maternal anxiety on emotionality in young rats. *Science* 125, 698 (1957).
20. De Fries, J. C., Prenatal maternal stress in mice. *J. Heredity* 55, 289 (1964).
21. Joffe, J. M., Genotype and prenatal and premating stress interact to affect adult behavior in rats. *Science* 150, 1844 (1965).

DISCUSSION

Goldfoot: Since this conference has been dichotomizing in some ways 'genetic' from environmental and hormonal effects, I'd like to briefly comment on your finding of penile insensitivity to androgens in the adult rats which were castrated just after birth. There is a syndrome in man, testicular feminization, which, as you know, is characterized by essentially normal levels of androgen production by the testis in adulthood, but by the relative or complete absence of external male genitals and wolffian duct structures. The literature treats this as a genetic mistake, implying that the 'anlagen' for these structures are incapable of responding to early androgen. Couldn't it be the case, alternatively as your findings and others as well suggest, that the early androgens were absent, and therefore these peripheral structures were later incapable of normal activation, just as is the case for neural organization in the studies which you cited?

Levine: You see, David, it could still be a genetic mistake. If you say it is a genetic mistake it does not tell you anything about the mechanisms. By some enzymatic deficiency the tissue becomes unresponsive to androgen and by virtue of its unresponsiveness to androgen all of those changes, which normally should occur as a consequence of the presence of androgen in that system do not occur, and therefore the system then remains essentially female. Because that is the primordial system which normally would have gone on in the absence of these things.

It is still indeed, you know, a genetic defect in the sense that there is something that is chromosomally caused. But that is only one level of the explanation. To start with that level of the explanation: it simply does not give you all of the intricacies, the exclusiveness of the phenomena which you are observing. I really do believe that there are ingenious ways in which you use genetic material. All I'm trying to say is not an explanatory device. It does not explain anything. I mean, it may tell you the loci of something. It does not tell you all of the sets of intervening processes.

Baum: One possible interpretation of testicular feminization is that an insensitivity to androgen develops in adulthood because an insufficient amount of androgen was present at the critical postnatal period. I think Dave was thinking of the experiments with male pseudohermaphroditic rats which had a completely analogous syndrome in adulthood to the human case of testicular feminization (Bardin, C. W., Bullock, L., Schneider, G., Allison, J. E. and Stanley, A. J., *Science* 167, 1136, 1970). A simple experiment would be to take these young pseudohermaphroditic male rats at birth and give them some testosterone and then look to see whether in adulthood the accessory organs of these animals are responsive to testosterone. One other question. Have you systematically compared the adult receptivity of neonatally castrated male rats with that of littermate females ovariectomized at the same time the males were castrated? Is there in fact no difference in the receptivity of these animals?

Levine: Not so far as we can detect. Davidson and I have shown that progesterone sensitivity was also very different (Davidson, J. M. and Levine, S., *J. Endocr.* 44, 129, 1969). The neonatally castrated males have the same progesterone sensitivity as ovariectomized females, but very different from intact males. Davidson has been able to get some of these animals to show lordosis, a very low level of lordosis, but they do show it. And progesterone has no effect on this. Whereas if you do this in the neonatally castrated male you have very interesting progesterone effects. The progesterone sensitivity is changed. The important thing to us is not so much that we cannot discriminate this. It is really the behavior of the adult male that discriminates these neonatally castrated males when they are given estrogen or progesterone. And they will not show it to a male given the same estrogen and progesterone, or to a weanling given estrogen and progesterone. So that the stimuli can be very complicated. It need not only be odour, but obviously whole sets of behaviors. The female does have all of this darting, and all of these movements are indeed important releasing stimuli for the male behavior. The neonatal castrate shows all of this, whereas though the male may show some lordosis, it does not have any of this behavior in terms of having the appropriate releasing stimuli to elicit this behavior.

Baum: I was thinking of a paper by Thomas and Gerall where they are claiming that you have to castrate the male rat literally at birth, as opposed to say 24 hours after birth, in order to get the full-blown female type of behavior in later life (Thomas, C. N. and Gerall, A. A., *Psychonomic Science* 16, 19, 1969).

Levine: This may be true. In our hands 12 hours works fine. I suspect that the timing of this is really less important than the fact that it does occur.

De Wied: I would like to ask you about that very elegant study you only mentioned very briefly, with the ACTH secreting tumor. You said before you mentioned this that the injection of corticosteroids in the early days of life is rather toxic. Now what about the toxicity of the steroids produced by this tumor?

Levine: We don't find any evidence of toxicity in the fetuses except what you see in the adrenal system. There are no weight differences. All of these animals were cross-fostered to normal lactating females. We've been doing another preparation which is going to be intriguing and that is: we have been putting small amounts of crystalline hormone into the general area of the median eminence of the new-born. If you put a blob of hormone in, about 2 or 3 micrograms at the most, you get none of these toxic effects by the way. And you get some interesting differences in adulthood. This is a very preliminary sort of experiment, but it seems to work in a similar manner. You do the same thing with testosterone as you know. You put very small amounts into the brain and you will see the same effect. You will see all the effects of androgen.

Akiyama: I think this is a very fascinating study particularly from the standpoint of the cyclic phenomena that you have observed. I would like to ask questions in regard to the castrated male with the ovarian transplant: were the corpora lutea cycles similar to those of the normal female? Also, I believe you showed a slide on activity cycles. Were these also similar to the cycles of non-treated animals?

Levine: As far as we know, the ovarian cycles are almost identical, indistinguishable from any normal four-day cycle. They are receptive at exactly the time you would get the pro-oestrus/oestrus smear. Fortunately they don't become pregnant. I am not sure they could not. I mean, Prof. Harris has had this dream for years really. What he wants to do now is to transplant a uterus and he is convinced that he can get these animals to deliver. At least to carry on to term. It is in fact a fascinating question because now you could look at the function of the denervated uterus. The uterus will have no innervation in this preparation. They have a free-floating uterus and it would be marvellous to see what would happen. Some day somebody will do that.

I see no reason why they could not conceive and could not become pregnant as they have all the other apparatus.

Baum: Van der Schoot in our lab replicated some of Harris's early work looking at transplanted ovaries in neonatally castrated males. He finds nice cycles in these males as you also found. But after a long period of time he invariably finds persistent oestrus phenomena in vaginas transplanted in these animals. So somehow cyclic function in the transplanted ovaries seems to disappear after a period of normal function.

Levine: This may have something to do with the maintenance of the ovarian tissue. The only way to really test that is to retransplant another ovary and then you can very easily see whether something has happened to the cyclic mechanisms or whether something has happened to the ovary. And that is a very simple experiment to do. I think that an ovary will take anywhere you put it. You can do it much simpler by just putting in subcutaneous tissue, as long as you get good vasculature. It is easy enough to test that as to whether there is something happening to the cyclic mechanism. You have the same thing in early androgen treated animals, a period of cyclicity followed by a-cyclicity. The same thing may be happening here.

Van der Werff ten Bosch: Since the problem has been raised, I think the findings that Baum refers to confirm earlier work by Yazaki who found that in ovaries implanted in males the ovarian cycles stop sooner than in the normal female. I think this has nothing to do with the transplantation. I think it is the ageing of the cyclicity mechanism. And I think it really fits very nicely into your picture, where you show that even at birth there is already an established effect of androgens on the brain. So that if you remove the testes at birth you may get some of the let's say normal female phenomena, but not all of them.

Levine: I think the point that you are making is a very good one. What I was going to say is very simply that one of the reasons why we see this difference in sensitivity is very obviously because we are not catching that animal before it has seen androgen. Androgen secretion begins at about 17 days of age and then stops essentially right after birth. So there is a period of time when the testes are producing high amounts of androgen. The brain is already seeing androgen, and you may be having some priming effect.

THE EFFECTS OF EARLY HYPOTHYROIDISM ON IQ, SCHOOL PERFORMANCE, AND ELECTROENCEPHALOGRAM PATTERN IN CHILDREN

J. J. VAN GEMUND AND M. S. LAURENT DE ANGULO

Congenital hypothyroidism in man offers a naturally occurring biological model for the study of brain-thyroid relationships during the formative period of the central nervous system.

Thyroid deficiency early in life has long been known to give rise to a severe and frequently irreversible mental retardation whose underlying cause is not well understood (1). A better understanding of what may take place in man emerged from the investigations based on experimental thyroidectomy in the rat performed by Eayrs *et al.* since 1951 (2, 3, 4, 5, 6) and by Legrand and Jost (7). The rat is especially suitable for such investigations because its nervous system is exceedingly immature at birth and in this respect is comparable to that of man during gestation. Furthermore, thyroid activity in the rat starts one or two days before birth.

Important consequences of neonatal thyroidectomy in the rat observed by Eayrs *et al.* include a retardation in structural and neurochemical maturation of the brain leading to a decrease in the average size of the constituent nerve cells, a reduction in the ramification and outgrowth of dendrites and axons, a hypoplasia of the vascular pattern of the cerebral cortex, a retardation of myelination (8) and a reduction in the activity of glutamate decarboxylase, the enzyme concentrated in the synaptosomal fraction of the nerve ending (9). This situation as a whole is reflected in the delayed appearance of conditioned reflex activity and of certain EEG characteristics and in an impaired capacity to respond adaptatively to changes in the environment (10).

The early and scarce histopathological studies of congenital hypothyroidism in man (11, 12) indicate a similar underdevelopment of cerebral structures.

About a decade ago, Eayrs *et al.* showed in the rat that the effects of neonatal thyroidectomy may be reversible and that the degree of recovery is directly related to the age at which hormone substitution is started. If substitution is provided before the age of 10 days, recovery appears to be complete, but if delayed until the 24th day, recovery is only partial. These authors saw the correlation between neuro-morphological, bio-electrical, and enzymic abnormalities on the one hand and the thyroxine-deficient rat's corresponding aberrant innate and adaptive behaviour on the other, in terms of a reduction in the probability of functional interaction of neurons (Fig. 1) (13). Their tentative interpretation may be relevant with respect to

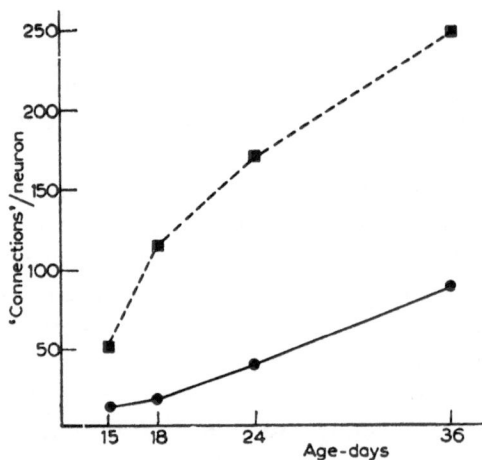

Fig. 1. Differences in probability of axo-dendritic interaction in normal (broken line) and hypothyroid (solid line) rats with advancing age derived from quantitative histological data. (From: J. T. Eayrs (13)

the effects of congenital hypothyroidism in man, in view of the positive effects of thyroxine on human protein synthesis (14), the time of onset of thyroid activity in the human foetus (about the 14th week), the inadequate transplacental passage of thyroxine (15, 16), and the time-courses of brain development in man (17, 18).

Most of the studies done to evaluate the effects of substitution therapy on the mental prognosis of children with hypothyroidism have led to conclusions only indicating the attainment of stratified IQ levels (19, 20, 21, 22). IQ levels do not, however, give much information about the neurological status of the individual child or about the efficiency with which the intelligence is used.

As part of the continuation of an earlier follow-up study (23), this paper presents the evaluation of the mental prognosis of 64 children (age range 4-28 years) with hypothyroidism, in relation to nosological classification, age of onset, neurological maturation, school performance, and familial mental endowment.

The practical classification of thyroid dysgenesis in aplasia (athyreosis) and in the more common hypoplasia has prognostic significance for the clinician. Aplasia is associated with lack of thyroxine during the prenatal period of rapid brain growth, and may consequently result in irreversible distortion of cerebral morphogenesis. Due to the severity of the effects of thyroxine deficiency, the diagnosis is generally made within the first six months of the infant's life.

A dystopic thyroid remnant (usually located sublingually), to the contrary, may produce enough hormone during foetal and early postnatal life to give considerable protection against permanent mental retardation. Children with this less severe form of hypothyroidism show the earliest clinical signs later in life, e.g. between about 6 months and 4 years of age, depending on the functional capacity of the underdeveloped gland (24, 25).

PATIENTS AND METHODS

All children with the main diagnosis of hypothyroidism seen in the Leiden Department of Paediatrics since 1952 were considered for this survey. Young children with adequate hormone substitution for less than two years were not included.

Diagnostic classification was based on conventional criteria such as those deriving from the clinical picture, radiological findings, serum protein bound iodine (PBI) values, radio-iodine uptake, and the scintigram (Table I).

Table 1. Patient groups according to diagnosis

I	congenital athyreosis (n = 9, including 1 boy)
II	congenital dystopic hypoplasia (n = 27, including 7 boys)
III	congenital dyshormonogenesis (n = 10, including 4 boys)
IV	auto-immune hypothyroidism (n = 2, both girls)
V	pituitary hypothyroidism (n = 16, including 3 girls)

For some of the older patients (age > 12 years), most of whom were referred before modern routine methods of clinical chemistry became available, diagnostic classification could be accomplished by combining the available data about onset of the clinical symptoms and the stage of prenatal ossification (femur, foot, dentition) with the outcome of recent diagnostic studies after the withdrawal of hormone substitution for 4 weeks or longer (24, 25).

A total of 46 children showed a congenital type and 18 children an acquired type of hypothyroidism. Treatment was started as soon as the diagnosis was confirmed.

The treatment with the well-standardized desiccated thyroid preparation Thyranon® was considered adequate when evidence of normal PBI (5-8 µg/100 ml), normal statural growth, and normal skeletal maturation was obtained. An audiogram was made in almost every case with disturbed speech development.

School performance of each patient was compared with that of the siblings and the educational history of its parents. Psychological and EEG examinations were performed regularly in most of the cases. Depending on the child's age, the psychometric tests used were the Griffith, the Bühler-Hetzer, the revised Stanford-Binet, the WISC, and the Wechsler-Bellevue I. Within the given age range, the obligatory WISC was usually combined with the Dutch non-verbal test of Dr Snijders-Oomen (S.O.N.).

Tabel 2. IQ distribution in relation to diagnostic groups.

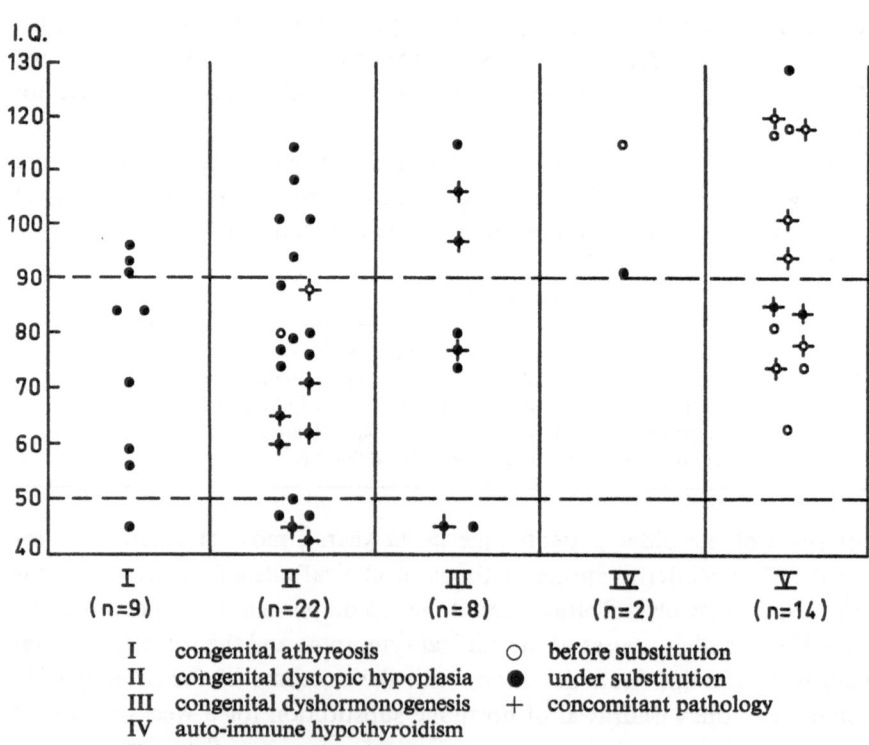

I   congenital athyreosis   ○   before substitution
II   congenital dystopic hypoplasia   ●   under substitution
III   congenital dyshormonogenesis   +   concomitant pathology
IV   auto-immune hypothyroidism
V   pituitary hypothyroidism

We are well aware of the shortcomings of comparing IQ values obtained with different tests. From the age of five years we usually relied on the Wechsler scales. All psychometric data will be tabulated in a final report. For this communication, most emphasis will be laid on actual school performance.

INTELLIGENCE QUOTIENT FINDINGS

It was not possible to classify all cases on the basis of PBI values or radio-iodine uptake studies due to gaps in the data of the older patients. Since the age of onset of clinical hypothyroidism reflects the amount of functioning thyroid tissue available during foetal and postnatal life and therefore the ultimate mental prognosis, the IQ findings were considered in relation to diagnostic groups (Table 2) and the age at which thyroxine substitution was instituted (Table 3). An IQ ⩾ 90 was found in 28% (11/39) of the cases of the congenital types (I, II, III); if we include those patients who were only submitted to gross testing, this percentage rises to 34 (16/46). In only 56%

Table 3. IQ distribution in relation to age at initiation of thyroxine substitution.

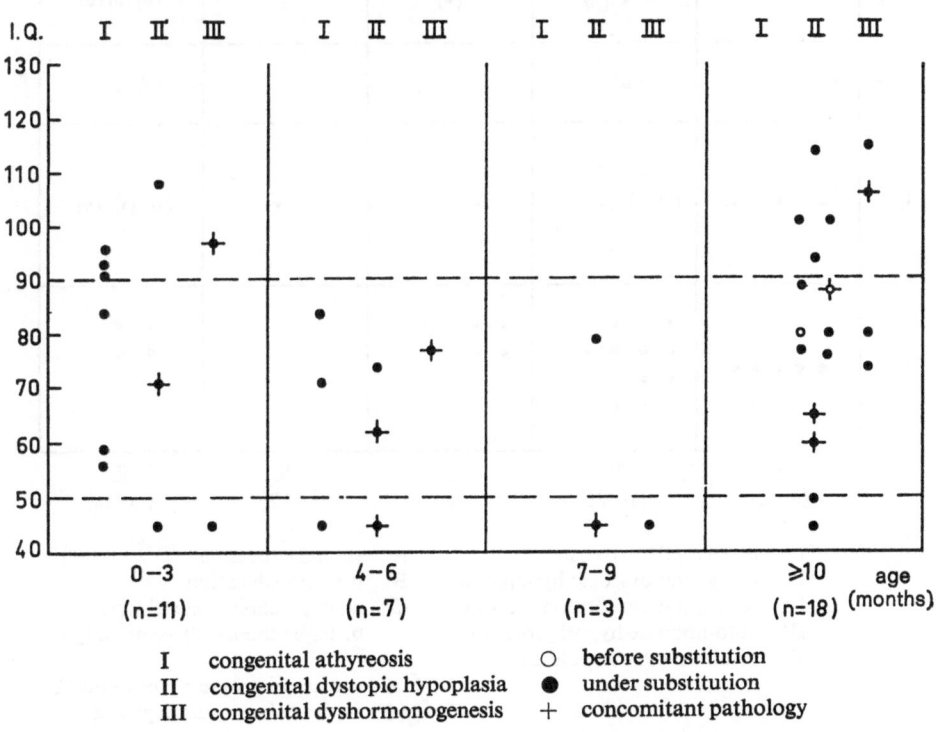

	I	congenital athyreosis	○	before substitution
	II	congenital dystopic hypoplasia	●	under substitution
	III	congenital dyshormonogenesis	+	concomitant pathology

(9/16) of the cases of the acquired types (IV, V) was an IQ ⩾ 90 found. This latter percentage is low due to the additional central nervous system pathology (e.g. neonatal asphyxia associated with predominantly breech presentation) associated with group V.

For the congenital types (I, II, III), a mean IQ of 71 was reached when thyroxine substitution had been started before the age of 10 months (cases of early diagnosis with severe deficiency) and of 83 when substitution had been started later in mildly affected cases with a later onset of clinical deficiency. This differentiation increases in value when the corresponding findings on the achievements in primary school are taken into consideration.

SCHOOL READINESS AND SCHOOL PERFORMANCE
The general and very complex concept of school readiness comprises such aspects as intellectual development ('mental age') and the development of

Table 4. Educational levels in relation to diagnostic groups.

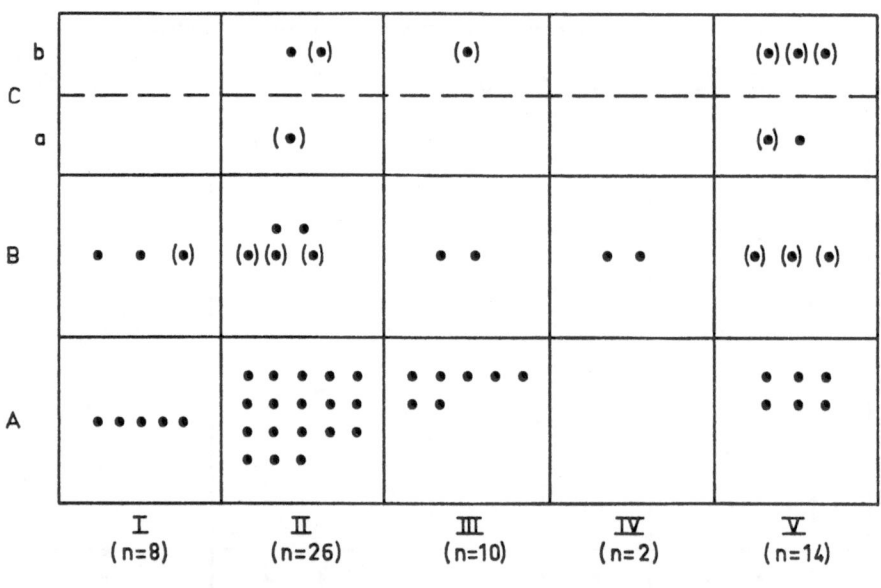

		I (n=8)	II (n=26)	III (n=10)	IV (n=2)	V (n=14)
C	b		● (●)	(●)		(●) (●) (●)
	a		(●)			(●) ●
B		● ● (●)	●● (●)(●)(●)	● ●	● ●	(●) (●) (●)
A		●●●●●	(many dots)	(dots)		(dots)

I	congenital athyreosis
II	congenital dystopic hypoplasia
III	congenital dyshormonogenesis
IV	auto-immune hypothyroidism
V	pituitary hypothyroidism

A	special education
B*	primary education
C* a.	high school-general type
b.	high school-college prep. type

$$* \left\{ \begin{array}{l} \bullet \quad \text{successful progress accomplished} \\ (\bullet) \quad \text{successful progress expected} \end{array} \right.$$

visual and auditory discrimination. Since it thus reflects the state of neuro-psychological organization, it may be used for group comparisons.

Only 31% (13/42) of the children with the congenital types of the disease (I, II, III) were found to be ready for schooling at the age of 6 years.

School performance and progress were also considered in relation to diagnostic groups (Table 4) and to the age at which thyroxine substitution was instituted (Table 5). Normal progress through primary school (including

Table 5. Educational levels in relation to age at initiation of thyroxine substitution.

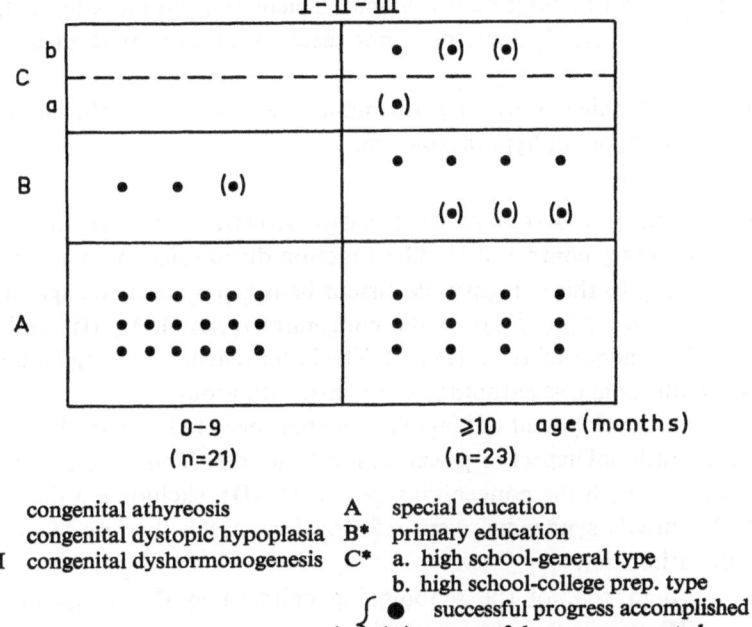

I congenital athyreosis
II congenital dystopic hypoplasia
III congenital dyshormonogenesis

A special education
B* primary education
C* a. high school-general type
 b. high school-college prep. type
* { ● successful progress accomplished
 (●) successful progress expected

repeating one class) was accomplished by only 38% (9/24) with the congenital types (I and II: 6/17; III: 3/7). If we include children still in primary school and doing poorly, the expected percentage of successful children would amount only to 32 (14/44). None of the 8 children with congenital athyreosis (I) qualified for secondary school.

Referral to special schools occurred for 57% (25/44) of the children belonging to the congenital types (I, II, III). If we include the children who obviously required special schools but whose parents refused to follow advice to this effect, the percentage would amount to 68 (30/44).

The prognostic significance of the age of onset of thyroid failure is more clearly demonstrated if we again classify these children according to the age of initiation of thyroxine substitution:

0-9 months: special education 86% (18/21)⎫
⎬ mean: 68% (30/44)
≥ 10 months: special education 52% (12/23)⎭

Characteristic learning disabilities proved to be high distractibility and short attention span as compared with the age-mates. In primary school poor performance is especially marked in arithmetic (related to concept formation) and in subjects for which efficient imprinting is needed, for instance geography. Dyslexia does not seem to be an important anomaly in this group.

In general, this pattern of performance was not seen in the children with the acquired types of hypothyroidism.

MATURATIONAL ASPECTS OF PSYCHO-MOTOR FUNCTIONS

The involuntary control of bladder function during sleep may be considered as belonging to this category. Persistent bedwetting after the age of 4 years was found in 44% (17/39) of the congenital types (I, II, III) and in 36% (4/11) of the acquired types (IV, V). The latter percentage is again influenced by the additional CNS pathology associated with group V.

Like the development of language, the mastery of clear speech articulation is a maturational aspect of psychomotor functions. Thirty percent (10/33) of the children with the congenital types (I, II, III), excluding 2 deaf children with Pendred's syndrome, were referred for speech therapy by the school health authorities.

More than 50% of the schoolgoing children in the congenital groups (I, II, III) were strongly retarded in mastering the motor-coordination needed for swimming and cycling.

FAMILIAL INTELLIGENCE

For practical reasons, it was not possible to give members of our patients' families formal IQ tests. Instead, data on educational and vocational training were used. Of the 84 parents involved, only 3 (3.6%) had been in special classes and 4 (4.8%) were university graduates. The other parents were spread over primary and secondary education in accordance with the national distribution for their generation. Of the 109 siblings of schoolgoing age, only 6 (5.5%) were in special schools. On the other hand, 30 (68%) of

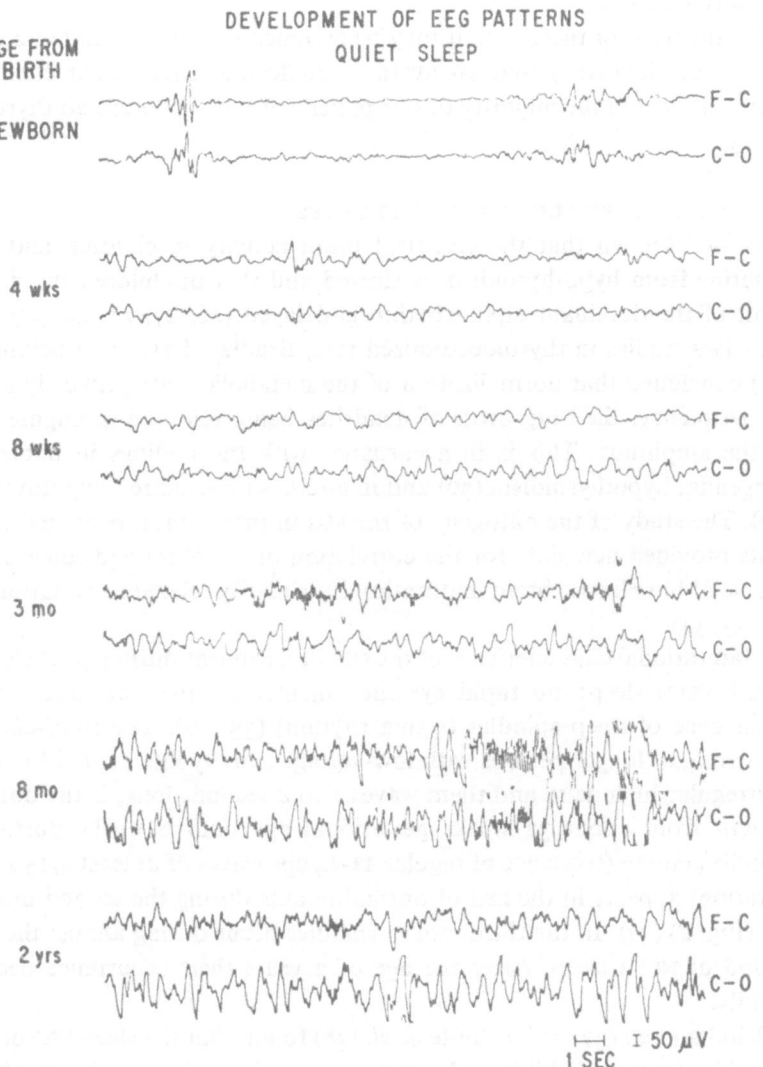

Fig. 2. **Development of** EEG **pattern during** NREM **sleep at successive ages from birth to 2 years. Spindles appear at the age of 3 months; thereafter they decrease in duration and frequency. (From: M. A. Schultz** *et al.* **37)**

our 44 children with congenital hypothyroidism (types I, II, III) qualified for special education.

On the basis of these data it may be assumed (as far as social and genetic factors are involved) that an average intellectual endowment could have been expected in the majority of our patients if they had not had thyroid defiency.

ELECTROENCEPHALOGRAPHIC STUDIES

It is well known that the electrical brain activity in children and adults suffering from hypothyroidism is slowed and that in children the development of the dominant alpha-rhythm is delayed (26, 27, 28, 29, 30). From their EEG studies in thyroidectomized rats, Bradley, Eayrs and Schmalbach (31) concluded that normalization of the metabolic state primarily restores the frequency, the outgrowth of dendrites being reflected in augmentation of the amplitude. This is in accordance with the findings in babies with congenital hypothyroidism (30) and in adults with acquired hypothyroidism (29). The study of the ontogeny of the EEG in prematures, neonates, and infants provided new data for the correlation of structure and function. The course of bio-electric brain maturation is primarily related to gestational age (32, 33, 34).

Maturational characteristics of the EEG of newborns during quiet sleep (so-called NREM sleep: no rapid eye movements) are the tracé-alternant and occurrence of sleep spindles (sigma rhythm) (35, 36). The tracé-alternant, consisting of longer periods with low-voltage activity interrupted by periods of irregular high delta and theta waves 1 to 4 seconds long, is the dominant pattern from about 32 weeks gestational age until 6 weeks postnatally. Spindle activity (sequence of regular 11-14 cps waves of at least 4/15 seconds duration) appears in the EEG of normal infants during the second month of life (Fig. 2) (37). In the third month spindles occur during almost the whole period of NREM sleep. After the age of 2 years their occurrence decreases rapidly.

Schultz et al. (37) and Schulte et al. (38) found that the sleep EEG of hypothyroid infants and children showed a strongly retarded and incomplete development of sleep spindles during quiet sleep without eye movements (NREM), but there was no correlation with the corresponding serum parameters of thyroid function, such as PBI, T_3, and T_4. The development of sleep spindles proved to be strongly retarded as compared with the normalization of these serum values and remained incomplete in children damaged by long-standing hypothyroidism.

The following case will serve as an illustration of the foregoing:

Case report: Baby B.N., male, born at term after uneventful pregnancy. Birth weight 4080 g. Symptoms of hypothyroidism assumed to have become manifest at the age of six months.
Laboratory findings at the age of 10½ months.

Serum-PBI: 0.4 μg/100 ml. ^{131}I-uptake: 19%/24 hr.
Scintigram: dystopic sublingual hypoplasia.
EEG (Fig. 3) before treatment, at the age of 10½ months: quiet sleep; sleep spindles in leads 1, 2, 5, 6 and 7.
EEG (Fig. 4) after 2 months of treatment, at the age of 13 months: quiet sleep; sleep spindles in leads 2, 3, 6, and 7. There is an increase in the duration and amplitude of the spindle activity, and spindles occur more frequently in the record. Correspondingly, the background activity shows a greater amount of activity in the beta and alpha frequencies.

Unequivocal data concerning the correlation between disappearance of EEG

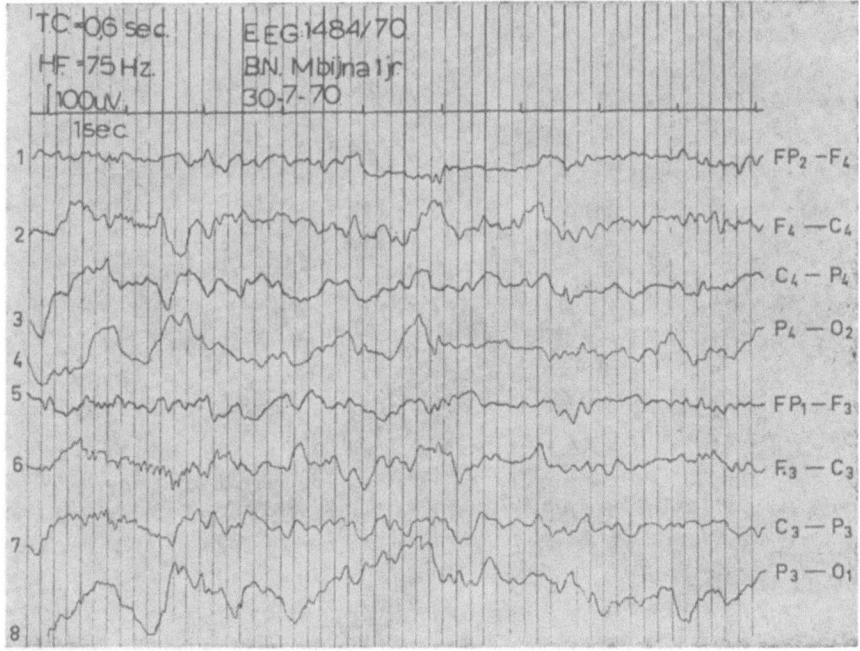

Fig. 3. EEG infant B.N. before treatment at the age of 10½ months. Quiet sleep. Sleep spindles in leads 1, 2, 5, 6 and 7.

abnormalities and mental development is still needed. Catch-up improvement in bio-electrical maturity into adulthood after hormone substitution may be less complete than is the rule for the corresponding skeletal maturation.

It is hoped that quantitative analysis of these changes will offer a basis for the objective evaluation of the long-term effects of treatment.*

DISCUSSION

Our findings in general confirm the data obtained in earlier comparable studies (19, 20, 21, 22, 39, 40, 41, 42, 43), the most noteworthy of which is the comprehensive study done by Smith, Blizzard and Wilkins in 1957 on 128 infants and children with hypothyroidism (19). In 1956, Money reported a related study of the concomitant psychological aspects in 70 children of the same group of 128 (44). Smith *et al.* reported that out of 79 severely affected 'cretins' (onset of symptoms between 0 and 6 months) on adequate treatment, only 15% attained an IQ > 90; of 32 mildly affected 'cretins' (onset of symp-

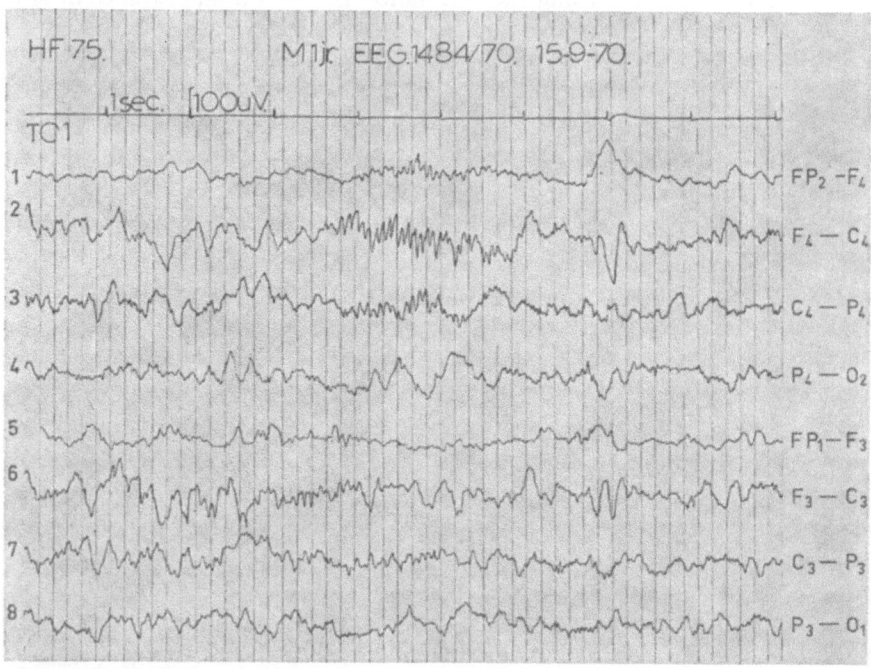

Fig. 4. EEG infant B.N. after 2 months of treatment at the age of 13 months. Quiet sleep. Sleep spindles in leads 2, 3, 6 and 7.

* The results of the EEG studies in this survey will be published separately.

toms between 6 and 18 months), 41% reached an IQ > 90; and of 17 children with 'acquired' hypothyroidism (onset of disease after 2 years), 77% passed the 90 level. These authors suggested that hypothyroidism acquired after the second year of life has little or no serious irreversible effect on mental development. They also demonstrated clearly that adequate therapy started within the first six months of life may fail to establish normal mentality (12 out of 22 patients so treated did not attain an IQ > 90) in those patients who could be assumed to have suffered from thyroid insufficiency in utero (diagnosis supported by signs of retarded prenatal ossification). Their findings concerning concomitant neurological impairment such as shuffling gait and clumsiness, are in good agreement with histopathological studies on cerebellar structure in thyroidectomized rats (7) and with the known occurrence of ataxic syndrome in children with congenital hypothyroidism (45). The cognitive dysfunctions, e.g. perseveration, paraphasia, and periphrasis, as reported by Money (44), present another example of cerebral impairment associated with congenital hypothyroidism.

Medical supervision aimed only at keeping the patient somatically in a euthyroid state is basically inadequate.

The parents should be prepared in good time to accept special education if necessary. In spite of early treatment, children with a history of congenital hypothyroidism continue to be at a disadvantage with respect to their educational prognosis and social situation. The IQ can be expected to become stabilized after two to five years of euthyroidism (22, 46).

The paediatrician should convince the school health officials of the necessity for preventing educational failure of the children with a nearly normal IQ level by removing them from the overcrowded classrooms in our standard primary school (about 40 children to a class in the 1st and 2nd grades).

Interrelated physical, intellectual, social, and emotional factors are operative on this kind of handicapped child, and the child with his abilities, as an integral whole, is in continuous interaction with his environments. Psycho-social, educational, and vocational guidance are therefore imperative throughout the entire period of childhood and adolescence.

ACKNOWLEDGEMENTS

The authors are indebted to Dr F. J. Bekker (Department of Psychology, University of Leiden) for supervising most of the testing procedures as well as to Miss W. M. Bodar, clinical psychologist (Department of Paediatrics, Leiden University Hospital); to Dr K. Mechelse (Department of Electroneurology, Leiden University Hospital) for reading the EEGs; and to Miss Eveline D. Veraart for helpful co-operation throughout the study.

REFERENCES

1. Siegert, F., Myxödem im Kindesalter. *Ergeb. inn. Med. Kinderh.* 6, 601 (1910).
2. Eayrs, J. T. & Taylor, S. H., The effect of thyroid deficiency induced by methyl-thiouracil on the maturation of the central nervous system. *J. Anat.* 85, 350 (1951).
3. Eayrs, J. T., The cerebral cortex of normal and hypothyroid rats. *Acta anat.* 25, 160 (1955).
4. Eayrs, J. T., The status of the thyroid gland in relation to the development of the nervous system. *Anim. Behav.* 7, 1 (1959).
5. Eayrs, J. T., Influence of the thyroid on the central nervous system. *Brit. med. Bull* 16, 122 (1960).
6. Eayrs, J. T., Thyroid and central nervous development. In: *The scientific basis of medicine,* London 1966.
7. Legrand, J., Kriegel, A. & Jost, A., Déficience thyroïdienne et maturation du cervelet chez le rat blanc. *Arch. Anat. Microsc. Morphol. Exp.* 50, 507 (1961).
8. Balázs, R., Brooksbank, B. W. L., Davison, A. N., Eayrs, J. T. & Wilson, D. A., The effect of neonatal thyroidectomy on myelination in the rat brain. *Brain Res.* 15, 219 (1969).
9. Balázs, R., Kóvacs, S., Teichgräber, P., Cocks, W. A. & Eayrs, J. T., Biochemical effects of thyroid deficiency on the developing brain. *J. Neurochem.* 15, 1335 (1968).
10. Eayrs, J. T. & Levine, S., Influence of thyroidectomy and subsequent replacement therapy upon conditioned avoidance learning in the rat. *J. Endocrinol.* 25, 505 (1963).
11. Marinesco, M.G., Contribution à l'étude des lésions du myxoedème congénital. *Encéphale* 19: 265 (1924).
12. Lotmar, F., Histopathologische Befunde in Gehirnen vom kongenitalen Myxödem (Thyreoplasie). *Z. ges. Neur. Psychiat.,* 491 (1929).
13. Eayrs, J. T., Functional correlates of modified cortical structure. In: *Structure and function of the cerebral cortex,* Tower, D. B. & Schadé, J. P. (eds.), Amsterdam 1960.
14. Sokoloff, L., Roberts, P. A., Januska, M. M. & Kline, J. E., Mechanisms of stimulation of protein synthesis by thyroid hormones in vivo. *Proc. Nat. Acad. Sci.* 60, 652 (1968).
15. Fisher, D. A., Lehman, H. & Lackey, C., Placental transport of thyroxine. *J. Clin. Endocrinol.* 24, 393 (1964).
16. Pickering, D. E., Maternal thyroid hormone in the developing fetus. (Observations on Macaca Mulatta). *Amer. J. Dis. Child.* 107, 567 (1964).
17. Dobbing, J. & Sands, J., Timing of neuroblast multiplication in developing human brain. *Nature* 226, 639 (1970).
18. Winick, N., Changes in nucleic acid and protein content of the human brain during growth. *Pediat. Res.* 2, 352 (1968).
19. Smith, D. W., Blizzard, R. M. & Wilkins, L., The mental prognosis in hypothyroidism of infancy and childhood. *Pediatrics* 19, 1011 (1957).
20. Bernheim, M., Berger, M., Bertrand, J. & Frederich, A., Le pronostic du myxoedème congénital. *Presse méd.* 69, 2182 (1961).
21. Andersen, H. J., Studies of hypothyroidism in children. *Acta paed.* 50, suppl. 125 (1961).
22. Andersen, H. & Skinhøj, K., Longitudinal studies of I.Q. in hypothyroid children during treatment. *Proc. intern. Copenhagen congress on the scientific study of mental retardation,* vol. II. 1964.
23. Chorus, A., Bekker, F. J., Kuipers, A., Koornstra, M. & Gemund, J. J. van. On the occurrence and prevention of mental deficiency in hypothyroidism. *Proc. intern. Copenhagen congress on the scientific study of mental retardation,* vol. I. 1964.

24. Wilkins, L., *The diagnosis and treatment of endocrine disorders in childhood and adolescence*, Springfield (Ill.) 1965.
25. Hutchison, J. H., Diseases of the thyroid gland. In: *Paediatric endocrinology*, Hubble, D. (ed,), Oxford 1969.
26. Ross, D. A. & Schwab, R. S., The cortical alpha rhythm in thyroid disorders. *Endocrinology* 25, 75 (1939).
27. d'Avignon, M. & Melin, K. A., The electroencephalogram in congenital hypothyreosis. *Acta Paed.* 38, 37 (1949).
28. Nieman, E. A., The electroencephalogram in congenital hypothyroidism: a study of 10 cases. *J. Neurol. Neurosurg. Psychiat.* 24, 50 (1961).
29. Lansing, R. W. & Trunnell, J. B., Electroencephalographic changes accompanying thyroid deficiency in man. *J. Clin. Endocrinol.* 23, 470 (1963).
30. Harris, R., della Rovere, M. & Prior, P. F., Electroencephalographic studies in infants and children with hypothyroidism. *Arch. Dis. Child.* 40, 612 (1965).
31. Bradley, P. B., Eayrs, J. T. & Schmalbach, K., The electroencephalogram of normal and hypothyroid rats. *Electroenceph. Clin. Neurophysiol.* 12, 467 (1960).
32. Dreyfus-Brisac, C., Samson-Dollfus, D. & Fischgold, H., L'activité électrique cérébrale du prématuré et du nouveau-né. *Sem. Hôp. Paris* 31, 1783 (1955).
33. Dreyfus-Brisac, C., The electroencephalogram of the premature infant and full-term newborn. In: *Neurological and electroencephalographic correlative studies in infancy*, Kellaway, P. & Petersén, I. (eds.), New York 1964.
34. Samson-Dollfus, D., Forthomme, J. & Capron, E., EEG of the human infant during sleep and wakefulness during the first year of life. In: *Neurological and electroencephalographic correlative studies in infancy*, Kellaway, P. & Petersén, I. (eds.), New York 1964.
35. Lenard, H. G., Sleep studies in infancy. *Acta Paed. Scand.* 59, 572 (1970).
36. Lenard, H. G., The development of sleep spindles in the EEG during the first two years of life. *Neuropädiat.* 1, 264 (1970).
37. Schultz, M. A., Schulte, F. J., Akiyama, Y. & Parmelee, A. H., Development of electroencephalographic sleep phenomena in hypothyroid infants. *Electroenceph. Clin. Neurophysiol.* 25, 351 (1968).
38. Schulte, F. J. & Parmelee, A. H., Thyroid hormone and brain development. An analysis of polygraphic data of hypothyroid babies before and during treatment (abstr.). *Electroenceph. Clin. Neurophysiol.* 29, 212 (1970).
39. Lewis, A., A study of cretinism in London, with special reference to mental development and problems of growth. *Lancet* I, 1505 (1937).
40. Topper, A., Mental achievement of congenitally hypothyroid children. *Amer. J. Dis. Child.* 81, 233 (1951).
41. Harnack, G. A. von & Wallis, H., Zur Psychopathologie der Hypothyreose im Kindesalter. *Monatsschr. Kinderheilk.* 108, 373 (1960).
42. Neimann, N., Pierson, M. & Berthier, X., Le pronostic mental du myxoedème infantile. *Arch. Franç. Pédiat.* 20, 147 (1963).
43. König, M. P., *Die kongenitale Hypothyreose und der endemische Kretinismus*, Berlin 1968.
44. Money, J., Psychologic studies in hypothyroidism. *Arch. Neurol. Psychiat.* 76, 296 (1956).
45. Hagberg, B. & Westphal, O., Ataxic syndrome in congenital hypothyroidism. *Acta Paed. Scans.* 59, 323 (1970).
46. Money, J. & Lewis, V., Longitudinal study of intelligence quotient in treated congenital hypothyroidism. In: *Brain-thyroid relationships*, Ciba Foundation Study Group nr. 18, London 1964.

DISCUSSION

Widdowson: Thank you Dr Van Gemund. Dr Dobbing had to leave but I am sure, if he could have been here he would have been the first to agree that there is more to brain function than the number of cells and nuclei, and I am glad you brought one aspect of this so clearly.

Croughs: Dr Van Gemund, your early treatment group had a worse mental prognosis than your late treatment group. Now, of course this must be because your early treatment group has mainly children with complete thyroid deficiency and your late treatment group has mainly children with partial thyroid deficiency. Why did you not completely separate these two groups? I think your study would have gained much importance if you had done this, because now you suggest that it is better to postpone treatment. And of course this is not your intention.

Van Gemund: Well, I hope I made it clear that the group in which substitution was instituted after the 10th month was the better-off group, that had remnants of thyroid gland activity at the lingual level. We were not able at the time to classify all our cases in terms of iodine uptake, scintigram appearance and serum free thyroxine. We have patients, who are now 25 years of age, in which the original data were scant and at best contained information on PBI-levels. We could, however, reconstruct their proper classification by looking at the bone-age patterns of prenatal centres, like the distal centre of the femur, foot-centres etc.

Akiyama: In your abstract you mentioned a delay in the maturation of the alpha rhythm. Did you see any other delays in EEG maturation at an older age, e.g. hypnogogic (four cycles per second) activity in sleeping children.

Van Gemund: We have just made our first steps towards analysing by means of a computer programme the conventional characteristics of EEG's and we have not yet been able so far to study this phenomenon with proper monitoring of the state.

PITUITARY-ADRENAL HORMONES AND BEHAVIOR

D. DE WIED

After the introduction of ACTH and corticosteroids into the clinic, a great deal of data suggesting an effect of these hormones in the central nervous system has accumulated. These data were in line with observations on electroencephalographic alteration, convulsions and mental changes in patients suffering from hypo- and hypercorticism. Experimentally, it was found that corticosteroids alter the excitability of the brain. Glucocorticosteroids and ACTH were shown to decrease the threshold for electric shock in animals. Other studies revealed electroencephalographic changes, in the hypothalamus, the mesencephalic reticular structures and in the thalamus following administration of ACTH or glucocorticosteroids. These and similar investigations demonstrated that the central nervous system contains areas which are sensitive to steroids not only with respect to feed back regulation of pituitary function but to other regulatory mechanisms like the modulation of behavior as well.

Relatively little is known about the influence of the pituitary-adrenal system and its hormones on behavior but recent developments in this area have revealed that the pituitary-adrenal system is involved in the acquisition and retention of conditioned avoidance behavior. Removal of the pituitary gland has been shown to retard the acquisition of a shuttle box avoidance response in rats (1, 2, 3, 4). An adrenal maintenance dose of ACTH restores the rate of acquisition of the avoidance response of hypophysectomized rats toward nearly normal levels (4). These results suggested that lack of adrenocortical hormones causes a behavioral deficiency in hypophysectomized rats. Treatment of these rats with either thyroxine, testosterone or dexamethasone, however, revealed that glucocorticosteroids are not essential for the restoration of avoidance behavior in hypophysectomized rats. Dexamethasone failed to improve avoidance learning but thyroxine as well as testosterone significantly facilitated the rate of acquisition of the avoidance response in hypophysectomized rats (Fig. 1).

Treatment with thyroxine induced a substantial increase in intertrial response activity suggesting a nonspecific influence on avoidance acquisition. Behavioral deficiency of hypophysectomized rats is certainly linked to some extent to metabolic derangements in and physical weakness of the hypophysectomized organism (3). In fact, the beneficial effect of testosterone on avoidance acquisition may be explained in this way since this steroid markedly inhibited loss of body weight as normally occurs in hypophysectomized rats (Fig. 2).

Accordingly, the effect of ACTH on avoidance acquisition in hypophysectomized rats is not mediated by the adrenal cortex but due to an influence of this polypeptide on other structures, presumably located in the central nervous system. This extra target effect of ACTH was demonstrated with the use of structurally related peptides like α-MSH, ACTH 1-10 and ACTH 4-10 which are devoid of corticotrophic activities. These peptides are capable of restoring the rate of acquisition of the avoidance response in hypophysectomized rats (Fig. 1). Studies of the effects of these peptides on endocrine and metabolic functions, on motor capacities and sensory function and on the

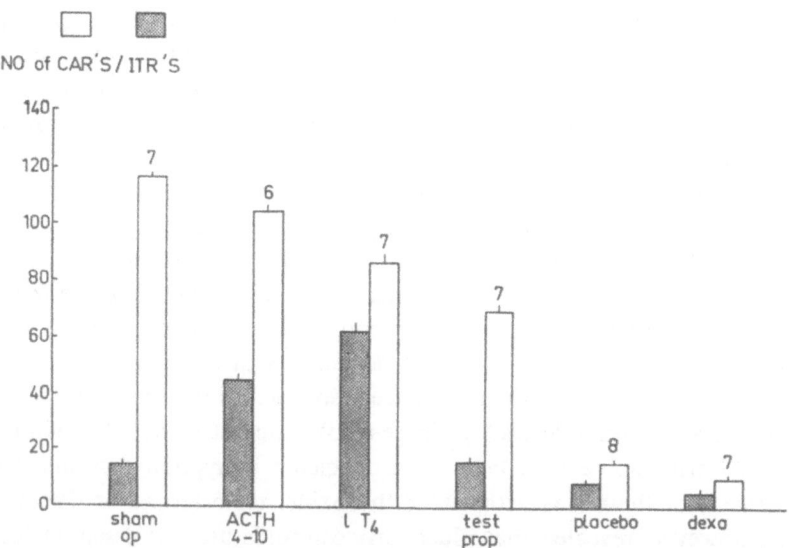

Fig. I. Effect of various hormones on the rate of acquisition of a shuttle box avoidance response in male hypophysectomized rats. Treatment was started 1 week after operation. (ACTH 4-10) ACTH 4-10 was given in long acting form as a zinc phosphate preparation in a dose of 20 μg per 2 days. (sham op) Sham operated controls; (l T4) l-thyroxine 10 μg per 2 days; (test prop) testosterone propionate 0.2 mg per 2 days; (placebo) zinc phosphate complex 0.5 ml per 2 days; (dexa) dexamethasone 10 μg per day.
All substances given subcutaneously.

general health and condition of the hypophysectomized rat did not indicate that the behavioral effect of the heptapeptide ACTH 4-10 is due to any of these functions (4) (Fig. 3).

It was therefore postulated that peptides like ACTH 4-10 or closely resembling this heptapeptide normally operate in the development of learned behavior patterns. Such peptides with neurogenic activities may be synthetized by the pituitary gland and released upon adequate stimulation to affect central nervous structures involved in learning processes. In fact, evidence for the existence of such peptides in the pituitary has been obtained and recently a peptide has been isolated in pure form from hog pituitary tissue

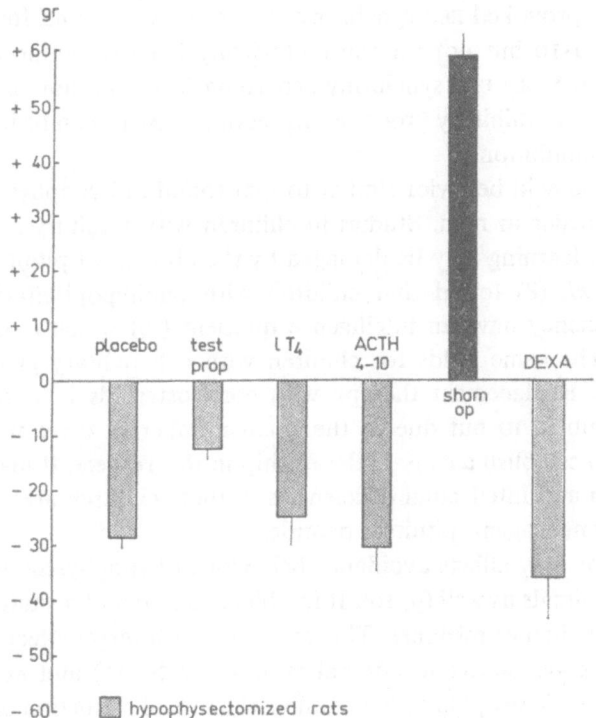

Fig. 2. Influence of treatment on body weight of hypophysectomized rats. See legend to figure I.

	4	5	6	7	8	9	10
H –	Met –	Glu –	His –	Phe –	Arg –	Trp –	Gly – OH

Fig. 3. Amino acid sequence of ACTH 4-10.

which is capable of restoring the deficient behavior of hypophysectomized rats. This peptide is 10 to 20 times more active than ACTH 4-10 (5). Amino acid analysis of this peptide revealed that it is closely related to vasopressin (6). Other active fractions have been found which contain peptides which may be more related to MSH or ACTH.

This extra target effect of ACTH has been recently demonstrated in humans on EEG (7). Presentation of a novel stimulus like sound or light elicits both behavioral and EEG arousal. Repetition of this stimulus results in elimination of the arousal reaction and leads to habituation. Prolonged repetition of the stimulus is associated with enhancement of alpha activity and bursts of slow waves, a situation designated as synchronized EEG activity. ACTH markedly suppresses provoked EEG synchrony. The same was found for the decapeptide ACTH 1-10 but not for the biologically inactive amino acid sequence ACTH 11-24. Since EEG synchrony according to the authors indicates a predominance of inhibitory processes, the action of ACTH can be interpreted as a kind of disinhibition.

A deficiency in behavior similar to that found in hypophysectomized rats may also occur in man. Studies in children with pituitary insufficiency indicate that learning may be damaged by the absence of pituitary hormones. Laron et al. (8) found that children with panhypopituitarism including ACTH deficiency have an intelligence quotient (IQ) which is well below the average. The same holds for children with a hereditary growth hormone deficiency. Replacement therapy with corticosteroids is associated with a distinct gain in IQ but due to the small number of cases it has not been possible to establish a causal relationship in this respect. It may well be that behavioral and intellectual deficiencies in these children are also caused by the lack of neurogenic pituitary peptides.

ACTH not only affects avoidance behavior in hypophysectomized rats but in intact animals as well (9, 10). It inhibits extinction of a shuttle box or pole jumping avoidance response. This too is an extra target effect of ACTH. This hormone is also active in adrenalectomized rats (11) and ACTH analogues devoid of corticotrophic activities affect the rate of extinction of the avoidance response. In fact the heptapeptide ACTH 4-10 is nearly as potent in this respect as the synthetic ACTH β 1-24 molecule (12).

Glucocorticosteroids do not inhibit extinction of the avoidance response. On the contrary, they facilitate extinction (13, 14). Since the glucocorticosteroids inhibit the release of ACTH as a consequence of the negative feed back action, the facilitating effect of corticosterone on extinction might be explained by blockade of pituitary ACTH-release. However, corticosterone as

well as dexamethasone also facilitate the rate of extinction in hypophysectomized rats indicating that these steroids act independently of pituitary ACTH
(13). This is supported by experiments with implantation of cortisol in the
median eminence of the hypothalamus, which inhibits ACTH-release and at
the same time facilitates the rate of extinction of an avoidance response; the
more the release of ACTH is suppressed the stronger the effect on extinction
(15). However, implantation of cortisol in the mesencephalic reticular formation which hardly reduces ACTH-release, also facilitates extinction of the
avoidance response. This indicates that steroids may have a dual effect on
extinction of an avoidance response: through inhibition of ACTH-release and
through a direct action in the central nervous system.

In a structure activity relationship study, Van Wimersma Greidanus (16)
found that the pregnene or pregnadiene type steroids facilitate extinction of
conditioned avoidance behavior while the cholestene, androstene, estratriene
and pregnane types are ineffective. Common features of the active steroids
are double bond(s) in ring A or B and their ketogroup or hydroxy-group at
C_3 (Fig. 4). The keto-group at C_{20} is important for the strength of the effect

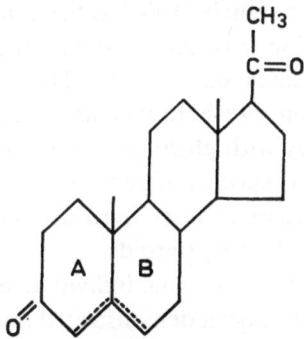

Fig. 4. A steroid with 21 C atoms, a double bond in ring A or B, a keto or hydroxy group
at C_3 and a keto group at C_{20} is required for facilitating the rate of extinction of the
avoidance response.

but not essential. The action of the steroids on extinction of conditioned
avoidance behavior, therefore, is not directly related to their glucocorticoid
activity. For example, progesterone and pregnenolone are as potent in
facilitating extinction as corticosterone. Interestingly, the production of
these steroids is like corticosterone increased during stress (17, 18).

The site of action of ACTH analogues and of the steroids is in the central
nervous system. This was suggested from studies with lesions in the nucleus

parafascicularis and adjacent areas. Such lesions prevent the inhibitory effect of α-MSH on the rate of extinction of a shuttle box avoidance response (19). Implantation of small amounts of dexamethasone, corticosterone or progesterone in the mesencephalic reticular formation or in the posterior thalamic area facilitate the rate of extinction of an avoidance response (15, 20). Implantation of the heptapeptide ACTH 1-10 in the same area inhibits extinction (21).

Accordingly, an important locus of action of the steroids and the peptides on avoidance behavior is the nonspecific thalamic reticular system. This system is thought to have important integrative functions (22, 23) since all incoming information converges in this area. Implantations and lesions are, however small, effective in disturbing the output of this system by interfering with impulse transmission. Since the nonspecific thalamic system acts as a filter for ascending information to other areas in the brain (24), the behavioral effects of implantation of ACTH analogues and steroids indicate that these substances may be acting to modulate neural transmission in this nodal point of sensory integration in the central nervous system.

Removal of adrenocortical hormones in man and lower animals increases the ability to detect sensory signals. This has been shown for taste, olfaction, audition and proprioception (25). At the same time the ability to integrate sensory information decreases significantly. Thus, the detection threshold decreases as the recognition threshold increases. Treatment of patients with adrenocortical insufficiency with glucocorticosteroids returns sensory detection to normal. Conversely, surplus of adrenocortical hormones as found in Cushing's syndrome decreases sensory detection and this is restored after removal of the excess of circulating steroids.

Such changes are found in the normal individual as well. Reciprocal alteration in sensory detection has been demonstrated during circadian alteration of adrenocortical function. When the glucocorticosteroid activity is at its lowest (during late afternoon and evening) taste detection is highest and vice versa. There are indications that other (presumably pituitary) hormones are involved. When all adrenocortical hormones are absent as in untreated Addison's disease or total adrenalectomy there is little or no detectable circadian variation in taste detection. However, circadian alteration in sensory detection is observed again following treatment with glucocorticosteroids (25).

The organism possesses a complex adaptive apparatus which is needed to integrate extrinsic and intrinsic information. The pituitary-adrenal system plays an essential role in this respect. In addition to the metabolic effects of

ACTH and glucocorticosteroids they profoundly affect sensory integration and consequently adaptive behavior. Disturbances in the function of the pituitary-adrenal system and in the production and release of its hormones and related agents may therefore affect the adaptive capacities of the organism. It is even possible that disturbances in the pituitary-adrenal system and its hormones may precipitate or underlie certain kinds of behavioral disorders. A more sophisticated analysis of the activity of this complex neuroendocrine system may eventually lead to a better understanding of the development of psychosomatic and neurotic disturbances for which the term disorder of adaptation may be used.

ACKNOWLEDGEMENT

The ample supply of hormones as used in this study, by N.V. Organon, Oss, Holland, is gratefully acknowledged.

REFERENCES

1. Applezweig, M. H. & Baudry, F. D., The pituitary-adrenocortical system in avoidance learning. *Psychol. Rep.* 1, 417 (1955).
2. Applezweig, M. H. & Moeller, G. The pituitary-adrenocortical system and anxiety in avoidance learning. *Acta Psychol.* 15, 602 (1959).
3. De Wied, D., Influence of anterior pituitary on avoidance learning and escape behavior. *Amer. J. Physiol.* 207, 255 (1964).
4. De Wied, D., The anterior pituitary and conditioned avoidance behaviour. In: *Progress in endocrinology*, Exc. Med. Int. Congress Series No. 184, 310 (1968). Proceedings Third International Congress of Endocrinology Mexico, D. F., 30 June – 5 July, 1968.
5. De Wied, D., Witter, A. & Lande, S., Anterior pituitary peptides and avoidance acquisition of hypophysectomized rats. In: *Progress in Brain Research* 32, 213. De Wied, D. & Weijnen, J. A. W. M. (eds.), Amsterdam 1970.
6. Lande, S., Witter, A. & de Wied, D., Pituitary Peptides: an octapeptide that stimulates conditioned avoidance acquisition in hypophysectomized rats. *J. biol. Chem.* 246, 2058 (1971).
7. Endröczi, E., Lissák, K., Fekete, T. & de Wied, D., Effects of ACTH on EEG habituation in human subjects. In: *Progress in brain research* 32, 254. De Wied, D. & Weijnen, J. A. W. M. (eds.), Amsterdam 1970.
8. Laron, Z., Karp, M., Pertzelan, A. & Frankel, J., ACTH deficiency in children and adolescents (clinical and psychological aspects). In: *Progress in brain research* 32, 305 De Wied, D. & Weijnen, J. A. W. M. (eds.), Amsterdam 1970.
9. Murphy, J. V. & Miller, R. E., The effect of adrenocorticotrophic hormone (ACTH) on avoidance conditioning in the rat. *J. comp. physiol. Psychol.* 48, 47 (1955).
10. De Wied, D., Inhibitory effect of ACTH and related peptides on extinction of conditioned avoidance behavior in rats. *Proc. Soc. exp. Biol.* 122, 28 (1966).
11. Miller, R. E. & Ogawa, N., The effect of adrenocorticotrophic hormone (ATCH) on

avoidance conditioning in the adrenalectomized rats. *J. comp. physiol. Psychol.* 55, 211 (1962).

12. Greven, H. M. & de Wied, D., The active sequence in the ACTH molecule responsible for inhibition of the extinction of conditioned avoidance behaviour in rats. *Europ. J. Pharmacol.* 2, 14 (1967).

13. De Wied, D., Opposite effects of ACTH and glucocorticosteroids on extinction of conditioned avoidance behavior. In: *Exc. Med. Int. Congress Series* No. 132, 945 (1967). Proceedings Second International Congress on Hormonal Steroids, Milan, May, 1966.

14. De Wied, D., Bohus, B. & Greven, H. M., Influence of pituitary and adrenocortical hormones on conditioned avoidance behaviour in rats. In: *Endocrinology and human behaviour*, 188. Michael, R. P. (ed.), Proceedings of a conference held at the Institute of Psychiatry, London, 9-11 May, 1967. Oxford 1968.

15. Bohus, B., Pituitary ACTH release and avoidance behavior of rats with cortisol implants in mesencephalic reticular formation and median eminence. *Neuroendocrinology* 3, 355 (1968).

16. Van Wimersma Greidanus, Tj. B., Effects of steroids on extinction of an avoidance response in rats. A structure-activity relationship study. In: *Progress in brain research* 32, 185. De Wied, D. & Weijnen, J. A. W. M. (eds.), Amsterdam 1970.

17. Resko, J. A., Endocrine control of adrenal progesterone secretion in the ovariectomized rat. *Science* 164, 70 (1969).

18. Holzbauer, M. & Newport, H. M., The effect of stress on the concentration of 3β-hydroxypregn-5-en-20-one (pregnenolone) in the adrenal gland of the rat. *J. Physiol. (Lond.)* 193, 131 (1967).

19. Bohus, B. & de Wied, D., Failure of α-MSH to delay extinction of conditioned avoidance behavior in rats with lesions in the parafascicular nuclei of the thalamus. *Physiol. Behav.* 2, 221 (1967).

20. Van Wimersma Greidanus, Tj. B. & de Wied, D., Effects of intracerebral implantation of corticosteroids on extinction of an avoidance response in rats. *Physiol. Behav.* 4, 365 (1969).

21. Van Wimersma Greidanus, Tj. B. & de Wied, D., Effects of systemic and intracerebral administration of two opposite acting ACTH-related peptides on extinction of conditioned avoidance behavior. *Neuroendocrinology* 7, 291 (1971).

22. Cardo, D., Rôle de certains noyaux thalamiques dans l'élaboration et la conservation de divers conditionnements. *Revue Psychologie Française* 10, 344 (1965).

23. Cardo, B., Effects de la stimulation du noyau parafasciculaire thalamique sur l'acquisition d'un conditionnement d'évitement chez le rat. *Physiol. Behav.* 2, 245 (1967).

24. Korányi, L. & Endröczi, E., Influence of pituitary-adrenocortical hormones on thalamo-cortical and brain stem limbic circuits. In: *Progress in brain research* 32, 120. De Wied, D. & Weijnen, J. A. W. M. (eds.), Amsterdam 1970.

25. Henkin, R. I., The effects of corticosteroids and ACTH on sensory systems. In: *Progress in brain research* 32, 270. De Wied, D. & Weijnen, J. A. W. M. (eds.), Amsterdam 1970.

DISCUSSION

Van den Brande: Do you have any data on the effect of growth hormone replacement on the avoidance behaviour?

De Wied: Yes sir. Growth hormone in the hypophysectomized animal will also substitute for the behavioural deficiency. But since I have never used pure or synthetic growth hormone I'm very hesitant to say that growth hormone plays an essential role in this respect. As you have seen, a small peptide can substitute for this deficiency, and it is possible that other closely related peptides from the pituitary may have the same effect. In fact, we have found a peptide in the pituitary which has an effect which is about 20-30 times as strong as the effect of the peptide ACTH 4-10. We think that there are small peptides in the pituitary which are essential for this kind of behaviour, avoidance behaviour or at least adaptive behaviour, if you want to call it that way. That's the reason why I thought that this audience should know this and look for this kind of behavioural disturbances in children, in particular in children with a damaged pituitary.

Visser: You have shown that there is some dose-response effect relationship after giving several doses of ACTH. Is that a qualitative or a quantitative effect, is it a permissive effect? If you give more of this will the effect go up?

De Wied: There is a dose response relationship. However, if we give too high a dose the effect becomes less. If we give the proper amount, that is the amount which maintains the size of the adrenal cortex in the hypophysectomized rat, the effect is optimal.

Visser: So there is maximum effect then.

De Wied: Yes, if one increases the dose the effect on avoidance learning diminishes. We never knew what this meant, till we found that the administration of a corticosteroid also reduces the already reduced acquisition behaviour of hypophysectomized rats.

Slob: There is also a difference in the sham-operated groups.

De Wied: That's true. I can assure you that there is a quantitative effect. We have shown this with the smaller peptides which are devoid of corticotrophic activity, because the glucocorticosteroids counteract the effect of ACTH.

Levine: You talk in terms of adaptive significance. Could you just elaborate on this question: which are the various functions that have been shown to be sensitive to these parameters of adrenocortical and pituitary function. At this point in addition to avoidance conditioning which is very well established, there seems to be a variety of things which are involved in the adaptive sequence of the animal, beginning with alterations in sensory function.

De Wied: This is the last point I tried to make, in order to show the importance of the pituitary-adrenal system for sensory function, by referring to Henkin's experiments.

Levine: Well, the point I'm trying to make is that there is an interesting sequence. Not only do you get the sensory changes, but then you get the whole process involved in orientation and habituation, the ways in which the organism deals with its environment. Then you get the processes involved in learning, then you get the processes involved in distinction, and all of these really make a very nice sequence of events, all indicating the role of the pituitary-adrenal system in the whole adaptive mechanism of the organism.

HORMONAL AND SOCIAL DETERMINANTS OF SEXUAL BEHAVIOR IN THE PIGTAIL MONKEY (MACACA NEMESTRINA)

D. A. GOLDFOOT*

INTRODUCTION

Ovarian hormones have been recognized as controlling agents for the expression of female sexual behavior in an extremely wide range of animals for many years (1, 2, 3). With few exceptions, sub-primate female mammals demonstrate behavioral patterns during the pre-ovulatory phase of the ovarian cycle which are never shown at any other time. These responses, collectively defined as *behavioral estrus*, include the display of opisthotonus and/or lordosis in response to the stimulation of a mount, the acceptance of the mount without escape or threat responses, an increase in running behavior and general locomotor activities, and, for several species, the display of mounting behavior by the female. Behavioral estrus begins abruptly in the hours or days immediately preceding ovulation, and normally ends shortly after ovulation (2). At any other time in the ovarian cycle, none of these responses is displayed, and any attempt by the male to mount is met with escape or aggression by the female.

The sexual behavior of higher primates does not readily conform to this definition of estrus. Earlier investigators reported that Catarhine monkeys and apes copulate throughout the entire menstrual cycle in captivity (4, 5, 6, 7, 8). Later work showed that although copulatory sequences do occur throughout the cycle, the number of intromissions and ejaculations by the male progressively increases in frequency during the follicular phase and reaches a peak near the time of expected ovulation. Copulations then diminish in frequency, and 'ejaculation latencies' become longer in the luteal

* New data reported in this paper are part of an unpublished Ph. D. thesis by D. A. Goldfoot presented to the Department of Medical Psychology, University of Oregon Medical School, Portland, Oregon, USA. The work was supported in part by grants FR-00163 and MH-08634 from the National Institutes of Health, and in part by GM-01495, a General Medical Sciences Traineeship.

phase of the cycle in chimpanzee (9, 10), in rhesus (11, 12, 13) and in the pigtail macaque (14).

Individual variance is a major problem in all of these studies, however, and the question of direct ovarian effects on the behavior of the female during the menstrual cycle is still in question to some extent. Michael (15) reports, for example, that only 50% of the intact monkey pairs he has observed display behavioral cycles related to ovarian states, and that a given pair displaying such rhythmicity for one cycle may not display the same pattern for the following cycle. Moreover, given a pair of monkeys which do demonstrate increased copulatory behaviors near ovulation, responses by the *male* rather than the female are decidedly better indicators of the ovarian status of the female. Indeed, no laboratory pair-test study has found statistical evidence for reliable cyclicity of the major primate posture of female sexual receptivity, 'presenting' (15, 14, 10).

Nonetheless, several other lines of evidence demonstrate that ovarian hormones do influence the sexual behavior of the female monkey. First, ovariectomy significantly reduces not only male copulatory behaviors, but also female presenting (16). Second, estrogens, given to the ovariectomized female either systemically or as hypothalamic implants, reinstate sexual behaviors of both the female and her male partner to preoperative levels (17).

On the one hand, then, studies employing ovariectomy and replacement therapy clearly reveal statistically significant changes in the sexual behavior of the female monkey. In contrast, laboratory studies of intact females observed in pair-tests show indications of female changes in receptivity, but, at best, can only demonstrate statistically significant changes in the behavior of the male partners. These two circumstances clearly suggest that factors other than ovarian influence on the CNS of the female might be involved in the control of female sexual responses.

In recent years, three possible mechanisms besides an ovarian hormone-brain relationship have been proposed. First, Michael and Keverne (18) have presented evidence that peripheral cue systems affecting the male, such as hormone-dependent odor or sex-skin changes of the female, have a decided influence on the sexual activities of the pair. Michael (16, 17) suggests that these peripheral alterations, which are under ovarian control, render the female more attractive to the male, and therefore directly influence his behavior. Everitt and Herbert (19), in turn, have drawn attention to the adrenal as an additional factor which is involved in the control of female sexual behaviors. These authors show that adrenal androgens influence both presenting behaviors and toleration of the males' mounts. Suppression of adrenal function by dexamethasone treatment or adrenalectomy with cortisol replacement both lead to depressed levels of these behaviors in ovariectomized females given estradiol. A third factor, the social environment itself, might be a very potent variable affecting sexual activities of the female. Contrary to the findings of laboratory pair-test investigations, results from studies of monkeys in the field indicate that definite changes in the behavior of females occur near the time of ovulation, including increased frequencies of presenting, increased behaviors which bring the female in close proximity to the male, and increased incidences of aggression in rhesus monkey (20, 21, 22, 23, 24), in baboon (25, 26), in pigtail macaque (27) and Japanese macaque (28). Carpenter (22) describes the preovulatory rhesus female in the troup as follows.

The estrous female, furthermore, is the vortex of stressful relationships in her group. During her receptive period, her social status in the group shifts and she becomes a sexual incentive for the groups' males. She actively approaches males and must overcome their usual resistance to close association. Hence she becomes an object of attacks by them. Even other females attack her as a result of her shifted social status.

These observations from the field suggest that receptivity in primates may manifest itself as a complex change in social interactions rather than as a simple postural change in response to a male. A social environment involving several animals may be necessary for the occurrence of behavioral changes which females might display at midcycle, but which are not recognized or cannot be elicited in isolation with a single partner. The laboratory pair-test might, therefore, be an inappropriate technique for detecting changes in the behavior of receptive females.

The hypothesis that social influences play a role in determining the sexual behavior of the monkey is also supported by several laboratory investigations. Rowell (29) observed small groups of male and female baboons in captivity and found that females displayed higher levels of sexual and aggressive behavior when in phases of maximum perineal turgescence associated with the preovulatory state. Herbert (30) reported that differences between individual females in a group situation heavily influenced sexual behavior: when two ovariectomized females given identical estrogen replacement treatment were presented simultaneously to a male, the male demonstrated decided preferences for one of the two females, despite their equivalent endocrine conditions. In a second report, Everitt and Herbert (31) confirmed this observation and found that withdrawal of estrogen from the

'preferred' female depressed but did not completely reverse preference behavior by the male. Further, estrogen withdrawal from the preferred partner
stimulated sexual presentations to the male by the 'non-favorite'.

Laboratory studies such as these reveal that social as well as endocrine
factors strongly influence the behavior of primates. The following study, reported in depth, was designed to identify specific social variables as well as
hormonal influences in intact females which determine the patterns of
sexual behavior in a group situation.

METHODS

General design summary

Fifteen adult, intact female pigtail macaque monkeys (Macaca nemestrina)
were observed for menstrual bleeding and daily perineal sex-skin changes
over a six-month period. In addition, plasma progesterone determinations
were made 4-6 days after the beginning of menstruation, and 7-9 days following the beginning of perineal deturgescence. With these measures, it was
possible to make an accurate estimation of the stage of the cycle, including
the approximate day of ovulation (14, 32).

Based on these measures, two types of temporary groups were formed
during restricted phases of the cycle. In one type of group, 3 females were
combined when all were in the same stage of the cycle: all were early follicular or all were mid-luteal. These groups were referred to as *monophase triads*.
The second type of group, referred to as a *multiphase triad*, consisted of 3
females, each in a different phase of the cycle: one animal was early follicular, the second preovulatory, and the third mid-luteal. A given triad was
observed for a variety of behavioral interactions in a large testing cage for
5-15 minutes, and then a vasectomized male was brought to the group. Observations continued for an additional 15 minutes with the male present. The
male was then removed and testing was continued with a second male. This
procedure was repeated for a third male, and the triad was then disbanded.
New triads were formed over a six-month period until all fifteen females had
been observed in each of the three ovarian phases in the *multiphase triads* and
had also been in both an 'all follicular' and an 'all luteal' *monophase triad*.
These two types of groups made it not only possible to assess behavioral
patterns of a female in a group situation during three different ovarian conditions, but also to identify those social factors in a group setting that influenced sex behavior when females were in equivalent endocrine states.

Determination of the phase of the ovarian cycle

The distance between two tattooed marks placed at the lateral extremities of the perineum, directly in line with the superior margin of the ischial callosities, was measured daily for each of the 15 females. From these measures, and knowledge of the first menstrual day, three conditions of sex-skin swelling were defined. The phase of early turgescence (T) was defined as the degree of turgescence seen between days 2-6 of the menstrual cycle, provided that maximal turgescence and deturgescence occurred during that cycle. This stage was assumed to be related to early follicular activity of the ovary. Maximal turgescence (M) was defined as the three-day period during which the largest successive sex-skin diameters were reached, immediately before the onset of rapid and continued deturgescence. The M condition was thought to reflect a pre- or immediately postovulatory period. Deturgescence (D) was defined as days 7-10 following the onset of rapid and continued deturgescence, and was taken as the mid-luteal period. Plasma progesterone determinations were used to confirm the occurrence of ovulatory cycles. All triads formed were made up of various combinations of animals as they attained these defined states. Thus, each multiphase triad was made from a T, M and D animal, and each monophase triad was made from three T animals or three D animals, but never three M animals.

Behavioral testing procedure

A. Dominance ratings

Monophase and multiphase triads were treated identically for all behavioral determinations, as follows: dominance orders were rated independently by two observers before the introduction of the first male. Since overt aggression was very rare among females, dominance ranks were based on the maintenance of central or peripheral areas of the room, eye aversion, displacement of one female by another, and the overt display of threats, aggression, fear grimaces, and withdrawals. Triads were excluded from consideration of dominance relations when both observers did not completely agree on the dominance order or when no clear dominance hierarchy was discerned.

B. Scoring in the presence of the male

A total of 6 adult vasectomized males were used for this study. Three males were randomly selected to be tested with a given triad. The first male to be used was brought to the triad immediately after the female dominance hierarchy was determined. Behavioral interactions which occurred among any of the animals (male-female or female-female) were recorded during the test period according to the definitions summarized in the Appendix. The scoring system was such that the initiatior and recipient(s) of any behavior were identified. A tape recorder was used to facilitate scoring and to verify behaviors tallied on score sheets. Both experimenters participated in observations for each triad studied. Observations were conducted with each of three males on a given day, but there was never more than one male at a time placed with the triad.

RESULTS AND DISCUSSION
The multiphase triads
A. Relation of ovarian condition to sexual behavior

When in the presumed preovulatory condition (M), females in multiphase triads received and displayed significantly more sexual and social behaviors

Table 1. Changes in behavior of females observed in multiphase triads during three different phases of the sex-skin cycle in Macaca nemestrina.

Behavior	Early turgescent (T)	Maximally turgescent (M)	Deturgescent (D)	Statistical comparison (F values)
Sex pout	0.00	0.87	0.00	4.67*
Present near	2.07	5.60	0.73	5.92**
Present far	18.20	36.80	10.40	8.51**
Present to approach	0.40	5.20	0.67	15.11**
Present to contact	0.67	6.60	0.53	15.46**
All presents	21.34	54.20	12.33	15.26**
Approach	2.87	9.93	1.93	10.79**
Proximity	0.40	1.80	0.20	10.06**
Vicinity	1.07	6.07	0.67	10.42**
Follow	0.73	6.07	0.13	10.67**
Closeness	2.20	13.93	1.00	17.10**
Groom	1.67	9.07	0.80	9.17**
Fear grimace	0.93	0.87	0.80	0.00

Data composed of mean frequencies per 3 males for 15 females tested once in each of the three sex-skin conditions. Females were observed with 3 males successively in each condition.

*   p < .05
** p < .01

with the male than at any other time in the cycle (Table 1). All four classes of presenting were displayed significantly more by females when they were observed in the M condition. In addition, several females displayed certain behaviors exclusively during the M condition (i.e. sex pout, proximity, vicinity and follow). Most grooming was also done by M females, quite contrary to reports obtained in pair-tests (33). Since each female was evaluated in each of the three defined stages of the ovarian cycle in a multiphase triad, these results represent true increases in the sex behavior of individual females as they attained the M state.

In turn, males observed in the multiphase triad situation responded differentially to the M female on all measures of social and sexual activity. Males ejaculated exclusively with M females, and pouted at them, groomed them, sat near them, approached, contacted and mounted them, all with frequencies of obvious statistical significance (Table 2). Males approached M

Table 2. Responses of the male to females observed in multiphase triads during three different phases of the sex-skin cycle.

Behavior	Early turgescent (T)	Maximally turgescent (M)	Deturgescent (D)	Statistical comparison (F values)
Sex pout	3.27	22.47	1.93	61.60*
Approach	4.20	22.60	2.93	35.59*
Contact	6.33	32.67	2.60	87.04*
Mount	4.07	27.47	1.73	67.83*
Intromission	2.47	20.87	0.73	58.79*
Ejaculation	0.00	2.20	0.00	25.42*
Proximity	0.13	0.47	0.13	2.33
Groom	0.27	1.40	0.33	5.79*
Threat	0.73	0.67	2.60	1.70

Data composed of mean frequencies per 3 males for 15 females tested once in each of the three sex-skin conditions. Females were observed with 3 males in each condition.
* $p < 0.01$

females on 90% of the occasions that a present-far was displayed, whereas they responded to less than 25% of the presents-far shown by T or D females in multiphase triads. Although no statistical differences were found between the T and D states for any social or sexual behavior in multiphase triads, females tended to display somewhat higher levels of each behavior when in the T condition than they did in the D condition.

B. Relation of ovarian condition to the dominance hierarchy
One of the few behavioral patterns which did not vary significantly with the cycle was the female threat. In addition, female dominance ratings, successfully determined for 16 of 21 multiphase triads before the introduction of the first male, were not associated with any particular ovarian condition

(Table 3). Moreover, threat behaviors among females reflected no change in dominance after the male was with the group (Table 4). In other words, an M female who was rated most dominant (α), second in dominance (β) or

Table 3. Distribution of dominance ranks among three conditions of sex-skin swelling before the introduction of the male (16 multiphase triads).

	Early turgescence	Maximal turgescence	Deturgescence
Alpha	5	7	4
Beta	4	4	8
Gamma	7	5	4

Table 4. Mean frequency of threats displayed by females after the introduction of the male (16 multiphase triads).

Triads in which M female was Alpha*			Triads in which M female was Beta*			Triads in which M female was Gamma*		
Alpha	Beta	Gamma	Alpha	Beta	Gamma	Alpha	Beta	Gamma
20.1	4.3	0.71	9.25	0.75	0	18.8	2.4	0

* All dominance ratings (i.e. alpha, beta, gamma position) made before male was introduced.

least dominant (γ) before the male was brought to the group, maintained that position in the hierarchy after the male was present.

C. Relation between dominance and sex behavior

A complicated but very real interaction between dominance position and endocrine state was found to affect the degree of sexual behavior displayed by females. Fig. 1 demonstrates that dominance relationships among females definitely influenced the sexual behavior displayed in the multiphase triad condition. In all triads in which the M female was also most dominant (α) (N=7 triads), the M female displayed and received the highest levels of behavior within her group (Fig. 1A and 1B; only two behaviors are illustrated, but these are representative of most of the behaviors studied). This situation produced the highest over-all mounting performance in any social condition.

In triads in which the M female was β in the hierarchy (N=4 triads; fig. 1C and 1D) the M female also displayed the highest level of sexual behavior within her group, even though the α female would often 'compete' with her and even aggress her.

In triads in which the M female was γ, (N=5 triads; fig. 1E and 1F) an entirely different pattern emerged. The α animal, and *not* the M female, displayed the highest levels of sexual behavior in spite of the fact that the α female was not preovulatory and was in the presence of another female who *was* in the M condition. However, males did not ejaculate with the α female,

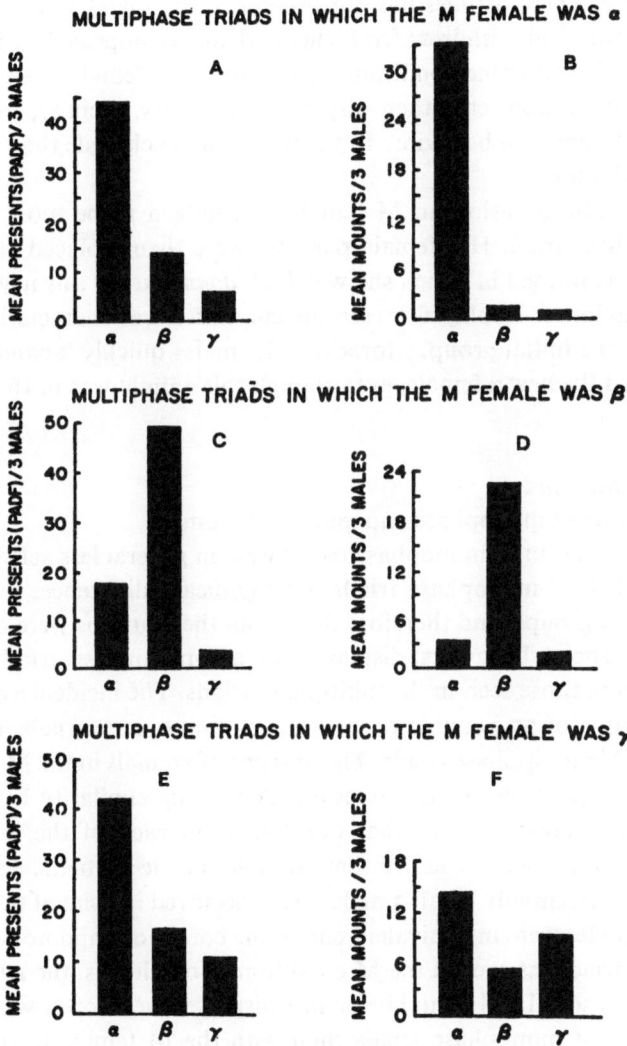

Figs. 1A-F. Mounts received and presents displayed by maximally turgescent females of differing positions of dominance in multiphase triads.

even though they were mounting and achieving repeated intromissions with her.

The following observations further demonstrated that social relations strongly influenced the sexual behavior of the females. On two separate occasions, an M female who was rated as least dominant in the triad situation was tested individually with a male immediately after their multiphase test was over. These females did not present to the males when in their respective triads, and withdrew from them whenever approached in spite of their favorable endocrine condition. When the other females were removed, the M female in each case then displayed proximity, vicinity, follow, presenting, and approach behaviors to the male, and each male then ejaculated within 10 minutes.

On a separate occasion an M female was judged to be most dominant in a multiphase triad. Her female partners were then replaced such that a new triad was formed in which she was *least dominant*. In this new triad the M female no longer displayed presenting etc. which was characteristic of her behavior in the initial group. Moreover, the males quickly 'abandoned' her and mounted the new α female, even though this animal was in the D condition.

The monophase triads
A. Comparison of monophase and multiphase tests

Although animals in D-monophase triads were in general less active sexually than animals in T-monophase triads, no significant differences were found between these groups, and therefore data from these groups were combined. Sexual and social behaviors displayed in all monophase triads differed markedly from those seen in the multiphase triads. The incidence of ejaculation was only 2 of 27 possible occurrences in monophase triads, compared with 33 of 45 in multiphase triads. The absence of animals in the M condition was clearly responsible for these results. A striking similarity between the two situations, however, was that one female in each of the monophase triads was invariably more active than her two female partners, and was responded to differentially by all 3 males. This occurred in spite of the fact that all of the females were in equivalent endocrine conditions and no female in a monophase triad was ever in the M condition. Nonetheless, the average frequencies of all social and sexual behaviors displayed were lower with the preferred female in monophase triads than with the M female in multiphase triads for 23 of 24 measures studied. Both the preferred female in monophase triads and the M female in multiphase triads displayed significantly more presenting towards the male, and both approached the male more than other females. However, only the M female displayed significantly more presenting which was done within inches of the male's face (present near), and significantly higher frequencies of behaviors which maintained close physical proximity to the male (proximity, vicinity, follow, groom).

B. Relation of dominance to sex behavior in monophase triads

The fact that males did respond preferentially toward one female in each monophase triad suggested that non-endocrine determinants were influencing the display of sexual activities. The data revealed that males invariably spent most time with the most dominant (α) member of each monophase triad (Table 5). For all 9 of the monophase triads in which dominance was

Table 5. Behaviors displayed by males towards females in monophase triads.

Behavior	Female dominance position			Statistical comparison (F values)
	Alpha	Beta	Gamma	
Sex pout	5.33	4.78	6.33	0.31
Approach	9.89	6.22	10.00	0.98
Contact	23.56	6.89	11.56	6.12**
Mount	20.44	4.89	7.78	6.29**
Intromission	15.33	3.44	5.44	4.02*
Ejaculation	0.22	0.00	0.00	0.00
Proximity	0.44	0.00	0.56	1.09
Groom	0.89	0.56	0.00	1.29
Threat	1.67	0.44	1.00	0.57

Data composed of mean frequencies per 3 males for 15 females in 9 triads in which dominance ranking was possible.
* $p < .05$
** $p < .01$

successfully determined, the α female demonstrated the most sexual behavior and received the most mounts, contacts, and intromissions from the males. The females rated β and γ in dominance in monophase triads displayed only low levels of sexual behavior relative to the α member of the group (Table 6).

Thus a non-gonadal factor, associated with the social rank of the female in a group situation, is definitely involved in the mediation of sexual behavior of the pigtail macaque, even at times in the cycle when conception is impossible.

Table 6. Behaviors displayed by females towards males in monophase triads.

Behavior	Female dominance position			Statistical comparison (F values)
	Alpha	Beta	Gamma	
Sex pout	0.22	0.00	0.00	0.00
Present near	2.78	0.56	1.11	1.38
Present far	30.33	12.22	10.89	3.25
Present to approach	2.56	1.44	2.78	0.65
Present to contact	4.89	0.78	2.11	5.10**
All presents	43.89	15.78	15.11	4.30*
Approach	5.67	1.67	1.00	5.27**
Proximity	1.00	1.33	0.33	0.58
Vicinity	5.00	0.67	2.44	2.30
Follow	2.89	0.67	2.00	0.84
Closeness	8.89	2.67	4.78	1.24
Groom	2.89	4.11	2.78	0.24
Fear grimace	0.11	0.33	0.33	1.09

Data composed of mean frequencies per 3 males for 15 females in 9 triads in which dominance ranking was possible.
* $p < .05$
** $p < .01$

CONCLUSION

Sexual behaviors of the female pigtail macaque are clearly influenced by ovarian cyclicity. When seen in a small group situation, females responded during the presumed preovulatory phase of the cycle with a variety of behaviors which had in common the effect of increasing the probability of receiving ejaculations with the male. Several behaviors were displayed almost exclusively at mid-cycle, while others were significantly more frequent near the time of ovulation.

Of equal or greater interest was the finding that sexual behaviors of the female were influenced by the social dominance structure of the group. This was most clearly seen when all three females in a triad were in the equivalent endocrine condition (monophase triads) well removed from the day of expected ovulation. Dominance position in the group was then an excellent predictor for selecting the female who would obtain the highest scores of sexual behaviors and would be responded to differentially by the males. In the presence of a preovulatory female in the group (multiphase triads), dominance factors were also exerting a decided influence on the patterns of sexual behavior which were displayed, and a definite interaction between endocrine and social factors could be seen. In monophase triads, only the α female was sexually active to any pronounced degree. In multiphase triads, the preovulatory female would display and receive most of the sexual behavior even if she was β, suggesting that ovarian conditions were 'over-riding' dominance factors. If the preovulatory female was γ, then she did not show high sex behavior scores, and dominance factors could 'over-ride' the normally potent endocrine condition.

The specific ways in which the dominance position was related to events controlling sexual behavior could not be discerned in this study. The complex relationship between animals in this social environment excluded the possibility of determining, for example, whether the behaviors of sub-ordinate females in monophase triads were actively depressed by the α female, or alternatively, that these sexual behaviors did not occur with high frequency because the male did not vigorously pursue the subordinate females. Neither was it possible to identify the behavioral or physiological aspects of 'being dominant' which resulted in the males' ultimate preference for the α female as a sexual partner. Can males recognize these characteristics in a female when they are placed alone with her? If so, can this explain some of the experimental variance and lack of positive evidence for female behavioral cyclicity reported in studies using the pair-test situation?

The female primate is unique among mammals in that sexual behavior can be displayed at times during the cycle when conception is impossible. She is also unique in that the occurrence or non-occurrence of sexual behavior can be determined by social dynamics, independent of the state of the ovary. Although the mechanisms whereby these social factors exert their in-fluence are not understood, it is clear that social pressures can affect the amount and kind of sexual behavior which is seen in a group. This suggests that while gonadal factors are always operative, their actions occur upon a background of individual and group extra-gonadal factors which together determine the nature and degree of sexual behavior which is displayed.

SUMMARY

The influences of both social factors and ovarian states were studied in Macaca nemestrina in relation to the display of sexual behavior. Results of the study may be summarized as follows:

1. In *multiphase triads*, composed of one early follicular, one preovulatory, and one mid-luteal female, the preovulatory animal displayed significantly more sexual and social behaviors directed towards the male than either of her female partners, and in turn received the most sexual behavior from the male. However, the probability that a preovulatory female would show in-

creased sexual activity in a group was also a function of her dominance status.

a. The preovulatory female who was most dominant or second in dominance among her group always received and displayed significantly more sexual behavior.

b. Preovulatory females who were lowest in dominance among their group did *not* copulate with the male, and did not show high frequencies of presenting or other sexual behaviors normally characteristic of the preovulatory condition. In this situation, the most dominant female in the group, even though she was not in a preovulatory condition, showed the most sexual activity.

2. In triads in which all females were in the same endocrine condition (*monophase triads*) the most dominant animal always showed the highest frequencies of sexual behavior, although ejaculation rarely took place. Both of her female partners, in turn, displayed relatively low frequencies of sexual behavior.

3. Social dominance among females, measured before the introduction of the male to the group, was unrelated to ovarian condition. Moreover, dominance positions, measured by threats displayed among females, did not change after the male was placed with the group.

4. The results indicated that both endocrine and social factors interacted in determining the display of sexual behavior. Endocrine factors increased the probability that insemination occurred at an optimum time for conception, while social factors operated to decrease the probability of conception with females who were in positions of very low dominance.

ACKNOWLEDGMENTS

Dr R. W. Goy is thanked for his continued guidance and advice during the course of this investigation. Mr C. A. Paris and Mr J. Jensen provided great assistance throughout the study. Drs Bullock and Resko are thanked for their determinations of plasma progesterone. Dr W. Montagna, director of the Oregon Regional Primate Research Center, and all personnel at the Center who assisted with this work are acknowledged for their excellent cooperation. A special note of appreciation is expressed to Dr Charles Phoenix for his interest in this study.

DEFINITIONS OF BEHAVIORS

All categories of behaviors were scored for males and females with the exception of 'vicinity' and 'follow' which were specifically scored for females interacting with a male.

THREAT. Includes gape, ear retraction, feint lunge, and/or brief bouts of biting, shaking, or tugging.
AGGRESSION. Severe biting, and severe shaking and tugging.
APPROACH. Animal A moves directly towards animal B and stops in immediate vicinity of B.
PROXIMITY. Animal A sits down next to animal B within touching distance.
VICINITY. Animal A stands or paces within touch of animal B.
FOLLOW. Animal A follows B, and stops when B stops.
SEX POUT. Facial expression seen only with M. nemestrina. Lips pursed in flat expression, head extended towards another animal. Scored only in situations devoid of threat expressions, and including immediately preceding or subsequent behaviors of sexual nature.
FEAR GRIMACE. Lips are retracted to expose teeth with mouth slightly opened. Remotely resembles human smile.
PRESENTING. Stereotyped posture of receptivity with quadrapedal immobility, orientation of perineum towards partner, moderate extension of fore and hind limbs. Presenting postures were categorized as follows:

a. Presenting in response to another animal's APPROACH.
b. Presenting in response to another animal's CONTACT.
c. Presenting 'spontaneously' within 1 foot of partner (PRESENT NEAR).
d. Presenting 'spontaneously' further than 1 foot from partner (PRESENT FAR).

CONTACT. Animal A lightly touches perineum or hips of animal B. Forceful contact with lifting is scored as POSITIONING.
MOUNT. An erect stance in which the hands are placed on partner's hips, perineum or back, and one or both feet are clasping partner's ankles or legs. Thrusting may or may not occur.
INTROMISSION. Penile insertion, recognized by deep and regular thrusting.
EJACULATION. Recognized by deep thrust which is accompanied by immobility and slight quivering. Anus often dilates and contracts rapidly.
GROOM. Stereotyped spreading and picking of hair of partner. May include slaps.

REFERENCES

1. Young, W. C., Observations and experiments on mating behavior in female mammals. *Quart. Rev. Biol.* 16, 135, 311 (1941).
2. Young, W. C., The hormones and mating behavior. In: *Sex and internal secretions*, 2, 1173, Young, W. C. (ed.), Baltimore 1961.
3. Beach, F. A., *Hormones and behavior.* New York 1961.
4. Hartman, C. G., The period of gestation in the monkey (Macaca rhesus): First description of parturition in monkeys, size, and behavior of young. *J. Mammal.* 9, 181 (1928).
5. Eckstein, P. & Zuckerman, S., The oestrus cycle in the mammalia. In: *Marshall's physiology of reproduction. 1*, Parkes A. S. (ed.), London 1956.

6. Maslow, A. H., The role of dominance in the social and sexual behavior of infra-human primates: III. A theory of sexual behavior of infra-human primates. *J. Genet. Psychol.* 48, 310 (1936).

7. Yerkes, R. M., Sexual behavior in the chimpanzee. *Human Biol.* 11, 78 (1939).

8. Rowell, T. E., Behaviour and female reproductive cycles of rhesus macaques. *J. Reprod. Fertil.* 6, 193 (1963).

9. Yerkes, R. M. & Elder, J. H., Oestrus, receptivity and mating in chimpanzee. *Comp. Psychol. Monog.* 13, 1 (1936).

10. Young, W. C. & Orbison, W. D., Changes in selected features of behavior in pairs of oppositely sexed chimpanzees during the sexual cycle and after ovariectomy. *J. Comp. Psychol.* 37, 107 (1944).

11. Ball, J. & Hartman, C. G., Sexual excitability as related to the menstrual cycle in the monkey. *Am. J. Obst. Gyn*, 29, 117 (1935).

12. Michael, R. P., Herbert, J. & Welegalla, J., Ovarian hormones and the sexual behaviour of the male rhesus monkey (*Macaca mulatta*) under laboratory conditions. *J. Endocr.* 39, 81 (1967).

13. Phoenix, C. H., Goy, R. W., Resko, J. A. & Koering, M., Probability of mating during various stages of the ovarian cycle in *Macaca mulatta*. *Anat. Rec.* 160, 490 (Abst.) (1968).

14. Bullock, D. W., Paris, C. A., Resko, J. A. & Goy, R. W., Sexual behavior and progesterone secretion during the menstrual cycle in rhesus and pigtail macaques. *Proc. VIe Cong. Intern. Reprod. Anim. Insem. Artif.* II, 1657, Paris 1968.

15. Michael, R. P., Gonadal hormones and the control of primate behaviour. In: *Endocrinology and Human Behaviour*. Michael, R. P. (ed.), p. 69, London 1968.

16. Michael, R. P. & Welegalla, J., Ovarian hormones and the sexual behaviour of the female rhesus monkey (*Macaca mulatta*) under laboratory conditions. *J. Endocr.* 41, 407 (1968).

17. Michael, R. P., Neural and non-neural mechanisms in the reproductive behaviour of primates. *Progress in Endocrinology*, Gual, C. & Ebling, F. J. G. (eds.), p. 302, Amsterdam 1969.

18. Michael, R. P. & Keverne, E. B., Pheromones in the communication of sexual status in primates. *Nature* 218, 746 (1968).

19. Everitt, B. J. & Herbert, J., The maintenance of sexual receptivity by adrenal androgens in female rhesus monkeys. *J. Endocr.* 48, xxxviii (1970).

20. Altmann, S., A field study of the sociobiology of rhesus monkeys, *Macaca mulatta*. *Ann. N.Y. Acad. Sci.* 102, 338 (1962).

21. Carpenter, C. R., Sexual behavior of free ranging rhesus monkeys (*Macaca mulatta*). I. Specimens, procedures and behavioral characteristics of estrus. *J. Comp. Psychol.* 33, 113 (1942).

22. Carpenter, C. R., Sexual behavior of free ranging rhesus monkeys (*Macaca mulatta*). II. Periodicity of estrus, homosexual, autoerotic and nonconformist behavior *J. Comp. Psychol.* 33, 143 (1942).

23. Conaway, C. H. & Koford, C. B., Estrous cycles and mating behavior in a free-ranging band of rhesus monkeys. *J. Mammal.* 45, 577 (1964).

24. Vanderbergh, J. G. & Vessey, S., Seasonal breeding of free-ranging rhesus monkeys and related ecological factors. *J. Reprod. Fertil.* 15, 71 (1968).

25. DeVore, I., Male dominance and mating behavior in baboons. In: *Sex and behavior*, Beach F. A. (ed.), p. 266, New York 1965.

26. Hall, K. R. L. & DeVore, I., Baboon social behavior. In: *Primate behavior: field studies of monkeys and apes*, DeVore I. (ed.), p. 53 New York 1965.

27. Bernstein, I. S., A field study of the pigtail monkey (*Macaca nemestrina*). *Primates* 8, 217 (1967).

28. Tokuda, K., A study on the sexual behavior in the Japanese monkey troop. *Primates* 3, 1 (1961).
29. Rowell, T. E., Female reproductive cycles and the behavior of baboons and rhesus macaques. In: *Social communication among primates*, Altmann, S. A. (ed.), p. 15 Chicago 1967.
30. Herbert, J., The social modification of sexual and other behavior in the rhesus monkey. In: *Neue Ergibnisse der Primatologie (Progress in Primatology)*, Stark, D., Schneider, R. & Kuhn, H. J. (eds.), p. 232-246. First Cong. Int. Primat. Soc., Frankfurt (a.M.) 26-30 juli, 1966. Stuttgart 1967.
31. Everitt, B. J. & Herbert, J., The role of ovarian hormones in the sexual preference of rhesus monkeys. *Anim. Behav.* 17, 738 (1969).
32. Zuckerman, S. & Parkes, A. S., The menstrual cycle of the primates. V. The cycle of the baboon. *Proc. Zool. Soc. London*, Part I, 139 (1937).
33. Michael, R. P., Herbert, J. & Welegalla, J. Ovarian hormones and grooming behaviour in the rhesus monkey (Macaca mulatta) under laboratory conditions. *J. Endocr.* 36, 263 (1967).

DISCUSSION

Snow: In terms of a natural situation, what does this mean? Do gamma females or omega females as they would be in a large troop, copulate?

Goldfoot: The omega female does copulate in natural troop situations but almost never with the alpha male (Hall & DeVore, 26). Obviously the interactions in a natural troop are much more complicated than those of the present study; it appears for several species of Old World monkeys that females copulate with peripheral males during early follicular stages of the cycle, but that they usually copulate with the alpha male during the periovulatory period. By restricting our study to just one male and three females for any given observation, we've created an artificial situation probably much different from the social dynamics of a natural troop.

Levine: What are the factors concerned in establishing these various dominance hierarchies?

Goldfoot: Factors which contribute to the development of dominance status are almost entirely unknown, although the complexity of the problem is obvious. In Japanese macaques, for example, the status of the mother in the troop influences the dominance position of her offspring, and kinship support during dominance encounters is often reported among siblings, 'aunts' etc. However, the particular genetic, hormonal and environmental factors which might influence dominance relations are still largely unexplored. Part of the problem is that no single definition of dominance serves all purposes. Food and water competition tests, often used to measure dominance, are clearly influenced by deprivation states of the animals involved, and results are often quite different from rankings of aggressions. In addition, different dominance orders are often obtained for a given group of monkeys if they are tested in all possible combinations of pairs in contrast to testing them all together in one group. The problem is extremely complex and much research is needed.

INDEX OF SUBJECTS